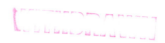

SOCIAL PSYCHIATRY

SOCIAL PSYCHIATRY

Theory, Methodology, and Practice

Edited by
Paul E. Bebbington

With a foreword by
J. L. T. Birley

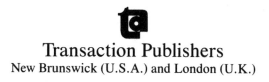

Transaction Publishers
New Brunswick (U.S.A.) and London (U.K.)

Library of Congress Catalog Number: 90-11304
ISBN: 0-88738-403-X
Printed in the United States of America

Library of Congress Cataloging-in-Publication Data

Social psychiatry : theory, methodology, and practice / edited by Paul
    Bebbington ; with a foreword by J. L. T. Birley.
      p.   cm.
    Discusses social psychiatry within the context of the work of the
  Medical Research Council Social Psychiatry Unit.
    Includes index.
    ISBN 0-88738-403-X
    1. Social psychiatry.   2. Medical Research Council (Great
  Britain).   Social Psychiatry Unit.   I. Bebbington, Paul.
    [DNLM: 1. Community Psychiatry.   2. Mental Disorders.
  3. Social Behavior.   4. Social Environment.   WM 30.6 S677 1991]
  RC455.S622   1991
  616.89—dc20
  DNLM/DLC
  for Library of Congress   90-11304
                                                                CIP

Contents

Foreword

The essays in this volume make up a series of variations upon one of the basic themes of human existence—the interaction between human beings and their environment. As the authors are concerned with social psychiatry, their attention is focused on those aspects of the environment that affect psychological states, whether of persons previously healthy or already suffering from some form of psychiatric illness or disability. Humans are social animals, whose social behavior is as "biological" as many other human functions. Consequently, an important element of the environment that requires investigation is the nature of a person's relationships with other human beings.

Social relationships and psychiatric disturbances are swampy ground for investigators, many of whom have become lost or have returned with nothing but truisms or unvalidated assertions. It is hardly surprising, therefore, that one of the reasons for the MRC Social Psychiatry Unit's success is its long-standing attention to methodology. A painstaking attention to detail, though essential to the enterprise, is only a minor feature. Of far greater importance is attention to theory. Karl Popper pointed out over fifty years ago that it is impossible to "observe" in a theoretical vacuum. All observations are based on theory, on the schemata of the observing individual. (DSM III, although naively claiming to be "atheoretical," is no exception.) It follows that theory must inform and dictate both what is to be observed, and how. The Unit's most significant activity has been to develop theories and methodology constructed to test them.

The Unit's first two directors, Aubrey Lewis and John Wing have provided notable leadership to this enterprise, both by their own writings and by their encouragement of others. The quality of the research has led to its international recognition both for its scientific standards and for its applicability. The Unit has always been interested in very real clinical and social problems; its finds have suggested new approaches both to prevention and treatment and to the assessment of the effectiveness of psychiatric services. In terms of humanity and power, this set of variations on a theme may well stand comparison with Diabelli and Haydn.

J.L.T. BIRLEY

Introduction

The MRC Social Psychiatry Unit and the World of Social Psychiatry

Paul E. Bebbington

The Medical Research Council (MRC) and its predecessor the Medical Research Committee recently celebrated its seventy-fifth anniversary. The establishment of this body was an explicit recognition of the role of governmental funding in the encouragement of medical research, based on an acknowledgement of the worth of such research for society as a whole.

The first Annual Report (MRC, 1915)—it actually cost three pence which seems good value—reveals an awareness of the value of supporting competent bodies of investigators working together in the permanent employ of the MRC, thus foreshadowing the development of Research Units. Setting up centers of this type indicates recognition of the long time span required for progress in some fields of research; work that may or may not produce results that are applicable in the short term. It also demonstrates the consciously pro-active approach of the Council toward medical research. The council identifies an area for encouragement and fosters research in the area, but relies only on the broadest stipulations. It sends "fleets out in several directions and in different seas, hoping that individuals will seize any prize of discovery that shows itself in any quarter" (MRC, 1939).

This method of engendering research is peculiarly British, and builds on the tradition of research in the eighteenth and nineteenth centuries, when gifted amateurs wealthy enough to support themselves gave British science, pure and applied, an enviable reputation by following their own inclinations. In this age of audit, it may look old fashioned, and it carries the risk of supporting occasional mediocrities by mistake. On the other hand, it can lead to outstanding success, often in unexpected ways.

The policy has certainly borne fruit in many branches of medical research. Social psychiatry may be less glamorous than some of the MRC's children, but it exemplifies the worth of the approach as well as any. Indeed, the MRC Social Psychiatry Unit might be taken as an ideal type of the way lines of research should evolve.

Evolution is an apposite term: as the evolutionary tree grows, some branches fluorish, others wither. This capacity for evolution is a major justification for the establishment of research units. They are well placed to take advantage of opportunities that flow from their own research findings, as from others in the field.

Looking backwards, the logic of development is clear, but the end-point cannot entirely be predicted from the outset: "it is impossible for any organization to foresee its needs for more than a few steps ahead" (MRC, 1962).

An MRC Unit and its director therefore ideally functions as an umbrella, a shelter under which researchers of intellect and scholarship may develop the direction of their research with substantial freedom. They are given time to think in a way denied to many researchers elsewhere—as those who have moved on from such Units well understand. Nevertheless, many who do move on have been able to use their time in the employ of the MRC as a launchpad. Many careers have taken off as a consequence.

The origins of the current MRC Social Psychiatry Unit go back to the association in 1942 of Sir Aubrey Lewis with work carried out by Dr. Russell Frazer on the prevalence of neurosis in industry and its cost to the nation. The consequence of this work included the setting up of an MRC Unit under Lewis's honorary direction in 1948. It was then called the Occupational Psychiatry Research Unit, changed three years later to the Unit for Research in Occupational Adaptation. It was finally named the Social Psychiatry Research Unit in 1958. This was entirely reasonable, as the Unit had moved from its early studies of rehabilitation in mental retardation and aspects of occupational psychology into the field of social psychiatry in its broadest sense.

This breadth of interest has been maintained to the present day, and looking backwards from 1990, it is possible to see how an underlying philosophy has guided the various lines of Unit research. Crucial to this progression has been the ability to formulate conceptual issues in clear terms, and, in consequence, to develop the practical methods needed to test the resulting hypotheses. Without this intellectual approach, opportunities are missed, developments stillborn.

By following these lines, the Unit has become a significant influence on the way social psychiatry has developed throughout the world. In the process, distinction has become attached to the names of those who have at various times worked within the Unit—Tizard, O'Connor, Hermelin, Carstairs, the Wings, Brown, Rawnsley, Rutter, Hirsch, Leff. Moreover, the reputation of the Unit encouraged others to take up temporary attachments and to spend sabbatical periods in it.

The point of origin of work in the Unit has always been a concern with basic scientific principles—theory testing, method and measurement and these scientific preoccupations have also been closely linked with practical applications of the results.

The early history of the Unit has been covered in six chapters of the book edited by Shepherd and Davies (1968) to commemorate the retirement of Sir Aubrey Lewis. Since that time, work of distinction has been carried out under the direction of John Wing. Looking back, it is sometimes difficult to see how innovative much of this work was, precisely because it has gained such wide acceptance. In consequence, the way we view aspects of mental illness has changed radically. Although the approach to research was evolutionary, its impact was revolutionary.

A measure of this process of assimilation into everyday usage is the number of terms coined in the Unit or given new currency by Unit research that are now used without perhaps appreciating their origins: institutionalism, social disablement, primary and secondary disability, negative syndrome, poverty of the social environment, psychiatric rehabilitation, new longstay, life events, Expressed Emotion, social impairment, autistic spectrum, the PSE.

This is illustrated by the work on the influence of the environment on the course of schizophrenia. It is now accepted that symptoms, disabilities, and attitudes can be markedly influenced by different aspects of the social environment and that the severity and type of social disablement in any particular patient cannot be fully understood and influenced unless the pattern of causes is investigated. It is forgotten that at the time the first paper on the Three Hospital's Study was published many in the psychiatric profession had the greatest difficulty, not merely in accepting such conclusions, but in believing the findings on which they were based.

This research and the more detailed experiments on rehabilitations and resettlement that accompanied it had a major influence on attitudes towards practical clinical issues. There had always been professional people who felt that longstanding mental disablement was not immutable, that therapeutic efforts should never be abandoned. But many clinicians in the 1950s and 1960s had very pessimistic views. The work on environmental influences, both harmful and therapeutic, gave empirical backing to this optimism. It is so much a part of history that it is taken for granted.

For many patients with schizophrenia, the family is, in these days of community care, the major component of the social environment. Work on the influence of the family environment has been carried out over the last thirty years, following a logical programme of development. Establishing that family circumstances had a considerable influence on the course of schizophrenia, like much work in the Unit, set up the possibility for a novel intervention, even if this might seem over-optimistic, as it did to some unit members at the time—at least the hypotheses can be tested. The success of this experimental intervention has again revolutionized views of how the course of schizophrenia is determined, and, in particular, how the clinician should go about managing the condition.

The research on autism carried out in the Unit has also had a major impact on how we see that condition. At the time when the Unit's autism research was begun, the disorder was seen very much as a discrete entity. The fact that some autistic people showed relatively high, if patchy, intellectual capacity was over-emphasized. Interestingly, aetiological thinking was at that time dominated by social theories.

The Unit research broke new ground in a number of ways. First, by looking at features of autism over the whole range of intellectual abilities, it became clear that autism represented more of a spectrum than a category, and that in spite of the inclusion of Asperger's syndrome, its features were strongly associated with restricted intellectual ability. Those with areas of superior intellectual functioning were in a minority. Secondly, it became apparent that the disabilities of autism were relatively immune from social influence. In consequence, the central principle of management was not so much in modifying the symptoms as in evaluating them and using them to choose the environment most suitable for the management of the sufferer. In particular, the implications are crucial for the development of services.

The Unit's approach to these most difficult psychiatric conditions, schizophrenia and autism, can be used to emphasize the underlying logic. In both cases, the rather fatuous question of whether the conditions exist or not was dealt with by a close delineation of their features and of their relation to external circumstances. The result has been progress at a theoretical level, but also the illumination of important clinical issues. This has suggested innovations in services, and, in turn, the necessity for service evaluation. The researchers in the Unit have above all remained clinicians, with clinicians' interests.

The research in affective disorders, albeit of a later inception, has followed a similar line. Once more, there has been an interest in the relationship between the features of the condition and the influence of the social environment. This has led to an interest in the way the environment/disorder interaction is affected by "host factors," such as biological or psychological attributes of the sufferer. These studies have led to suggestions for practical intervention, which will be implemented and evaluated in studies in the successor Unit, the MRC Social and Community Psychiatry Unit.

Providing a solid foundation for these various lines of research, and indeed uniting them, has been the Unit's interest in instrumentation. The Unit has been very good at generating a range of reliable and useful measures for quantifying the "soft" data that characterize social research. Once more, the novelty of this endeavor is now hard to grasp. The PSE, for example, was the first attempt to standardize the examination of the mental state in order to provide a reliable description of clinical phenomena. Its later editions were linked to computerized algorithms designed to give a classification in terms of a range of ICD categories. The PSE-ID CATEGO system as a whole includes a range of facilities that comprise a flexible bottom-up approach to the classification of mental phenomena and disorders. However, this is just one of many innovative techniques developed under the Unit's umbrella, and now used in social psychiatry research all over the world—the contextual rating of life event threat, the Camberwell Family Interview and the Expressed Emotion measure, the HBS and its congeners, measures of social performance, relatives' burden, patients' needs, social networks and so on. The establishment of the Camberwell register was another venture that originated in concerns over method, in this case a method of recording high quality service data to be used for epidemiological studies. It too has been used for both basic scientific and evaluative purposes.

This insistence on the most accurate measurement possible is the natural consequence of an adherence to clear theoretical positions, which both informs and demands such an approach. It also underlines the fact that the broad range of the Unit's activities are in truth all of one cloth.

This book is about the work of the Social Psychiatry Unit, but because of the range of the Unit's concerns over the years, it is also about the subject of social psychiatry. The research carried out here interleaves with work carried out in other centers all over the world.

References

Medical Research Committee. (1915). First Annual Report of the Medical Research Committee 1914-1915. London, HMSO.

Medical Research Committee. (1939). Report of the Medical Research Council for the Year 1937-1938. London, HMSO.

Medical Research Council. (1962). Report of the Medical Research Council for the Year 1960-1961. London, HMSO.

Shephered, M. and Davies, D.L. (1968). *Studies in Psychiatry,* London, Oxford University Press.

I

The Theoretical Foreground

1

Social Psychiatry

J.K. Wing

The adjective "social" is probably the most
confusing and misleading term of our whole polit-
ical vocabulary, a sort of verbal magic wand.
. . . It has in fact become the most dangerous
instance of what. . . . the Americans call a
"weasel word." As a weasel is alleged to be able
to empty an egg without leaving a visible sign,
so can these words deprive any term to which
they are prefixed of content, while seemingly
leaving them untouched. A weasel word is used to
draw the teeth from a concept which one is
obliged to employ, but from which one wishes to
eliminate all implications that challenge one's
ideological premises.
—Friedrich A. von Hayek, 1983

Biomedical and Psychosocial Models of Psychiatric Disorders

In the article in the *London Times* from which this quotation is taken, Friedrich A. von Hayek was concerned with the use of weasel words in politics: *social justice,* the *social market, social democracy,* the *social state.* In each case, he thought that the adjective diminished the meaning of the succeeding noun, instead of enhancing it.

Like many terms that contain both a social and a biological component, *social psychiatry* (or, more broadly, *social medicine*) seems to some to contain the seeds of its own contradiction—not so much a weasel term as an oxymoron. This position can be taken both by those who deny that the term *psychiatry* has any biological content or significance, that is, those who use an exclusively social model, and by those who use an exclusively

3

biological or so-called medical model, and therefore cannot see the point of the adjective *social*. Each side tends to talk about *the* social or *the* medical model, as though there could be only one of each, with no possibility of overlap. Psychological models tend to be divided in similar fashion into psychobiological and psychosocial.

In the following discussion, I shall first consider exclusively biological, then exclusively social, models before turning to formulations that are less confrontational.

Biomedical Models of Psychiatric Disorders

A respectable advocate for biological psychiatry is Samuel Guze (1989). He points out that evolution has shaped the development of the brain and its functions, including perception, learning, thought, memory, emotions, and communications: "A major portion of the approximately three billion nucleotides constituting the human genome is devoted to programming the brain." During the course of millenia, the interaction between genotype and environment has led to enormous variation in brain functions between individuals. According to Guze, a case against an exclusively medical model for psychiatry could only be made if it could be shown that "patients develop their disorders primarily, if not exclusively, through normal learning processes that are independent of brain variability." For example, if most individuals exposed to a specific pattern of social or cultural learning developed a particular disorder while others not so exposed did not, "psychiatry would have much less need for neuroscience and much more for cultural anthropology, sociology, and social psychology."

Since no such case has been made, Guze regards resistance to the adoption of this fully biological version of the medical model as explicable only in terms of a failure to understand that non-biological treatments such as psychotherapy, which he agrees can ameliorate symptoms, provide no clues as to necessary and sufficient causes. Once this is accepted, he thinks, acceptance of the fundamentally biological nature of psychiatry follows automatically.

This summary presents the core of the argument, which is based not on evidence for the thesis but on first principles. It is a manifesto of faith in what psychiatric knowledge will be like in the mid-twenty-first century. The evidence that a biological substrate is of overwhelming significance in causing (let alone in treating) the troubles that people bring to psychiatrists seems, at the moment, at best incomplete and at worst exiguous. A bio-ideology may provide motivation for mounting a research programme but scientists can test specific biological hypotheses without the aid of such grand theorizing. All such ideas have to be judged by their performance in tough competition with others.

Guze does accept that psychosocial theories and practices have their place in medicine and even suggests that he could accept a "biopsychosocial" model. He goes on to make the unexceptionable point that no "thoughtful and knowledgeable individual advocates an approach to psychiatry (or to the rest of medicine for that matter) that isolates it from its social and cultural context." But at the same time he can argue that "the religious, ethical and moral characteristics of humans have their roots in biology too." If this is more than a trivial circularity (*everything* we think, feel, and do depends on our being alive) it suggests that Guze, at heart, is a radical sociobiologist, though he does not list Edward Wilson's mammoth book in his bibliography.

Wilson (1975) sets out to restate and bring up to date the "modern synthesis" of evolutionary biology, to show how this will develop during the next thirty years and to formulate a theory of the biological basis of human ethics. He achieves the first of these aims with clarity, wit, and economy, not forgetting (in the extraordinary wealth of detail) that a group, troup, or band may consist of a murmuration of starlings, an exaltation of larks, a bouquet of pheasants, or a murder of crows. He misses only a shrewdness of apes.

He is also aware of the fact that the imprecise results of work in sociobiology and the multiplicity of explanations available for the adaptiveness or non-adaptiveness of traits, tend to lead too readily to grand theories, which are then remorselessly advocated and uncritically adopted until some other theory becomes fashionable. This is particularly true of theories purporting to explain human social behavior. Wilson regards the attempt to make hypotheses compete so that only the fittest survive as the key element in the transition from neo-Darwinism to post-Darwinism. Nevertheless, he gives very few examples of tests of evolutionary theories.

It is precisely at the point at which equivalents in animal behavior might have most evolutionary relevance for anthropologists, sociologists and psychiatrists ("selfishness," "altruism," "slavery," "deceit," "cuckoldry," "suicide") that sociobiological erudition tends to fail. The fact that inhibitory pheromones produced by termite kings and queens force most nymphs to develop into one of the sterile worker "castes" does little to illuminate the human caste system in India. In a final chapter, Wilson tries to derive human ethics from notions of genetic fitness. His few scraps of homespun wisdom, for example on how to prevent aggression among humans, are unlikely to impress most social workers or family doctors, to say nothing of policemen and magistrates. Genetic fitness is a postulated end-point in a process that has no ending. We can never know what it is; or we can know only a tautology.

These are reasonable men taking a reasonable case further than it can reasonably go. Most scientists like to do that, at least in private. None of this criticism is directed at the formulation of specific and testable hypotheses linking abnormal mental phenomena to biological processes that have themselves already been successfully linked to larger systematic ecological or evolutionary processes.

The social and the biological aspects of psychiatry are inextricably mixed in practice, as will be discussed later. But part of the relationship can be illustrated at once. Biomedical disease concepts can be misused if put into practice in the wrong social environment. The most recent example has occurred in the Soviet Union, where an unduly broad and uncritical assumption among psychiatrists that much social deviance is explicable in terms of disease entities, could be exploited within a society where those who dissented from promulgated norms of behavior and belief were liable to be locked away. The special hospital was even more convenient than the prison camp for this purpose, since the quality of the dissent was thereby devalued. The political nature of this exploitation is beginning to be understood in the new climate of *glasnost* but underlying attitudes are hard to change.

Another curious relationship is provided by the fact that the most rigidly biomedical of psychiatrists provide ammunition for their antagonists, who take as their starting point the "myth of mental illness." Szasz (1961, 1971), for example, is inadvertently on their side. For him, only organic pathology will do for disease status. Either there is a disease entity or there is nothing. Everything depends, in both cases, on whether "anxiety state," for example, is the name of a disease entity. But before analyzing the notion of disease it is necessary to consider attempts to formulate psychiatric disorders in purely psychological terms.

Social Models of Psychiatric Disorders

The chief advocates of *the* social model of mental disorders are, of course, sociologists. Edwin Lemert (1951), who started the tradition with his theory of social deviance, has much to say that is of keen relevance to psychiatry. He rejected earlier explanations of social pathology (crime, prostitution, alcoholism, and so on), which were couched in terms of a deviation from a past society less disorganized than ours, governed by "ideals of residential stability, property ownership, sobriety, thrift, habituation to work, small business enterprise, family solidarity, neighbourliness and discipline of the will." He also, though less explicitly (neither

Comte nor Marx is mentioned in the book), rejects the opposite kind of theory, which explained social pathology in terms of the disturbance caused by historical forces when they encountered resistance while driving towards a future millenium.

Lemert's formulation of "sociopathic" behavior has been influential. He begins with the same fact of behavioral diversity as do Guze and Wilson. When sufficiently unusual within a given society, this is called "primary deviation." An amplification of the primary deviation because of social penalties, rejection, and segregation, so that it becomes a way of life, is called "secondary deviation." The theory is amoral, in the sense that it would be socially as interesting to study exceptional beauty or musical talent, which can also lead to a "career" formed in part by a public reaction to deviation, as to study crime, poverty, or sexual delinquency. Nevertheless, like doctors, Lemert is concerned mainly with deviations defined by society as undesirable. He uses examples ranging from blindness through alcoholism and mental illness to political radicalism.

The theory behind secondary deviation may be stated in two forms, one moderate and one radical. In the moderate form there is an interaction between a primary deviation, which may be biological as in the case of blindness, and the societal reaction. In the radical form the primary element is trivial or non-existent; the societal label alone produces the deviation. Lemert generally inclines to the more moderate interpretation, leaving the explanation of the primary deviation open. However, his exposition of mental disorders tends towards the radical and has been enthusiastically developed by two of his followers, Erving Goffman and Thomas Scheff. Both inadvertently made a contribution to psychiatry as well as to sociology, but both tend, like most polemicists, to perpetuate stereotypes—to put up Aunt Sallies in order to knock them down again. Goffman (1961) is particularly good at this.

The strongest case for the radical interpretation of schizophrenia in terms of social deviance (or labelling theory, as it came to be called) is that of Scheff (1964, 1966). It is based in part on empirical evidence (Scheff, 1963). He studied the processes of admission to state mental hospitals in Wisconsin, at a time when all patients had to be admitted under compulsion. His conclusion was that the psychiatrist often acted as a legal, rather than a medical, agent, simply confirming the label of mental illness, which was more or less synonymous with schizophrenia.

In 1964, I interviewed all forty-five patients in a Wisconsin County Hospital who had been given a diagnosis of schizophrenia. All were under order, as there was no form of voluntary or nonstatutary admission. Only twenty-nine met the technically defined criteria used in the study, which was principally concerned with a comparison between three English hospitals characterized by very different environmental conditions (Wing and Brown, 1970, Chap. 9). The conditions in the Wisconsin hospital were markedly "institutional" and contact with the outside severely restricted.

The results of the U.S.-U.K. Diagnostic Project (Cooper, et al., 1972) and the International Pilot Study of Schizophrenia (IPSS, 1973) demonstrated without cavil that diagnostic methods could vary dramatically in different parts of the world. A very broad concept of schizophrenia was common in the United States, based on the non-biological psychoanalytic theories that were dominant at that time. In fact, the research results were responsible in part for the dramatic narrowing and sharpening of the rules for diagnosing schizophrenia that subsequently occurred in the United States. The IPSS results demonstrated that a very broad concept of schizophrenia was also used in Moscow. This time, however, it was based on vague organic theories.

Thus it has happened in the past, and may well happen again, that someone who is not severely disturbed, or whose disorder is transitory, has been committed to a mental hospital, given a diagnosis using vague criteria, and then kept in for years while secondary disadvantages and disabilities accumulated (providing a spurious confirmation of the diagnosis), so that he or she was no longer fit to leave and did not wish to do so. This would appear to confirm at least part of Scheff's version of labelling theory. The problem, however, is how far it can be generalized. In my view, for reasons specified in detail elsewhere (Wing, 1978, Chap. 5), the usefulness of the theory in its radical form, though undeniable, is limited and highly situational. It applies when such actions are based on current social ideas of "madness" (which can also be held by doctors).

An Attic parallel is provided by Bennett Simon (1978). He quotes, as an example of what was called "social psychiatry" in the *Laws* of Plato, who regarded madness as a lack of restraint of appetites, the opposite of intellect or sanity. He proposed the establishment of a *Sophronisterion,* or house of moderation, in which atheists who held their mistaken beliefs out of ignorance were to be held for five years in order to be given sound instruction.

> And when the time of their imprisonment has expired, if any of them be of sound mind, let him be restored to sane company, but if not, and if he be condemned a second time, let him be punished with death.

Dissent was equated with insanity: the state was made the arbiter of what was health and what was sickness. In this case, however, the attribution was not made in terms of disease concepts, at least not in any modern sense. This was a psychosocial model of deviance, but one that could have been operated in much the same way as happened more recently, with the aid of a biomedical model, in the USSR.

Another relevant historical example was the famous epidemic of witchcraft in Salem, Massachusetts, which ended only after nineteen "witches" had been hanged and more than a hundred suspects jailed. Marion Starkey (1949) explains this in terms of classical hysteria occurring in repressed teenagers brought up in a God-fearing Puritan community, whose ministers gave content to the epidemic and unconsciously guided it along its devastating course. Paul Boyer and Stephen Nissenbaum (1974) provide a more socio-economic interpretation. Hysteria is nowadays much under attack as a disease concept, but a curious twist to the story is provided by the fact that a doctor had been called to see the girls when they first became affected. Dr. William Griggs said that the problem was not medical.

Perhaps an application of the modern concept of "illness behavior" (Mechanic, 1968) might have enabled Dr. Griggs, without compromising his non-medical diagnosis, to suggest a course of action that would have helped events to take a more benign course. The moderate version of the theory of social deviance, which allows for an interaction between biological and social factors in causation and treatment, provides a similar frame of reference; though the contribution of biology towards explaining some of the personality traits of a few of the key actors, allowed by the social conditions of that time and place to play a key part in accelerating the progress of the tragedy, is no more understood now than it was in the late seventeenth century.

I conclude that social models of psychiatry that exclude any biological element are as unsatisfactory as biological models that exclude any social content. Both types of exclusivity tend towards tautology or triviality and both can be disastrous in practice.

Definitions

Epidemiology and Social Medicine

Michael Shepherd (1983) has attempted to solve the problem of defining social psychiatry (and, more broadly, social medicine) by absorbing it into epidemiology. His authority is Alfred Grotjahn (1923), who, like Lemert, called his book *Social Pathology*. In an interesting set of discussion papers, several authors made the point that such reductionism appears to deny any contribution to social psychiatry from the social and behavioral sciences, which are regarded as purely "humanistic." It also seems to assume, either that epidemiological methods are the only means of scientific investigation in medicine, or that all other techniques, from health economics to the double blind controlled trial, come exclusively within the province of epidemiology.

Since David Mechanic (1970) points out that epidemiology is something that people like himself "have been doing all their professional lives," Alan Williams (1979) argues that most of the topics of social medicine fall within the province of sociology, and Guze (1989), in his turn, claims epidemiology for biological psychiatry, the futility of these territorial claims is obvious. They are of little interest to most scientists, who cheerfully ignore the boundaries drawn by those whose horizons are limited by the way their departments or practices are funded and organized, and whose teaching may thus be channelled towards perpetuating, rather than challenging, tradition. What matters about epidemiology is that, whatever the field of application, the approach should be understood and the techniques used correctly to test interesting and potentially useful hypotheses. Pursuit of such research "is a more significant issue than whether social psychiatry, psychological medicine, or psychiatric epidemiology serves as a better overall theoretical framework" (Pardes, 1983).

Defining "Right to Left"

All the definitions of social and of biological psychiatry that have been considered so far have been, as Karl Popper (1945) puts it, from left to right. This is the natural way for everyday conversation, but it is highly restrictive when used in science. Aristotle was its most influential advocate. He taught that the term to be defined is "the name of the essence of a thing." The ultimate aim of all enquiry, therefore, is the compilation of an encyclopedia containing the names of all essences together with their defining formulae. These definitions would then constitute all our knowledge. Those who would like an assortment of such reifying formulae defining social psychiatry cannot do better than read Assen Jablensky's account (1990).

Popper points out that "these essentialist views stand in the strongest possible contrast to the methods of modern science," which cannot reach finality but can hope to discover whether or not a new hypothesis is superior to an old one. Scientific definitions "do not contain any knowledge whatever, nor even any 'opinion'; they do nothing but introduce new arbitrary shorthand labels; they cut a long story short." This is a different kind of labelling from Scheff's. To define one's terms scientifically means no more than to say that, for convenience, a term will be used in a particular way, using words and measurements as precisely as possible in order that other scientists who wish to do so can repeat the observation or experiment involved. The term does not have to be used in that way, and other people may legitimately use it to label a different concept or formula. Perhaps the most attractive feature of Popper's ideas is that they take the mystique out of scientific activities. Just as in everyday problem solving, it is a matter of trial and error, on the basis of previous experience, with the intention of eliminating error.

When Ernest Gruenberg (1983) commented on Shepherd's paper, he began by saying that he had never met a nonsocial psychiatrist and ended with a right-to-leftist manifesto: "For goodness' sake let those who wish to call themselves social psychiatrists decide what they want us to understand by the label."

Psychiatric Disorders

If asked to define psychiatry, most practitioners would be likely to say that it was the branch of medicine concerned with mental disorders. But what are mental disorders and how do they differ from "physical" diseases? For that matter, what is a physical disease? Such a sequence of left to right questions seems natural to start with but illustrates the inherent tendency towards an infinite regress or towards authoritarian definitions in terms of disease "entities," often nowadays couched in purely technical terms.

This latter is what moderate critics of biomedicine see as harmful. Leon Eisenberg (a professor of social medicine as well as of psychiatry) points to the way that its very success "has narrowed the physician's focus exclusively to the biology of disease." He is particularly concerned with the narrowing of the diagnostic process to focus on its technological aspects. "A gastroenterologist realizes a net hourly income from endoscopy that is more than six times greater than from the general management of the patient's illness. The disproportion between the fees paid for procedures and those for a thorough history and physical examination is transforming gastroenterologists into endoscopists and cardiologists into catheterologists." But this tendency is not due solely to the structure of payment for private medical services: "The fact is that medical education, far from being 'too scientific,' suffers from too much emphasis on memorizing evanescent 'facts' and too little on science as a way of framing questions and gathering evidence" (Eisenberg, 1988).

An exposition of the historical development of the two approaches to medicine has been given by Sir Henry Cohen (1961). The first, essentialist or rationalist, definition assumes that "when a healthy man A falls ill he becomes A *plus* B, where B is 'a disease.' " This view springs in part from the notion of demoniacal possession. In various forms (notably the Galenic humoral theory) it has been the main approach to medicine for two thousand years. It maintains that there are innumerable disease entities, each with its individual and recognizable characters and natural history.

> The concept of disease as a "clinical entity" still dominates much of our textbook descriptions, as illustrated by the so-called classical pictures of typhoid fever, influenza, disseminated sclerosis and the rest. Many of these are little more helpful in diagnosis than would be a composite portrait of a Cabinet or a Test Team in revealing whether a given individual is a member of either. And we will seek for pathognomonic signs as short cuts to diagnosis. . . . [especially when they] are revealed by the exact instruments of a clinical laboratory, by X-rays or by a whole gamut of electrical recording machines. This way lies simplicity and directness; this way labour, time and thought can be conserved. But this way lies also error and unreason.

The second, nominalist or empirical, approach defines "disease as a deviation from the normal; a healthy man A, through the influence of any number of factors (x1, x2, x3 . . . x)—physical or mental—is changed and suffers; he is dis-eased." This kind of medicine could hardly develop until theories of normal anatomical, physiological, and biochemical functioning had been tested and found useful. Simple quantitative deviations from the normal (hypertension, menorrhagia, hypoglycaemia, etc.) are interesting in themselves. Such deviations are also commonly combined in constantly recurring patterns, or syndromes. Cohen includes psychological dysfunctions (e.g., thirst as a symptom of impaired carbohydrate tolerance, or disturbances of sensation that may localize abnormality in the parietal lobe) under the heading of physiology. Because of their solid base in knowledge of normal functions, such syndromes or symptom complexes can be used to predict the site of abnormality, or associated functional disturbances, or disorder in some anatomical or physiological or psychological system, or more fundamental causes. "It is this concept which should dominate our teaching and our approach to medicine."

Aubrey Lewis (1953) has provided a precise discussion of "psychological dysfunctions" in terms of subjective experiences whose deviation from some postulated standard of normal functioning has led to their inclusion in the definition of a disorder. His use of the term does not depend on any accompanying physiological or anatomical dysfunctions, although they might be present or postulated, but on the subjective description of the phenomenon alone.

For example, a description of images or thoughts or impulses intruding into the mind against conscious resistance has long been familiar to psychiatrists who make a practice of listening in detail to their patients' complaints. The name "obsession" is a convenient label. The experience might well have social consequences, because of the resulting intereference with everyday activities, and be defined socially as abnormal because of its rarity and the difficulty most people would have in understanding it. For this reason, Lemert could fairly have included it as a "primary" social deviation. Nevertheless, it has no distinctively social content, and it is also reasonable to put forward the hypothesis that it has a biological basis. In fact, the evidence of post-encephalitic obsessions or those associated with Tourette's syndrome supports the idea. But the way the afflicted individual reacts will depend in part on the social effects of the dysfunction and on his or her own reaction. The sum of these factors will be expressed as social disablement and it is this, rather than a "disease entity" that the doctor will be faced with.

Other psychiatric phenomena can be described in similar fashion and given names: various kinds of hallucinations, "first rank" experiences, phobias, or affective or cognitive dysfunctions. Jaspers (1963) drew together many descriptive accounts in his *General Psychopathology* and provided a basis for later attempts at reliable discrimination, measurement, and classification. The phenomena are "valid" in their own right as observations. It is when they are assumed to be "symptoms" and "syndromes" representing disease entities (a beguiling vision for members of a specialty impatient to emulate the scientific status achieved by general medicine during the twentieth century, on the false premise that there is a short cut to that success) that claims for validity look pretentious. To seek for simple causes—a one-gene basis for some aspects of schizophrenia, for example—is a rational strategy, in view of the new options for prevention, therapy, and further extensions of scientific knowledge that would open if it turned out to be correct (MRC, 1987). But that would not be an entity either, simply a basis for further hypotheses and further testing.

Further consideration is given in chapter 7 to the way that many clinical "symptoms" and "syndromes" have been recognized and named before there was any possibility of testing hypotheses concerning their biological substrate.

Disease Theories

Cohen's preferred approach to medicine in general is thus fully applicable to psychiatric disorders in particular (Wing, 1978; Wing et al., 1981). Definitions are used as aids to testing theories. Dysfunctions are hypothesized to be "symptoms" of some underlying biological abnormality, itself specifiable in terms of deviations from some postulated cycle of normal functioning. In this way disease theories can be built and tested without reification.

Scadding (1982) has pointed out that, in medicine in general, it is possible to use the terminology of disease, if one is careful, without being essentialist. It is certainly convenient to do so; indeed, this is the point of right to left definition. Rather more care is necessary, however, when considering psychiatric disorders, where specific biological underpinning is often lacking, and terms like "disease" tend to be given greater weight than they deserve. With the term "disease theory," there can be no misunderstanding; evidence for the theory, or hypothesis if theory is too grand a word, has to be provided and to be at least as good as that for, say, diabetes. We are not there yet.

The rules laid down in the revised third edition of the APA's *Diagnostic and Statistical Manual* (APA, 1987), and those in Chapter F of the tenth edition of the *International Classification of Diseases* (WHO, 1990), do not have to be regarded as defining disease entities—though many people, including perhaps some of the authors of the systems, will accept them as doing just that. A recent book on DSM-IIIR contains examples of all shades of opinion (Robins and Barrett, 1989). The rules can be turned into reasonably reliable techniques for deriving constructs about which testable hypotheses concerning cause, treatment, and prognosis can be put forward and tested, thus allowing greater comparability between research groups across the world. This is a substantial justification. It is useful and convenient to have standard rules, representing an approximate consensus of professional opinion internationally, but that provides no guarantee of validity. The technical means of ensuring reliability, feasibility in use and adequate coverage of symptoms must be sufficiently flexible to allow researchers to test, at the same time, any other diagnostic formulation that they find scientifically interesting.

"Schizophrenia," for example, instead of being the biological entity that led some Soviet psychiatrists to treat social deviance (which later came to include political dissent) as a disease, is simply a name given to various technically definable patterns of subjective experiences and abnormal behaviors that have resulted in people being referred to caring professionals of many different kinds for at least two centuries. That experience (itself grounded in the experience of the people afflicted and their families) is precious. Which patterns will survive will depend on the results of research. When solid and quantitative links to deviations from normal psychophysiological or anatomical functions have been demonstrated, many of the "syndromes" tested will be found to need unpacking and their contents redistributed. Others will have to be amalgamated. The process of diagnosis will be refined in this way. Clinical experience and scientific investigation proceed in parallel.

To adopt a sceptical attitude both to the clinical syndromes that have been described up to now and to the theories so far put forward to explain them (most of which have been wrong) does not mean that the problems presented to psychiatrists are being treated lightly. On the contrary, this is the frame of mind most likely to reach and beneficially apply solutions to important parts of those problems.

The difficulty that adherents of rigid doctrines have concerning this approach is illustrated by three authors who started from the reasonable assumption that the concept of "schizophrenia" as a disease entity must be abandoned, but drew an unreasonable conclusion that no further attempts should be made to test theories (in particular biomedical theories) based on combinations of symptoms given this label. The only alternative they could think of was to substitute the "symptoms" for the "disease," without apparently realizing that they were falling into their own trap by regarding symptoms as entities (Bentall et al., 1988).

Nevertheless it is heartening to find psychologists who are interested in symptoms. (The term will be used conventionally from now on to denote observed deviations from normal psychological or physiological functioning, which singly or in combination can be used to test predictions of abnormality in biological systems.) Experimental psychologists have seemed unwilling to consider on their merits (not submerged into a "positive" syndrome) the extraordinary experiences described by many people diagnosed as having schizophrenia. For example, how can the experience of hearing one's thoughts aloud in one's head, so loud that one feels that someone nearby must be able to overhear them, have a cortical location? What are the neural factors that prevent most of us having this experience? An attempt to create neuropsychological structures intermediate between the phenomena of mental disorders and hypothetical biological abnormalities should potentially be fruitful. Perhaps a fear of becoming trapped in a circular mind-body dualism has been offputting. If so, the example of coronary heart disease, where often the only means of early diagnosis is a subjective experience—pain with a particular distribution—should be reassuring.

It is, of course, easier to get a diagnosis from a psychiatrist and then to compare and contrast groups with and without "schizophrenia." Some at least of the conclusions reached by Rudolph Cohen (1987), following a review of the psychological literature, that "the models and research that have been discussed in this paper do not give us immediate directions," must stem from the almost universal use of unstandardized, and therefore non-comparable, diagnoses. Peter Venables (1987) has summarized the substantial literature suggesting that there is a disorder of cognitive and attentional processes, which might—if valid and reliably specifiable—be of value to social and cognitive psychologists in formulating mechanisms of coping and, possibly, in the elucidation of symptom formation under different social conditions. Christopher and Uta Frith (1987, 1989, Frith and Frith, 1990, this volume) have put forward important hypotheses linking impairments to underlying brain malfunctions.

What is now needed is some firm empirical underpinning. Without it, such intermediate structures, if expressed operationally in terms of test results without firm attachment to the impairments that inspired them and to demonstrated deviation from biological norms, could be in danger of being misinterpreted as entities in themselves, instead of a different and potentially fruitful way of rephrasing the clinical observations. That would make confusion worse confounded.

Medical Role Models

Much of the foregoing discussion has centered on the role and signifi-cance of diagnosis in psychiatry, whichever adjective is used to qualify it. The term "medical model" seems to be most commonly used nowadays to denote a practice that is entirely dominated by diagnostic activities. The work of Eisenberg's endoscopist would perhaps deserve such an attribu-tion, but it is not a description of what most doctors actually do. Diagnosis and treatment are at the heart of the medical role—that is why, ostensibly at any rate—patients come, but these functions provide the occasion for others. Doctors should be able to understand, and many of them should be able to take on, something of the roles of counsellor, befriender, teacher, psychotherapist, social worker, and advocate. In fact, the right-to-left answer to the definition of "psychiatry" is that it is the label given to a discipline whose content can be described in terms of the activities of those who are officially licensed to call themselves psychiatrists. That allows a great deal of scope!

Moreover, diagnosis is at least as much to do with ruling out disease explanations as with establishing that one or other of them would prove useful for helping a patient. This is particularly true in psychiatric practice, where most disorders are recognized only by their manifestations and where disease theories are mostly rather fragile. The temptation to move to either extreme—no disease or all disease—is inherent in the use of entities but avoided by recognizing both the advantages and the limitations of current theories.

Concepts of Health and Normality

The more we know about the factors that maintain the structural integrity of the nervous system and regulate neurophysiological functioning, the better able we shall be to formulate theories that explain clinical disorders as manifestations of underlying disturbances in neural homeostatic mechanisms. Theories of normal biological functioning are very specific and limited. In open societies the results of tests can be replicated or criticized by anyone who has the competence to do so.

Social concepts of normality are different in kind. What is regarded as socially normal or deviant varies substantially from one culture or subculture to another and it is unsafe to generalize from the standards (themselves variable) of, say, a socially deprived area in south-east London to what might be expected elsewhere. The best way to avoid equating social nonconformity with mental disorder is to lay down as precise and reliable criteria as possible for defining impairments, using criteria with the least possible reliance on social definitions of abnormality. Nevertheless, local and personal attitudes do influence the choice of counsellor when people are looking for help with problems.

A useful starting point for all kinds of caring professional is "social disablement" (Wing, 1990), a term which expresses the extent to which an individual is unable to meet personal or social expectations of performance in various fields of action and responsibility, with a consequent loss of independence. Patients are likely to be referred to psychiatrists because of the possibility that psychological dysfunctions are the cause of at least part of the disablement. Practitioners cannot be frozen into inactivity while scientists carry out interminable tests. There has to be a "state of the art" consensus, constantly updated, as to what aspects of social disablement can usefully be regarded as remediable by specific or empirical treatments.

A convenient procedure is to divide the causes of social disablement into impairments, disadvantages and self-attitudes. The term "impairment" has been defined by the World Health Organization (1980) to mean loss or abnormality of biological or psychological functions (equivalent to Sir Henry Cohen's deviation from a normal biological standard). Examples include psychomotor slowness, perceptual disorders, abnormalities of mood, instability of autonomic reactions, and cognitive dysfunctions. Impairments can often be caused, precipitated, or amplified by environmental circumstances, both physical and psychosocial. If the impairment persists over a long period of time, in spite of the best care currently available, it is designated "intrinsic"—the hypothesis to beat being that it is likely to have a biological basis. Most such impairments are prolonged versions of acute symptoms.

Another type of cause of social disablement is environmental (and particularly long term) disadvantage: poverty, poor occupational or social skills due to lack of opportunity to acquire them, few or absent social supports. Physical and mental impairments, including those "minor" forms that may underlie "personality disorders" or predispose to major illness, are also potent causes. Amplification of such disadvantages (Lemert's secondary deviance) occurs when stigma, indifference, malpractice, ignorance, or destitution take away from those who already have little, even what they have. In a recent case of malpractice in a Greek hospital, the amplification was iatrogenic.

These two types of factor can be difficult to distinguish, the more so because disadvantage can cause impairment as well as being caused by it. The problem is compounded by the third factor: adverse attitudinal and behavioral changes that tend to accumulate in the presence of long term impairment and disadvantage. These include demoralization (Frank, 1973; Link and Dohrenwend, 1980), hopelessness, diminished self-esteem, underconfidence, and loss of motivation to use even functions that are unimpaired.

To all this must be added the social circumstances in which the patient is currently living: the family circle, the local housing situation, the level of unemployment, the availability of non-specialized sheltered settings for handicapped people, the social security arrangements, and the general level of development of the society.

The World Health Organization scheme does not identify these elements specifically, although the terms "disability" (restriction of ability to perform an activity, due to impairment) and "handicap" (the disadvantage resulting from disability) are recognized as complex biosocial constructs. The disadvantage of the WHO terminology for psychiatric (and perhaps even for general medical) practice is that it begins with impairment and derives disability and handicap from it. It is thus concentrated on the consequences of impairments and depends greatly on the ease with which these can be recognized and classified. The contributions made to "handicap" (what I prefer to call social disablement) by social and personal factors other than those stemming from impairment are not separately identified. The nature of the interaction between impairment, social deprivation, and self-attitudes can therefore only partially and vaguely be represented.

Psychiatrists often see patients at a point when all three factors have been combining and interacting for years. Each type has its own theories of causation and amelioration, its own battery of measuring instruments, and its own literature. In principle, they can be separated, and researchers assume this, but in practice the overall level of social disablement is difficult to resolve into neat components. Needs assessment systems based on these ideas require much further development (Mangen and Brewin, 1990, this volume).

Nevertheless, the intention to differentiate is important. One simple example, which could have serious consequences, may be sufficient to make the point. If someone with little apparent social responsiveness is regarded as "unfriendly," or someone who thinks and moves slowly is called "lazy," while the more likely explanation is that they are psychologically impaired, the probability that disablement will be amplified is substantially increased. The impairment is socially "invisible." Such behavior could be due to several kinds of impairment and be assigned to one of several syndromes, with different implications for treatment, care or coping advice. Whether this kind of psychiatry is labelled "social" or "biological" hardly seems to matter.

Research In Social Psychiatry

Members of the MRC Social Psychiatry Research Unit, even those who chose the title (O'Connor, 1968), never sought to restrict the use of the term to their own preoccupations or to suggest that it described everything they did. "Social impairment" (Frith, 1989), for example, can be regarded as a biological or as a social concept, depending on the context of the investigation.

The content of our research has included investigating the social precipitants and amplifiers of psychiatric disorders in order to devise methods of secondary and tertiary prevention; studying social influences on the course of these disorders in order to recommend techniques of treatment, rehabilitation and care and make a prognosis; and evaluating the success of various types of agent and agency so as to help plan the most effective, acceptable, and economic set of health and social services. The Unit has used ideas and techniques from phenomenology, nosology, psychophysiology, pharmacology, epidemiology, social and bio-statistics, health economics, social history, sociology, and social psychology (in particular an interest in the formation and measurement of attitudes and the structure of institutions). Members have been involved in promoting the efforts of voluntary organizations to help psychiatrists be as humane as they think they already are, and have kept a sympathetic though sceptical eye on the progress of efforts to enlarge knowledge of the biological basis of psychiatry, because that will enlarge its social basis as well.

Some examples of the kind of research we have been involved in are given in this book.

Conclusion

Health is a social concept, disease is a biological concept. Doctors are fundamentally concerned with both. They are not, and never have been, dealing with purely biological problems; much less so in psychiatry, in the present state of knowledge, than in other areas of medicine. To Samuel Guze's rhetorical question, "Biological psychiatry, is there any other kind?", the answer must be "No, of course not." By the same token, all psychiatry is social in nature. Both statements are trivial unless given content in terms of specific hypotheses that other workers can test and publicly criticize.

To end at the beginning, the reply to F.A. von Hayek came a few days later in a letter to the Times:

> A social market is one which supplies those needs of individuals which the market fails to provide. . . . For example, the income of the old is usually inadequate because they no longer have labour to sell. . . . The mentally handicapped are not only unable to sell their labour, but cannot use money to buy clothing, food and shelter even if they have any. . . . Admittedly the terminology is confusing, and if Professor Hayek wishes to change it, he has my support. But the underlying concepts are clear . . . (Parris, 1983)

This chapter is based in part on an unpublished lecture delivered at the Annual Meeting of the Royal College of Psychiatrists, Brighton, June 1988.

References

American Psychiatric Association (1987) *Diagnostic and Statistical Manual of Mental Disorders,* 3rd revision. Washington, D.C.: APA.

Bentall, R.P., Jackson, H.F. and Pilgrim, D. (1988) Abandoning the concept of schizophrenia. *British Journal of Psychology* 27: 303–324.

Boyer, P. and Nissenbaum, S. (1974) *Salem Possessed. The Social Origins of Witchcraft.* Boston: Harvard University Press.

Cohen, H. (1961) The evolution of the concept of disease. In: Lush, B. (ed.) *Concepts of Medicine,* pp. 159–169. Oxford: Pergamon.

Cohen, R. and Borst, U. (1987) Psychological models of schizophrenic impairments. In: Häfner, H., Gattaz, W.F. and Janzarik, W. (eds.): *Search for the Causes of Schizophrenia,* pp. 189–202. Heidelberg: Springer Verlag.

Cooper, J.E., Kendall, R.E., Gurland, B.J., Sharpe, L., Copeland, J.R.M., and Simon, R. (1972) *Psychiatric Diagnosis in New York and London.* London: Oxford University Press.

Eisenberg, L. (1988) Science in medicine. Too much or too little and too limited in scope? *American Journal of Medicine* 84: 483–491.

Frank, J.D. (1973) *Persuasion and Healing.* Baltimore: Johns Hopkins University Press.

Frith, C. and Frith, U. (1990) this volume, chapter 4.

Frith, U. (1989) *Autism: Explaining the Engima.* Oxford: Blackwell.

Goffman, E. (1961) *Asylums. Essays on the Social Situation of Mental Patients and Other Inmates.* New York: Doubleday.

Grotjahn, A. (1923) *Soziale Pathologie,* dritte Auflage. Berlin: Springer Verlag.

Gruenberg, E.M. (1983) Commentary on article by M. Shepherd. *Integrative Psychiatry* 1: 93–94.

Guze, S.B. (1989) Biological psychiatry. Is there any other kind? *Psychological Medicine* 19: 315–323.

Hayek, F.A. von (1983) Beware this weasel word. *The London Times,* 11 November.

Jablensky, A. (1990) Public health aspects of social psychiatry. In: Goldberg, D. and Tantum, D. (eds.) *Public Health and Social Psychiatry.* To be published.

Jaspers, K. (1963) *General Psychopathology.* Trans. from the seventh German edition by Hoenig, J. and Hamilton, M. Manchester: University Press.

Lemert, E.M. *Social Pathology.* New York: McGraw-Hill.

Lewis, A.J. (1953) Health as a social concept. *British Journal of Sociology* 4* 109–124.

Link, B. and Dohrenwend, B.P. (1980) Formulation of hypotheses about the true prevalence of demoralization in the United States. In: Dohrenwend, B.P., Dohrenwend, B.S., Gould, M.S., Link, B., Neugebauer, R. and Wunsch-Hitzig, R. (eds.) *Mental Illness in the United States: Epidemiological Estimates.* Heidelberg: Springer-Verlag.

Mangen, S. and Brewin, C. (1990) This volume, chapter 8.

Mechanic, D. (1968) *Medical Sociology: A Selective View.* New York: Free Press.

Mechanic, D. (1970) Problems and prospects in psychiatric epidemiology. In: Hare, E.H. and Wing, J. K. (eds.) *Psychiatric Epidemiology.* London: Oxford University Press.

Medical Research Council (1987) *Research into Schizophrenia.* London: MRC.

O'Connor, N. (1968) The origins of the Medical Research Council Social Psychiatry Research Unit. In: Shepherd, M. and Davies, D.L. (eds.) *Studies in Psychiatry.* London: Oxford University Press.

Pardes, H. (1983) Commentary on article by M. Shepherd. *Integrative Psychiatry* 1: 89–90.

Parris, H. (1983) The human needs of social justice. Letters. *The London Times,,* 15 November.

Popper, K.R. (1945) *The Open Society and its Enemies.* Volume II. *The High Tide of Prophecy.* Chapter 11. pp. 9–20. London: Routledge.

Robins, L.N. and Barrett, J.E. (1989) *The Validity of Psychiatric Diagnosis.* New York: Raven Press.

Scadding, J.G. (1982) Review of 'What is a Case?' *Psychological Medicine* 12: 207–208.

Scheff, T.J. (1963) The role of the mentally ill and the dynamics of mental disorder. A research framework. *Sociometry* 26: 436–453.

Scheff, T.J. (1964) The societal reaction to deviance. Ascriptive elements in the psychiatric screening of mental patients in a midwestern state. *Social Problems.* 2: 401–413.

Scheff, T.J. (1966) *Being Mentally Ill.* Chicago: Aldine.

Shepherd, M. (1983) The origins and directions of social psychiatry. *Integrative Psychiatry* 1: 86–88.

Simon, B. (1978) *Mind and Madness in Ancient Greece: The Classical Roots of Modern Psychiatry.* New York: Cornell University Press.

Starkey, M. (1949) *The Devil in Massachusetts.* New York: Knopf. Republished by Anchor Books, 1969.

Szasz, T. (1961) *The Myth of Mental Illness.* New York: Hoeber-Harper.

Szasz, T. (1971) *The Manufacture of Madness*. London: Routledge.

Venables, P. (1987) Cognitive and attentional disorders in the development of schizophrenia. In: Häfner, H. Gattaz, W.F., and Janzarik, W. (eds.): *Search for the Causes of Schizophrenia,* pp 189–202. Heidelberg: Springer Verlag.

Williams, A. (1979) One economist's view of social medicine. *Epidemiology and Community Health* 33: 3–7.

Wilson, E. (1975) *Sociobiology: The New Synthesis*. Cambridge, Mass: Belknap/ Harvard.

Wing, J.K. (1978) *Reasoning about Madness*. Oxford: University Press.

Wing, J.K. (1990) Meeting the needs of people with psychiatric disorders. *Social Psychiatry and Epidemiology*. 25: 2–8.

Wing, J.K. (1990) this volume, Chapter 7.

Wing, J.K. and Brown, G.W. (1970) *Institutionalism and Schizophrenia*. London: Cambridge University Press.

Wing, J.K., Bebbington, P. and Robins, L.N. (1981) What is a Case? The *Problem of Definition in Psychiatric Community Surveys*. Chapters 1 and 20. London: Grant McIntyre.

Wing, L. (1990) This volume, Chapter 6.

World Health Organization (1973) *The International Pilot Study of Schizophrenia*. Geneva: WHO.

World Health Organization (1980) *International Classification of Impairments, Disabilities and Handicaps*. Geneva: WHO.

World Health Organization (1990) *International Classification of Diseases,* tenth revision. Geneva: WHO.

2

Researching the Idea of Health

David Mechanic

Introduction

In a classic essay in the *British Journal of Sociology* in 1953, Sir Aubrey Lewis commenting on the World Health Organization's (WHO), definition of health as "a state of physical, mental and social well-being" noted that "a proposition could hardly be more comprehensive than that, or more meaningless" (Lewis, 1953). But being the scholar that he was, Sir Aubrey acknowledged the history and complexity of the idea linking health to the "ancient formula of unattainable wholeness of body, mind and soul." Given the difficulty of establishing empirical referents for the WHO definition, Lewis might have been surprised at its most recent expansion to include spiritual well-being as well. Whatever, Lewis' view of the expansive definition of health, the thrust of Sir Aubrey's focus and argument was that disease cannot be assessed in terms of social standards but rather must be adjudged by evidence of pathological function. As he noted:

> The physician is of course trained to relate signs of disturbed function and structure to the norm. His personal experience and the accumulated experience of others are at his disposal. For some organs he has much fuller and more exact information at his disposal than for others: he can, for example, with much more confidence judge the state of the heart than that of the liver. But for each organ and system he has a body of knowledge about the range of normal function and the evidences of normal structure, so that equally well-trained physicians would agree about whether a particular system is working normally.

I had the good fortune to be invited by John Wing to be a visiting scientist at the Social Psychiatry Unit in 1965 (Sir Aubrey's last year as Professor at the Institute). Lewis' and Wing's thoughtful work stimulated my exploration of the disease concept, the early results of which appear in the first edition of *Medical Sociology* (Mechanic, 1968, see particularly pp. 1–114). My thinking was also enriched by the perspectives of René Dubos, a microbiologist and discoverer of the source of the first commercially produced antibiotics. Dubos, seeking an enzyme to decompose the envelope protecting bacteria causing lobar pneumonia, turned his attention to the study of swamp soil where he began developing his appreciation for the richness of natural variability and its effects on the development of organisms. As he pursued his studies, Dubos became convinced that the "prevalence and severity of microbial diseases are conditioned more by the ways of life of the persons afflicted than by the virulence and other properties of the etiological agents" (Dubos, 1965).

As Dubos engaged the study of disease and environment and the extraordinary adaptiveness of organisms to changing conditions, he became critical of exaggerated claims about the effectiveness of solving health problems solely through medicine. While himself an eminent medical scientist, he understood that health cannot be an absolute or permanent value, however careful the social and medical planning. As he eloquently explained, "Biological success in all its manifestations is a measure of fitness, and fitness requires never-ending efforts of adaptation to the total environment which is ever changing" (Dubos, 1959).

In Wing's (1978) theoretical discussion of the bases of social psychiatry, *Reasoning About Madness,* he examined the compatibility between good, rigorous classification, and the broader dimensions of health and disease. As he observed,

> The fact that a disease theory is constructed on the basis of a syndrome of characteristics which are defined, as far as possible, in nonsocial terms and which are regarded as symptomatic of some underlying disturbance of biological functioning, does not mean that social factors can be ignored. (p. 25)

Simple categorical disease categories, he noted,

> give way to a more flexible approach based on an increasing knowledge of biological control mechanisms. Underlying every disease syndrome there are quantitative theories of normal biological functions. The more complete and interlocking these are, the less relevant are the categories, except as keys to unlock dimensional secrets. (p. 24)

Wing has laid special emphasis on the assessment of chronic impairments and their social management so as to alter the course of disease. He noted that whatever the source of intrinsic impairments, they may result in illness behavior,

> which may lead over a long period of time to extra personal and social handicaps that are not part of the disease process and that need not necessarily have accumulated at all if the context of treatment or rehabilitation had been different. (p. 26)

It is these types of conditions that increasingly account for the burden of disease as we have gained control over infectious disease and as longevity has increased. The AIDS epidemic should remind us that the notion of control, with its underlying assumption of equilibrium, is itself a mirage, conditioned by time and place. Medical history alerts us to how easily ecological balance can be disrupted (Grob, 1983).

There have been numerous efforts to define health both in general and psychological terms. Marie Jahoda (1958), for example, identified six primary themes recurring in definitions of positive mental health such as positive attitudes toward the self, integration of personality, autonomy, and environmental mastery. The difficulty is the lack of specificity in these criteria and their dependence on social values and social judgments which may vary widely by culture and social context. As she herself noted, "there is hardly a term in current psychological thought as vague, elusive, and ambiguous as the term 'mental health' " (Jahoda, 1958, p. 3). Yet the effort to study health as a global concept, whatever its difficulties and ambiguities, is not a fool's mission.

1. A number of important disease risk factors appear to have nonspecific effects on a wide range of disease conditions and mortality including broad factors such as socio-economic status, social networks and supports, and stressful life events as well as more specific patterns of behavior such as smoking, exercise, and intimate relations (Mechanic, 1982; Syme, 1986). It is conceivable that as we learn more we will be able to account for most of these influences through specific processes linked to each disease, but the nonspecific effects are robust. Moreover, the more we learn about biological processes, the more evident it becomes that while models of specific disease syndromes are pragmatic and essential for advancements, the syndromes are related and not discrete.

2. Self-reports of health status and subjective health assessments are among the best general predictors of mortality, morbidity, and use of medical care services (Ware, 1986). Various studies have found that such subjective assessments are not only significantly related to objective indicators such as physician assessments, medical record data and mortality (LaRue, Bank, Jarvik, and Hetland, 1979; Ferraro, 1980;

Eisen, Donald, Ware and Brook, 1980; Fillenbaum, 1979), but are independent predictors of mortality having controlled for objective assessments of health and known risk factors (Mossey and Shapiro, 1982; Kaplan and Camacho, 1983). Mossey and Shapiro (1982), in studying 3128 noninstitutionalized elderly, found a threefold difference in mortality over 6 years between those rating their health excellent and those rating it poor which persisted controlling for age, sex, residence, and health status indicators. Similarly, Kaplan and Camacho (1983) in a nine year follow-up of a large California adult sample found large differences in mortality associated with prior subjective assessments. These effects persist controlling for baseline measures of health practices, social networks, health indicators, and psychological status. The superiority of such self-assessments over objective medical assessments is an intriguing puzzle.

3. There is good statistical evidence that persons can "will" their survival or death over short time spans, and that for these limited time intervals social events can be powerful predictors (Phillips and Feldman, 1973; Phillips and King, 1988). Moreover, relatively modest social interventions among elderly institutionalized populations show effects not only on well-being but even mortality. Langner and Rodin (1976) assessed an intervention that gave nursing home residents more choices in their everyday lives. Follow-up after eighteen months found that those in the intervention group experienced improved health as well as a marginal improvement in longevity relative to the comparison group (Rodin and Langner, 1977; Rodin, 1986).

4. There is a large literature linking morbidity and mortality to patterns of industrialization, urbanization, migration, and acculturation (Dubos, 1959, 1965; Grob, 1983). Other powerful influences include schooling, patterns of marriage and divorce, religious and group affiliation, and participation and employment patterns (Mechanic, 1978, 1982, 1988). Many of these data are either cross-sectional or aggregated in ways making it impossible to differentiate cause and effect. But the literature in its totality is persuasive of the importance of depicting the role of broad processes by which the measured end results occur, and of the crucial intervening variables.

The challenge to the investigator is to dissect these enormously complicated patterns in ways that retain the meaningfulness of the original observations but with rigorous research procedures and measurement that allow testing alternative explanations. In this paper, I focus on only two areas which have been of research interest to me for many years: the meaning of subjective health concepts and the role of illness behavior in health outcomes.

Self-assessment of Health Status

The predictive value of simple health perceptions is remarkable, but their meaning remains uncertain. A number of studies indicate that individuals in making assessments of health adopt a holistic frame of reference which is influenced by appraisals of their ability to function and the extent to which health decrements interfere (Mechanic, 1978). Even when efforts are made to focus the individual's attention on the physical dimension of health, the rating reflects broader aspects of social function and not only measurable medical morbidity or lack of physical fitness. Furthermore, such assessments seem to be made typically in terms of some standard of comparison the respondent has in mind. For example, many studies have found that elderly respondents report more positive health assessments relative to objective indicators than younger adults (Maddox and Douglass, 1973; Linn and Linn, 1980; Friedsam and Martin, 1963; Cockerham, Sharp, and Wilcox, 1983). A number of researchers have suggested that elderly persons are health optimists, but this characterization simply renames rather than illuminates the issue. One possibility is that the elderly adjust their perceptions because of modified health expectations with age (Tornstam, 1975). A negative consequence of such altered expectations is that individuals may neglect remediable problems because they associate such deficits with aging rather than with disease.

In one analysis Richard Tessler and I (Tessler and Mechanic, 1978) examined four diverse data sets to ascertain the relationship between various independent predictors and persons' perceptions of their own health. Included were samples of persons participating in alternative health insurance plans, a large sample of students at a major state university, a sample of men in a state prison, and a sample of persons aged forty-five to sixty-nine in a southern state. In this analysis we were concerned with factors predicting perceived health status, controlling for measures of actual health status. The need to have a measure of objective health status, as well as some other variables, directed the choice of data sets. The particular measures used for the analysis in each of the data sets are generally comparable, although they vary somewhat. It was our view, however, that the diversity of samples and variations in measures employed were an advantage in that if the same results emerge across data sets in spite of the differences, we can have increased confidence in the generality of the basic processes under study.

In each data set the dependent variable is the respondent's assessment of his or her health status, and the independent predictors consist of (1) a measure of physical health status (in two data sets we had physician ratings, while in the other two we depended on reported measures of illness), (2) a measure of psychological distress, and (3) measures of age, marital status, sex, education and race whenever they were applicable. The main concern of the analysis was to assess the degree to which psychological distress influenced people's perceptions of their health, taking into account both sociodemographic factors and some measure of "objective physical health."

For each data set we constructed a multiple regression equation in which perceived health status was regressed simultaneously against the other variables. Psychological distress was the only variable other than the measure of physical health status that retained a statistically significant standardized beta coefficient in all four data sets. As we expected, physical health status had a larger influence on perceived health than psychological distress, although this was not true in the case of the prison sample, and the betas in the sample of older people for the two predictors were fairly close. It is worthy of note, however, that the measures of physical health status made by physicians were less powerful than those based on respondent reports of illness, suggesting that the latter are influenced by a certain degree of respondent subjectivity. This finding supported our basic contention that subjective reports of illness already reflect to some extent the psychological state of the person providing the data (see Mechanic, 1979).

I view the self-assessment of health as an active process involving cognitive and emotional strategies typically used in assessing the self. Thus, physical symptoms are only one of many building blocks for forming this conception. Particular symptoms may be given prominence or may be defined as peripheral to the person's judgments of self and health. The fact that young people have little serious morbidity (Haggerty, 1983) provided an opportunity to examine the constituents of health appraisals in a sample of 1193 adolescents using longitudinal data (Mechanic and Hansell, 1987). If serious illness is not a major constituent of the self-appraisal, how then do young people with little chronic disease or serious morbidity form a self-appraisal of their health? In this instance we predicted that psychological well-being and competence in age relevant areas would shape such self-conceptions.

We indeed found that adolescents who reported higher levels of school achievement and more participation in sports and other exercise assessed their health as better over a one-year period than those reporting lower achievement and less participation, controlling for self-assessed health at the beginning of the year. Other longitudinal results showed that adolescents who were initially less depressed assessed their health more positively. Our measure of common physical symptoms was associated cross-sectionally with self-assessed health, but its longitudinal effect was mediated by initial levels of self-assessed health. In short, for these adolescents health is truly a social concept which reflects psychological well-being and competence in age-appropriate activities. If we form conceptions about ourselves by observing our own behavior as Bem (1972) has suggested, then adolescents may conclude they are healthy in part because they are active and competent. Having only limited physiological feedback, they may depend on judgments of their competence and activity to appraise themselves.

If health appraisals develop in this way it becomes easier to understand why patients' presentations to physicians intermix physical symptoms, psychological distress, and psychosocial difficulties. Physicians are trained to apply a disease model that seeks discrete infirmities but patients do not typically respond to their health problems in accord with medical models. Understanding the source of these discordant definitions and how patients' conceptions are formed provides new opportunities for medical care interventions.

Illness Behavior

The study of illness behavior seeks to identify the socio-cultural, psychological, and situational determinants that make people aware of symptoms, the cognitive schemata they use to interpret them, and the ways the organization and financing of services facilitate or impede varying kinds of care-seeking. Illness behavior helps shape the formation and course of illness. Illness often serves a variety of social and personal objectives which have little to do with biological systems or the pathogenesis of disease. The boundaries of illness and its definitions are extraordinarily broad, and the illness process can be used to negotiate a range of cultural, social, and personal tensions. Illness behavior is one of many alternatives for coping with personal and social tensions and conflict.

There is now an extensive literature on illness behavior (Mechanic, 1978, 1982, 1983; Kleinman, 1986, 1988; McHugh and Vallis, 1985), and sufficient familiarity with the concept to reduce a need for general elaboration. Here I focus on just a few points continuous with the preceding discussion on health status assessment. While we take knowing about how our body feels as self-evident, such judgments are difficult because of the absence of objective guides to which we can compare our internal experiences. Because of the absence of standards, people look to their environment or popular theories for a reasonable accounting of their experiences (see Leventhal, 1985). People generally believe that stress elevates blood pressure, for example, and, thus hypertensives commonly believe that their blood pressure is high when they are under stress and adapt their medications accordingly. Expecting a relation between medication and symptom change, patients typically reduce prescribed medication as symptoms abate. Medication adherence requires overcoming commonly understood popular models of cause and effect.

Very popular theories are so widely shared that both patient and doctor understand the premises upon which judgments are being made. But in many instances there are no commonly accepted conceptions or the illness models people use are conditioned by subcultures or are idiosyncratic. Thus practitioners must explore the attributions and theories that help guide the patient's responses.

Illness behavior plays an intriguing role in pain response and disability particularly in respect to back pain (Osterweis, Kleinman, and Mechanic, 1987). Spitzer and Task Force (1986), in a Canadian study, found that less than eight percent of patients complaining of back pain not supported by objective findings became chronic. We have no adequate models that can predict which of these patients will have self-limited conditions and who will become chronic. Illness behavior plays an important role, contributing to work absenteeism, use of medical services, and demands on the disability insurance system, but the precise factors, and how they influence outcomes, are difficult to specify.

There is a number of studies demonstrating that when depression occurs concurrently with acute disease, patients may attribute to the acute disease symptoms associated with persistent depressed affect, thus prolonging the illness process (Imoden, Canter, and Cluff, 1959, 1961). Such studies alert us to the fact that many patients may have difficulty interpreting the origin of symptoms when illnesses occur concomitantly. While much of the existing literature is based on the assumption that chronicity is in some sense motivated by secondary gain, the opportunities for confusion in symptom appraisal exist independently of the uses of illness to achieve advantages not otherwise available.

In a study of back pain, we had an opportunity to analyze data from the United States Health and Nutrition Examination Survey (HANES) among a subsample of 2431 respondents for whom we had both self-report data and findings from an extensive medical examination (Mechanic and Angel, 1987). This allowed development of an index that depicted the extent to which reported back pain exceeded physical findings. As in other studies, we found that older patients and those reporting higher levels of psychological well-being were less likely to make invalidated complaints, controlling for age, sex, race, marital status, education, and income. Depressed mood was associated with both more complaints and more physical findings, suggesting that causal factors operated in both directions. Our most interesting finding was that the inclination of older persons to report less pain at comparable levels of physical status based on the examination was significant only among those with higher levels of psychological well-being. This supports the notion that subjective assessments of health are made in the context of self-and-other comparisons. As people age, they may attribute some of their discomforts to the aging process and, thus, are more likely to normalize bodily discomforts. Persons who, in general, are experiencing a sense of well-being may feel they are doing well relative to their reference groups. Those with depressed mood are less likely to feel so.

The tendency of patients to view their health holistically, and not in terms of discrete categories, also complicates the way they seek help and express their complaints. The association between psychological and physical symptoms are widely recognized (Eastwood, 1975), and psychiatric patients are large consumers of nonpsychiatric health services (Jones and Vischi, 1979) relative to the population. In a study comparing a sample of psychiatric outpatients with a representative sample from the same population from which they came (Mechanic, Cleary and Greenley, 1982), we found that the psychiatric patients made 100 percent more nonpsychiatric medical care visits in the year prior to the study and 83 percent more in the year following than those in the representative sample.

There are a variety of possible explanations. One is that the excess visit rate is largely due to physical symptoms and dysfunction concomitant with psychiatric disorder. A second is that a higher propensity to seek help contributes to both becoming a psychiatric patient and to using general medical services. A third possibility is that once a person enters the psychiatric system, access to other services is easier. We developed measures that allowed us to compare the strength of these alternative explanations. Among them, the hypothesis dealing with concomitant symptoms explained the most variance, but illness behavior propensities were also important. These results suggest that patients are often unclear about the origins of their symptoms, or the appropriate attributions and help-seeking behavior. Nor are physicians always helpful in clarifying such issues.

Conclusion

The sources of health and disease in societies are broad and complex. Communities will have different rates and patterns of pathology depending on demographic, economic, and psychosocial influences that interact with the biological potentials and limitations of people (Mechanic, 1986a, 1986b), and these patterns will be altered by changes in environmental ecology and social organization. The medical model offers a useful but limited perspective on the factors that affect the occurrence and course of disease and alternatives for prevention and control. The current AIDS crisis vividly reminds us of the influence of social organization and behavior on the transmission of disease and the role of social groupings and subcultures in its spread or control. From this perspective, the idea of health, and its broad conceptualization is hardly unimportant. Definition and measurement is central to the challenge but to allow the easily measurable to guide our definitions of what is important and our research efforts would be exceedingly foolish.

References

Bem, D. (1972) Self-Perception Theory, in: Berkowitz, L. (Ed.) *Advances in Experimental Social Psychology,* 6, pp. 2–62, (New York, Academic Press).

Cockerham, W.C., Sharp, K. and Wilcox, J.A. (1983) Aging and Perceived Health Status, *Journal of Gerontology,* 38, pp. 349–55.

Dubos, R. (1959) *Mirage of Health: Utopias, Progress, and Biological Change* (New York, Harper).

Dubos, R. (1965) *Man Adapting* (New Haven, Yale University Press).

Eastwood, M.R. (1975) *The Relation Between Physical and Mental Illness* (Toronto, University of Toronto Press).

Eisen, M., Donald, C.A., Ware, J.E. Jr. and Brook, R.H. (1980) *Conceptualization and Measurement of Health for Children in the Health Insurance Study,* R-2312-HEW (Santa Monica, CA., Rand Corporation).

Ferraro, K.F. (1980) Self-Ratings of Health among the Old and the Old-Old, *Journal of Health and Social Behavior,* 21, pp. 377–83.

Fillenbaum, G.G. (1979) Social Context and Self-Assessment of Health Among the Elderly, *Journal of Health and Social Behavior,* 20, pp. 45–51.

Friedsam, H. and Martin, H.W. (1963) A Comparison of Self and Physicians' Ratings in an Older Population, *Journal of Health and Social Behavior,* 4, pp. 179–83.

Grob, G. (1983) Disease and Environment in American History, in: Mechanic, D. (Ed.) *Handbook of Health, Health Care, and the Health Professions,* pp. 3–22 (New York, The Free Press).

Haggerty, R. (1983) Epidemiology of Childhood Disease, in: Mechanic, D. (Ed.) *Handbook of Health, Health Care, and the Health Professions,* pp. 101–19 (New York, Free Press).

Imboden, J.B., Canter, A., Cluff, L.E. and Trever, R.W. (1959) Brucellosis III: Psychologic Aspects of Delayed Convalescent, *Archives of Internal Medicine,* 103, pp. 406–14.

Imboden, J.B., Canter, A. and Cluff, L.E. (1961) Symptomatic Recovery from Medical Disorder, *Journal of the American Medical Association,* 178, pp. 1182–84.

Jahoda, M. (1958) *Current Concepts of Positive Mental Health* (New York, Basic Books).

Jones, K. and Vischi, T. (1979) Impact of Alcohol, Drug Abuse and Mental Health Treatment on Medical Care Utilization: A Review of the Research Literature, *Medical Care,* 17, Supplement, entire issue.

Kaplan, G.A. and Camacho, T. (1983) Perceived health and mortality: a nine-year follow-up of the Human Population Laboratory cohort, *American Journal of Epidemiology,* 117, pp. 292–304.

Kleinman, A. (1986) *Social Origins of Distress and Disease: Depression, Neurasthenia and Pain in Modern China* (New Haven, Yale University Press).

Kleinman, A. (1988) *The Illness Narratives: Healing and the Human Condition* (New York, Basic Books).

Langner, E.J. and Rodin, J. (1976) The Effects of Choice and Enhanced Personal Responsibility for the Aged: A Field Experiment in an Institutional Setting, *Journal of Personality and Social Psychology,* 34, pp. 191–198.

Larue, A., Bank, L., Jarvik, L. and Hetland, M. (1979) Health in Old Age: How Do Physicians' Ratings and Self-ratings Compare?, *Journal of Gerontology,* 34, pp. 687–91.

Leventhal, H. (1985) Symptoms Reporting: A Focus On Process, in: McHugh, S. and Vallis, T.M. (Eds.) *Illness Behavior: A Multidisciplinary Model,* pp. 219–237 (New York, Plenum).

Lewis, A. (1953) Health as a Social Concept, *British Journal of Sociology,* 4, pp. 109–24.

Linn, B.S. and Linn, M.W. (1980) Objective and Self-assessed Health in the Old and Very Old, *Social Science and Medicine,* 14, pp. 311–15.

Maddox, G.L. and Douglass, E.B. (1973) Self-Assessment of Health: A Longitudinal Study of Elderly Subjects, *Journal of Health and Social Behavior,* 14, pp. 87–93.

McHugh, S. and Vallis, T.M. (1985) *Illness Behavior: A Multidisciplinary Model* (New York, Plenum).

Mechanic, D. (1968) *Medical Sociology: A Selective View* (New York, The Free Press).

Mechanic, D. (1978) *Medical Sociology: (second edition)* (New York, The Free Press).

Mechanic, D. (1979) Correlates of Physician Utilization: Why Do Major Multivariate Studies of Physician Utilization Find Trivial Psychosocial Effects, *Journal of Health and Social Behavior,* 20, pp. 387–396.

Mechanic, D. (1982) Disease, Mortality, and the Promotion of Health, *Health Affairs,* 1, pp. 28–32.

Mechanic, D. (Ed.) (1982) *Symptoms, Illness Behavior and Help-Seeking* (New Brunswick, Rutgers University Press).

Mechanic, D. Cleary, P.D. and Greenley, J.R. (1982) Distress Syndromes, Illness Behavior, Access to Care and Medical Utilization in a Defined Population, *Medical Care,* 20, pp. 361–72.

Mechanic, D. (1983) *Handbook of Health, Health Care, and the Health Professions* (New York, The Free Press).

Mechanic, D. (1986a) Some Relationships Between Psychiatry and the Social Sciences, *British Journal of Psychiatry,* 149, pp. 548–553.

Mechanic, D. (1986b) The Role of Social Factors in Health and Well Being: The Biopsychosocial Model from a Social Perspective, *Integrative Psychiatry,* 4, pp. 2–11.

Mechanic, D. and Angel, R. (1987) Some Factors Associated with the Report and Evaluation of Back Pain, *Journal of Health and Social Behavior,* 28, pp. 131–139.

Mechanic, D. and Hansell, S. (1987) Adolescent Competence, Psychological Well-Being and Self-Assessed Physical Health, *Journal of Health and Social Behavior,* 28, pp. 364–374.

Mechanic, D. (1988) Social Class and Health Status: An Examination of Underlying Processes, *Conference on Socio-economic Status and Health* (Palo Alto, CA., Henry J. Waiser Family Foundation).

Mossey, J.M. and Shapiro, E. (1982) Self-rated health: a predictor of mortality among the elderly, *American Journal of Public Health*, 72, pp. 800–808.

Osterweis, M., Kleinman, A. and Mechanic, D. (Eds.) (1987) *Pain and Disability: Clinical, Behavioral and Policy Perspectives,* Committee on Pain, Disability, and Chronic Illness Behavior, Institute of Medicine, (Washington, D.C., National Academy Press).

Phillips, D. and Feldman, K. (1973) A Dip in Deaths Before Ceremonial Occasions: Some New Relationships Between Social Integration and Mortality, *American Sociology Review*, 38, pp. 678–696.

Phillips, D. and King, E.W. (1988) Death Takes a Holiday, Mortality Surrounding Major Social Occasions, *Lancet, ii*, 728–32.

Rodin, J. (1986) Aging and health: effects of the sense of control, *Science*, 233, pp. 1271–1276.

Rodin, J. and Langner, E.J. (1977) Long term effects of a control-relevant intervention with the institutionalized aged, *Journal of Personality and Social Psychology*, 35, pp. 897–902.

Spitzer, W.O. and Task Force. (1986) *Rapport du Groupe de Travail Quebecois sur les Aspects Cliniques des Affections Vertebrales Chez les Travailleurs, L'Institute de Recherche en Sante et en Securite du Travail du Quebec.*

Syme, S.L. (1986) Social Determinants of Health and Disease, in: Last, J. (Ed.) *Maxcy-Rosenau Public Health, Health and Preventive Medicine 12th edition* (Norwalk, CT., Appleton-Century-Crofts).

Tessler, R.C. and Mechanic, D. (1978) Psychological Distress and Perceived Health Status, *Journal of Health and Social Behavior*, 19, pp. 254–62.

Tornstam, L. (1975) Health and Self-Perception: A Systems Theoretical Approach *The Gerontologist*, 27, pp. 264–70.

Ware, J.E., Jr. (1986) The Assessment Of Health Status, in Aiken, L. H. and Mechanic, D. (Eds.) *Applications of Social Science to Clinical Medicine and Social Policy*, pp. 204–28 (New Brunswick, Rutgers University Press).

Wing, J. (1978) *Reasoning About Madness* (Oxford, Oxford University Press).

3

Aetiology of Depression: Something of the Future?

George W. Brown

Introduction

Research on depression has reached an exciting stage; important work is going on in many disciplines and there are already stimulating attempts to pull the work together (Gilbert, 1988). Such reviews make clear an impressive degree of convergence in ideas and findings. Research seems likely to become less narrow, and at times genuinely cross disciplinary. What is perhaps surprising, given the plethora of clinical, biological, and psychological reports, is that the case for the critical importance of social factors in aetiology and course remains strong. However, rather than deal directly with some of the possibilities that result from this convergence, I will discuss the future in terms of an altogether duller set of issues surrounding measurement. This choice reflects my concern that there is a real danger of methodological shortcomings stultifying profitable collaboration.

Inter-disciplinary work multiplies the amount of data to be collected, and this is bound to add to current pressure to collect psychosocial and clinical material as cheaply as possible. The pressure is I believe largely structural and relates not least to our methods of funding and organizing research, together with the increasing need for publications for professional advancement. The effect of these pressures can be particularly great in non-laboratory and non-experimental work where adequate preparation and sufficient time for analysis are essential—though infrequently openly recognized. Such pressures, for example, can be seen in the monumental

U.S. Epidemiologic Catchment Area (ECA) survey of mental disorder in five American communities. The launching of data gathering was premature and basic shortcomings in the highly standardized Diagnostic Interview Schedule (DIS) effectively rule out consideration of a number of key aetiological issues (Brown, in press(a)).

An Intensive Tradition of Measurement

Quality of data is the central methodological concern, something easily overlooked when faced by virtuoso performances in data analysis by microcomputer. It would be misleadingly reticent, particularly on such an occasion, if I did not to state my belief that during the late 1950s and early 1960s workers in the MRC Social Psychiatry Research Unit set off on the right lines. I will refer to the style of data collection that evolved as intensive, but it must be added at once that something like it has always had a place in behavioral research. It has, however, never been central and has in recent years been embroiled in tiresome debates about its scientific status. The alternative "harder" style, reflected in the use of "face-sheet" variables and the standardized questionnaires of survey research, has typically claimed superiority. It has been the approach of choice in epidemiology, the discipline that has done so much for the development of sociomedical research. Indeed, my essay can be seen as centering on the consequences of extending the style of measurement to population enquiries, and the resulting tension when cost is weighed against sensitivity. In fact, cost is more of an issue than the scientific status of the approach. The method's record in terms of reliability and validity is good—something often obscured by the rhetoric of the harder measurement tradition—aided, it must be added, by some muddled thinking on the part of its practitioners.

Looking back, it was this intensive approach that was critical in the early work of the Unit. The version developed resulted from the coming together of three different traditions—that of anthropology (Carstairs, Monck and myself), that of the clinical tradition of European psychopathology (reflected in Wing's admiration of Karl Jasper's *Allgemeine Psychopathologie*), and that of the more hard-nosed line of the psychologists (O'Connor, Tizard and Venables). We found that most people told us things in terms of stories, and we in turn usually pursued our questioning in terms of how they made sense to us as stories. Some respondents, with little questioning, provided full and coherent accounts, say, of how their son was admitted to mental hospital; others needed many prompts to fill in gaps and to iron out inconsistencies. When I arrived in the Unit, Morris Carstairs had already written up a series of interviews with families of discharged chronic patients. The very richness of such material meant that we had to rely on ourselves as the ultimate measuring instrument if we were to move beyond case descriptions and bring order to the material. This eventually led to concern with *how* things were said as well as *what* was said.

Concern with inter-rater reliability followed from this use of ourselves as measurement instruments. I mention this because it was only the success here that kept Unit members in some kind of loose alliance. If I were to sum it all up, there was a concern with encouraging talk, with seeing what people said in terms of stories that we did our best to understand, and with using ourselves to rate the resulting material. Yet for all of us there was the underlying awareness of how easy it would be to get things wrong if we did not hold fast to certain crucial conceptual boundaries—boundaries between external and internal worlds, boundaries between stimulus and response, and boundaries between symptoms and attitudes. The most important boundaries of all were set by time: nothing happening after onset or relapse should be held accountable for the clinical change. Out of this early period came, for example, versions of the Present State Examination (PSE), the Life Events and Difficulty Schedule (LEDS), and the Camberwell Family Interview (CFI). Michael Rutter's arrival in 1962 did nothing to lessen the concern, indeed obsession, with inter-rater reliability as more subtle judgments were attempted, between, for example, the expression of criticism, dissatisfaction, and hostility by family members (Brown and Rutter, 1966; Rutter and Brown, 1966). It was assumed (as I recall without question) that it would take time to produce the first "edition" of an instrument and that further versions would be required. It was also unquestioned that everyone would participate in development and data-gathering: there were no "hired hands" (Roth, 1966). This meant that it was difficult to hide from the nasty realities of data collection—something that undoubtedly contributed to the many revisions of the instruments during their development. It also meant that the business of data collection escaped the low status that is so often its fate.

Since this intensive method necessarily limited us to relatively small samples, and what was to be explained (e.g., relapse, handicap) often formed only a relatively modest subset of the sample, there was a further built-in impetus towards accuracy. The low margin of error often necessary with intensive material is easily illustrated with an example from a longitudinal enquiry in Islington. The data in the first column of table 3.1 suggest that low self-esteem may play a role in the development of depression (Brown et al., 1986a). Once those depressed at a case level had been excluded, a total of 130 of the women in the survey experienced a

TABLE 3.1
Onset of Depression for Islington Women with a Severe Event and Level of Self-Esteem in Terms of One Actual and Two Hypothetical Data Sets

Self-Esteem	Actual Result	Reallocation − 1 Onset	Reallocation − 2 Onsets
		% onset	
Low	(17/50)	(16/49)	(15/48)
	34%	33%	31%
High	(12/80)	(13/81)	(14/82)
	15%	16%	17%
X²	5.36	3.95	2.74
P	.02	.05	.10
	significant	significant	non significant

severely threatening event. For those who had initially been characterized as having low self-esteem, the subsequent experience of depression onset was doubled. This difference comfortably reaches statistical significance, but if one onset is moved from low to high self-esteem (column 2), it now only just does so, though the risk is still double. If a second woman is reallocated, as might easily occur with less valid measures, the result falls well below significance (column 3). It is unhelpful to point out that this is to make something of a fetish of such levels—the fact is that they are often demanded by our peers (and certainly by our criteria). And sadly, differences all too often move in and out of significance in this way.

Sample size will almost certainly need to be restricted because of the time-consuming nature of the intensive approach to measurement. Developmental work often takes years, and during this time the incorporation of a serendipitous insight in order to increase sensitivity often means that a set of rating scales has to be largely recast. Moreover, once the measures are developed, more time is needed to collect material than with the traditional standardized instrument. (Interviews are typically tape recorded and a good deal of transcript carried out before final ratings are made.)

But there are compensating advantages other than increased accuracy. Such material is open to reworking, if necessary years after it was originally collected. This is a considerable gain, given the importance of longitudinal designs and that theoretical insights and thereby relevance of measures can change. Despite this, it is bound to be tempting, not least in the current financial climate, to use a simpler approach. This in itself is entirely reasonable, particularly once more intensive measures have been developed as a basis for comparison. It would also be unreasonable to suggest that the contrasting standardized instruments are necessarily flawed, particularly for attitudinal material. But they frequently do have serious shortcomings, and such simpler methods are, as indicated, best evaluated by comparisons with the results of an intensive approach. For example, I think it possible to document that "standardized" questionnaire alternatives for instruments such as Expressed Emotion (Leff and Vaughn, 1985), Ainsworth Strange Situation assessment (Ainsworth et al., 1978), and the Type A Behavior interview (Friedman and Rosenman 1974), although on occasions promising, have fallen a good deal short of the predictive utility of the original intensive versions. In other words, with such an intensive approach it is unlikely to be possible to relax standards concerning measurement without a good deal of resulting trouble: the gap between what is statistically significant and non-significant is too often uncomfortably close. With large samples it is often accepted practice to use a measure with known shortcomings in terms of accuracy with the knowledge that the sample size will ensure statistical significance.

One bald question about the future of research on depression is whether intensive instruments will continue to be developed or even utilized. There are fashionable alternatives that promise just as much, and ones that fund-giving bodies have been ready to support. At this point it may therefore be useful to consider some of the consequences of employing such an approach. However, since the question is too broad for a short essay, I will concentrate on its relevance for the critical task of establishing boundaries between phenomena—depression versus non-depression, stressor versus non-stressor, and so on.

An earlier discussion (Harris and Brown, 1985) gave most attention to settling boundaries using "hard" data, a type of measurement that is not necessarily better carried out by intensive methods. It cites, for example, a study of attempted suicide in which those with a father dying in childhood appeared particularly susceptible to suicidal behavior in young adulthood (Adam et al., 1982). The inconsistency of this finding with work in London suggested that long-term separation from the mother following the death of the father should also be considered. This, in fact, radically changed the picture: the death of a father was only associated with suicidal behavior when there was also a separation from the mother. This suggested that the boundary concerning loss had been wrongly drawn, and that death of the father had been given misleading significance. However, the example is somewhat tiresome since there is no obvious way of getting things right other than by controlling for everything—although it is a reminder of how easy it is to miss the obvious, and such examples may serve as a useful spur to exploration . (I continue to be fascinated by my ability-and for the sake of expanding my sample I will add my colleagues' ability—to fail to notice for long periods in a data set what, when ultimately seen, appears unnervingly obvious.) It is also a reminder of the misplaced timidity of those who fail to move beyond prior hypotheses during analysis. A subsequent replication is all that is needed to make any finding scientifically respectable, and reluctance to test hypotheses not entertained prior to data collection may mean missing a chance to extend theoretical insights.

However, the question of boundaries is not only a matter of oversight. First, the boundaries mentioned earlier, such as that between the external and internal, stand a high chance of being confused in any study using only a respondent's account as a source of data. Moreover, appearances themselves may prove to be confusing. It is possible, for example, that questions about feelings concerning an activity may give a better indication of the nature of the activity itself than a non-probing direct question about this. Thus, a question about the perceived helpfulness of the emotional support offered by a close tie may illuminate its objective quality—in other words, the degree of genuine concern about the subject's problems exhibited by the other person. It is an obvious point. But it is dismaying how often we follow, apparently unthinkingly, the labels of our measures. Perhaps we do not question enough because some of our own measures are equally suspect, and none of us could get on with the job of research without some mutual tolerance about their verisimilitude. Furthermore, any such doubt is likely to push us into activity that some may see as equally suspect—that of using measures that deliberately fail to reflect the facts of a situation. But this is what I will argue for. Once measurement is in the hands of the investigator, he or she may withhold information from those involved in the rating process and so create "artificial" measures that seek to pull apart material into, say, what is "internal" and "external," or to create measures lying in some sense beyond the boundary of reporting bias.

Secondly, there are issues concerning the bringing together of measures in a causal model—particularly how far factors occurring at much the same point in time should be amalgamated under the same conceptual umbrella. Thirdly, still concerning casual models, the consideration of time raises a number of puzzling questions.

Contextual Measures

I will start with the problem of the highly detailed material that an intensive approach tends to produce. The most common way of dealing with this (and the one that conforms to conventional ideas about science) is to rate as accurately as possible fairly low-level features. Only when this has been done are they brought together in higher order indicators. This might be a matter of simple addition but could involve the use of complex statistical techniques. There is, however, an alternative: to deal from the start with a global judgment of a whole configuration of features. Kaplan contrasts the two approaches as follows:

> A man might choose a job or a house by first weighing separately a number of component desiderata (salary, working conditions, and prospects; or rental, size, and location), and then by somehow summing the results, as though the components were reducible to a common measure. But he does not choose his friends by summing his appraisals of component traits and habits; he reacts, rather to the personality as a whole. (Kaplan, 1964, p. 211)

Such a configurational approach has the bonus of offering one solution to the key issue of context. The meaning of something for a person will usually depend on the wider context; Hinde (1987), for example, points out that a given number of commands to a child from a mother who *also* expresses affection is likely to have a meaning for a child very different from the same number of commands from a mother who never expresses affection. This principle holds for the whole gamut of human behavior, and makes difficult any straightforward stimulus-response approach to human or (for that matter) animal behavior.

Such an approach has probably been taken furthest in social psychiatry in the contextual ratings of life events, developed to deal with the almost limitless range of circumstances that can affect the meaning of an event. In terms of, say, "the end of an affair" these would include the duration of the relationship, whether there had been a commitment to get married or live together, whether the relationship had been a sexual one, who had taken the initiative in bringing it to an end, the degree to which the person was insulted or rejected in any final crisis (the lover went off with their best friend), the extent to which it was expected, the social circumstances of the respondent (living alone, single parent), how far there was a possible replacement lover, and so on. (These down-to-earth features can all be put in more formal terms—say certainty/uncertainty of outcome or degree of change involved.) A contextual rating of severity of likely threat or unpleasantness would take such information (and more) into account. One attraction of the approach, as conveyed by Kaplan, is that such judgments are made most days of our lives and are perhaps the main trigger of emotional experience. But it is not a matter of rejecting the usefulness of systematic measurement of lower order features. The aspects of the affair I have just listed could (and perhaps should) all be rated systematically. The question is how to put such ratings together. This would obviously be a less daunting task if the investigator were dealing *only* with examples of "ends of affairs." But it is a task of a quite different order if many types of events are involved. In such circumstances, I believe, we should do our best to measure the components systematically but not to hesitate to use a configurational approach if this appears to be called for.

But contextual ratings are not just a matter of summarizing complex material. The approach makes it possible to assess likely meaning while ignoring anything said by the respondent about feelings resulting from the event. This artificiality has the advantage in aetiological research of enabling certain biases stemming from the respondent to be ruled out—say that the depression to be explained has influenced the reporting of what was felt about events. This methodological legerdemain is achieved by the interviewer giving only selected information to an independent panel of raters that is set the task of reaching a consensus about *likely* meaning (i.e., likely for most people in similar circumstances). Such control over the pabulum used for rating can be extended by filtering any information that might lead to bias on the part of the raters—it can exclude, say, whether or not the person subsequently developed a depressive illness. Creed (1981) in a study of appendicectomy and a comparison series was able to remain blind to whether the condition was "organic" or "functional" (settled later by referring to pathology reports), and then to keep the team rating events blind to whether or not the person belonged to the patient or the comparison series. Despite this curtailment of information a considerable association was found between the presence of a "severe event" and an onset of functional but not organic conditions. The whole exercise depended upon conceiving meaning in terms of the *most likely* response in the light of relevant aspects of a person's circumstances and biography. Thus for the rating of a long-term threat (relevant in onset of depression and functional appendicectomy), emphasis was placed on the likely impact of an event on significant plans and concerns in so far as these could be judged from the person's current circumstances and biography.

In parenthesis it should perhaps be added that in this way it has been possible to operationalize the influential concept of *Verstehen* (understanding). It is, for example, just this sensing of likely relevant plans and concerns that I suggest is behind Karl Jasper's interpretation of the concept:

> In any given case the judgment of whether a meaningful connection is real does not rest on its self-evident character alone. It depends primarily *on the tangible facts* (that is on the verbal contents, cultural factors, people's acts, ways of life, and expressive gestures) in terms of which the connection is understood, and which provide the objective data . . . but we can only assume the reality of such a connection to the extent that the objective data will allow. The fewer these

are, the less forcefully do they compel our understanding; we interpret more and understand less. (Jaspers, 1963: 303)

The "artificiality" of contextual ratings can also serve conceptual as well as methodological purposes. It is possible to exclude from consideration something that might well have affected the meaning of an event but which the investigator wishes to give separate consideration. It is now no longer a matter of avoiding possible bias in the sense of trying to push the balance of a rating from the internal towards the external—from, say, feelings about an activity to the activity itself. Let us assume we have managed to deal with social support in its external aspect. One possibility is that, in the measurement of threat of an event, the amount of support received in dealing with it is taken into account. If this was allowed to lower the contextual assessment of threat, it would be impossible to go on to show that support lowered risk since this effect would already have been taken into account in giving a low threat rating to the event; that is, the measurement procedure would not record a severely threatening event about which it could be protective. The answer therefore is again to hold back information from the rating team—this time any mention of support. Setting such a boundary can be effective in helping to sort out the protective role of support, even in instances where its impact has been so immediate that there has been no awareness on the part of the person of the potential threat of an event. It is then possible for the contextual rating to reflect high threat and for this to be juxtaposed with the fact of receiving support.

It should also be noted that contextual ratings need not be restricted to dealing with events. A rating of the security characteristics of a woman's role as wife can take account of the regularity of her husband's financial contributions, his general predictability and the like, and a judgment made of the *likely* feelings of most women in such a position, irrespective of the respondent's reported feelings.

Therefore, in dealing with "intensive" material, we have a choice of either making a configurative rating of various kinds or carrying out some kind of "summation" of component features. In either case, we will have to struggle to establish the traditional factors or variables of scientific enquiry: type of life event, qualify of support, form of coping, and so on. It is just such granular variables that, as Ernest Gellner (1985) points out, make the Popperian testing of ideas possible.

But configurative ratings are, as yet, not widely employed. Dohrenwend and his colleagues in New York have, for example, been articulate in their criticism. They note that although it is more precise than the checklist method of rating events which ignores context, "it is also more gross in that it involves collapsing into a single measure, in non-explicit ways, the social situation in which it occurs and the personal history of the individual involved. The resulting ambiguity is an obstacle to our understanding of statistical association, since there is no way to tell which of the components go into a rating account for a particular association" (Dohrenwend, et al., 1987, p. 113). However, it can be argued that it is in a "contextual" way that we probably in any case respond to events. Moreover, so far at least, there is no convincing alternative way of dealing with the variability of meaning within an event-category such as "end of an affair." Certainly the most recent efforts of the New York group appear to have taken them some way towards a contextual approach (Brown, in press(a)).

Extension of Contextual Ratings

The last few years have also seen the development of additional contextual dimensions of events designed to deal with specific qualities (such as loss, danger, challenge, intrusiveness, and goal frustration). These are of a different order from the original threat ratings so far discussed, in that they are far more specific about the kind of threat involved (Brown and Harris, 1989, especially Chap. 15). A range of positive (as against negative) scales for use in the study of recovery has also been developed. However, for some questions this may still not be enough, something perhaps best conveyed with an example. One unsolved problem in epidemiological psychiatry is the apparent, almost universally greater prevalence of depression among women. One possibility is that this is because men and women tend to experience different events. But here it is easy to beg the question of how to judge events as comparable. Diane Vaughan (1986) has pointed out that marital separation in the Western world is often preceded by a long period of discontent and tension when *one* of the couple is anticipating the eventual breakdown of the marriage and in this way works through some of the emotional problems relating to grief entailed by a separation. The other, meanwhile, although seemingly facing the same situation, is in fact confronting something different. She also makes clear that the person taking the initiative is more often the man, and that the woman is often unprepared emotionally for the breakdown. However, existing classificatory schemes using contextual ratings may well at times show the separation as an equivalent experience for such a couple , that is, a severe "loss" event, with the presence of "danger" depending on the circumstances surrounding it.

It is possible that the consideration of additional characteristics of the event—say its unexpectedness in the above example—would prove useful. But there are still more radical possibilities. It needs here to be borne in mind that the decision to exclude from consideration self-reports about feelings and motives was made in the setting of cross-sectional research in which the depressive episode to be explained would already have been experienced. Longitudinal research enables some modification of previous restrictions as "soft" material can be collected *before* the occurrence of the event or depression in question. In this way it has been possible to utilize ratings of a woman's commitment towards various domains of her life, and to show that severe events (in terms of context) roughly treble the chance of depression if they *also* match an area of high commitment. A woman highly committed to the role of mother would be considered to have such a matching event on discovering from her daughter's school that she had been consistently stealing from home and playing truant (Brown, et al., 1987). The heart of the approach is to compare in terms of congruence two configurative judgments made at *different* points in time.

It may well be possible in this way to establish that, say, the discovery of a child's truancy is not experienced by most husbands in the same way as by most wives, a result which in turn would have implications for issues of communication, sympathy and support in the marriage. It should be noted that this development is entirely within the spirit of the contextual approach. Instead of assessing commitment *indirectly* by consideration of current circumstances, plans, and concerns, it is established *directly*. Finally, now that the role of severe events in the aetiology of depression is well-established, it should also be possible to place some weight on the parallel ratings of self-reported feelings. These have been neglected and overlooked, and more sophisticated versions of the present measures would undoubtedly help to amplify results so far obtained.

To sum up: Contextual ratings have not been designed to reflect in any exact way a person's experience. On the one hand, they are made in terms of the likelihood of certain emotions being experienced. On the other hand, they attempt to assess likely response given a person's particular biography and current circumstances, leaving out, however, not only self-reports about feelings but likely contributory factors such as those of support, personality, and biological vulnerability which may dramatically change any such appraisal. The idea has some affinity to Lazarus' notion of primary appraisal defined by a person's immediate response to an event before other factors such as coping resources are taken into account, the latter represented by secondary appraisal (Lazarus, 1966). However, the notion of contextual rating is more complex. In the rating of long-term contextual threat (that has so far proved particularly useful) the situation some ten days after the occurrence of the event itself is considered. But this is a point when secondary appraisal, say stemming from support received, would be expected to have already taken place. Ratings are therefore thoroughly artificial, and it is just this that makes it possible to consider the influence of mediating factors such as quality of support.

It is of interest that Nico Frijda (1986) in his impressive general treatment of emotion emphasizes how the story defines the emotion. This leads him to suggest a dual system of categorizing emotions much along the lines of a contrast between contextual threat and self-reported experience, with both relying on the basic logic inherent in "stories." He also highlights a point not so far made about the intensive approach. The relating of such stories in a reasonably congenial setting is likely to evoke traces of the emotions associated with these very circumstances in "real" life, which in turn can be observed and utilized in measurement.

A central part of my argument will be that only by the kind of distinctions and boundaries made possible by contextual ratings are we likely to develop effective models to explain depression; and it is to a different illustration of this that I now turn.

Conceptualizing Support and the Problem of Time

Many studies have confirmed that lack of support, particularly with a husband or boyfriend, is a vulnerability factor (Brown and Harris, 1986a), that is, risk of depression associated with them is only activated in the presence of a stressor such as a severely threatening event. But most studies have been cross-sectional and have had to rely on retrospective questioning to establish time order of severe event and support. Moreover, two longitudinal studies that have measured support at time of first contact have not suggested (at least on first perusal) that support is protective (Henderson and Brown, 1988). A research group in Canberra utilized the standardized Interview Schedule of Social Interaction (ISSI), which takes about 45 minutes to administer, to explore both close, intimate relationships, and more diffuse ties, as with neighbors and casual daily contacts (Henderson et al., 1981). The items are assembled by "summation" into four principal indices, consisting of the availability and the adequacy of both close and diffuse relationships. It remains unsettled how far a more open mode of interviewing would improve the validity of ISSI. However, it is comprehensive in its coverage and it seems unlikely that shortcomings in the instrument itself provide sufficient explanation for its failure to find that support relates to the development of depression (although perceptions as to its adequacy *were* found to be associated.)

One possible reason is the way ISSI puts together its component parts. The distinction it draws between availability and adequacy is described as if the former gives an objective and the latter a subjective view of support. Closer examination suggests that the (subjective) adequacy measure may actually reflect the presence of high quality support much better than the (objective) availability measure which only takes account of quantity or quality (Henderson and Brown, 1988). In other words the boundaries of the concept "support" might have been located in a different place to include features of the supportiveness of the contact, not just its frequency. If this had been done, availability and adequacy might not have differed so markedly, and the expected association between onset and support might have emerged. The point follows from the argument about contextual ratings. It is unnecessary to see the likes of supportiveness merely as a perception by one individual. Like stressful events it can be judged contextually according to external criteria by consensus.

But unfortunately, in this instance at least, results from a second study suggest that such conceptual changes may not prove enough. The Bedford College Self Evaluation and Social Support schedule (SESS) is an instrument in the intensive tradition, and in the analysis of longitudinal material of women living in Islington made the kind of distinctions just suggested (O'Connor and Brown, 1984). Yet the situation it revealed at the time of first interview in terms of active emotional support from a core contact also failed to predict onset of depression in the following year. This is seen in the right-hand column of Table 3.2 showing onset among married women who had experienced a severe event. Those confiding in their husband at the time of the first interview had only a slightly lower risk of depression. However, as it turns out there is probably no need to reject the results of prior cross-sectional research.

The negative result appears to turn on the fact that confiding and emotional support are not stable commodities. As many as a third of the women (i.e., those experiencing a severe event in the follow-up year) who had confided in their husbands at the time of our first interview failed to confide *and* receive emotional support in a subsequent crisis. And, it was such *crisis support* that mattered (Brown et al., 1986a). It is just this support that is most likely to have been picked up in the earlier cross-sectional enquiries. Table 3.2 gives the basic results concerning support from husband. Cell "d" shows women with no support on either occasion, who as expected, had a high risk of depression. Cell "b" shows women who *did* confide in their husband at the earlier point, but who failed to obtain support from him in a crisis. Being "let down" in this way was associated with a particularly high risk. It is only those in cell "a" with support on both occasions that appeared to be protected.

Alloway and Bebbington (1987) show a certain scepticism about the Islington results on support on more specific grounds of likely error in the crisis support measure due to its retrospective nature; nonetheless, the results make a good deal of sense, and it will be shown later than it is, in

TABLE 3.2
Confiding in Husband at First Interview, Crisis Support During the Follow-Up Year
and Onset of Depression Among Those with a Severe Event
(98 Married Islington Women)

| Confiding in Husband at 1st Interview | CRISIS SUPPORT FROM HUSBAND DURING FOLLOW-UP | | TOTAL |
| | YES | NO | |
	% onset	% onset	% onset
YES	4 (1/23)[a]	40 (6/15)[b]	18 (7/38)
NO	29 (2/7)[c]	26 (10/38)[d]	27 (12/45)

Note: Crisis support not known for 3

any case, possible to predict depression equally well from psychosocial material collected *only* at first interview (the "Conjoint Index" to be described), thus avoiding any suggestion of bias. The issue I wish to underline at present is that of time. Stability of phenomena tends to be assumed by research workers, despite only modest "test-retest" correlations, on the grounds that these can be explained by measurement error. Yet instability of behavior appears to be the rule rather than the exception (Hinde, 1987, p. 45).

But this need to face the possibility of real change over time has an awkward corollary. One of the central points of recent work has been, following the definition of vulnerability, that absence of a supportive tie will only lead to greater risk in the presence of an aetiological agent. But, as just seen, such support may well change once an event has occurred; a woman, for example, at the death of her mother may receive support from her husband of a kind she has not known for years.

There has been a comparable problem with the measurement of Expressed Emotion (EE). A good deal of change is possible in family EE, with a tendency for it to lessen after a schizophrenic patient's discharge (Brown, Birley and Wing, 1972). One possibility is that high EE is a function of a relationship and at best represents a disposition to react to another person in a particular way; and whether this is actually expressed will depend (in part) on the setting. Its measurement in terms of overt behavior has probably proved effective because the expression of any propensity is likely to be somewhere near its maximum after a patient's admission (bearing in mind the trouble this is likely to have brought), and it is at this point that EE has typically been recorded. (One prediction here is that the present agreed criterion of 6/7 critical comments would need to be lowered for patients returning to relatives with whom they had not been living at admission as any predisposition to EE would not have been primed by pre-admission behavior. It follows that the overt behavior of relatives on which a rating of high EE has been based may be absent by the time attempts are underway to reduce EE. However, since such behavior may return with changing circumstances, such intervention is still justified if it is able to make a more fundamental change. Therefore overt behavior and disposition need to be distinguished.

The research on support and depression has faced a comparable problem, but with a reverse emphasis, given that it has been interested in onset rather than relapse. In studies of schizophrenia, EE has typically been first measured at the time of the crisis of the patient's admission, whereas, in studies of depression, support is first measured at a time when there is no depression and in a situation which is more often than not outside the context of a crisis. But this still leaves plenty of scope for quality of support to change when put to the test by a subsequent crisis, and such behavior would seem as good a candidate as any to represent any predisposition. But leaving the issue of predisposition aside, it is the depressogenic implications of any change for the worse in terms of support that appears to be important. Because of the need to keep track of such changes, the term "vulnerability" should be restricted to phenomena present immediately prior to any severe event. This has the advantage of making it possible to avoid the tricky task of amalgamating changing patterns of support. It also allows, as in the example of the husband's behavior at the death of his wife's mother, an empirical test of whether such improvement is able to lessen the impact of long-term neglect—apparently it does not (see cell "c", table 3.2).

Vulnerability Effects and Multivariate Statistics

I have argued that it is necessary to distinguish indicator (e.g., EE at one point in time) and underlying concept (e.g., predisposition to EE-type behavior), and causal models provide one way of testing such "epistemic correlations" (Blalock, 1968). However, further questions about boundaries have to be faced, since it is quite possible to keep indicators apart in terms of both definition and measurement, and then to treat them as equivalent at a conceptual level. Tennant and Bebbington's 1978 argument about vulnerability followed these lines on the basis of using a log-linear analysis. McKee and Vilhjalmsson (1986) have more recently taken a similar position and go over more fully the same statistical ground. In essence, the position of both is to suggest that the causal effects of aetiological agents (e.g., severe event) and vulnerability factors (e.g., low self-esteem) arise from a common component which they conceive as "strain" or "stress." I have discussed elsewhere why I think this is misleading on statistical grounds (Brown, 1986—see also Bebbington, 1986; Brown and Harris, 1986b; Rutter, 1981; Surtees, 1980). However, there is an alternative and persuasive non-statistical argument for keeping the "factors" distinct at a conceptual level. The logical implications of an argument in terms of a common factor such as "strain" is that the additivity (in terms of risk of depression) between two aetiological agents should be similar to that between aetiological agent and vulnerability factor. However, in studies where this has been examined, it has not held. In one, for example, two "unrelated" provoking agents (e.g., two severe events) had a resulting risk of depression of 8 percent compared with one of 24 percent for the presence of provoking agent and one vulnerability factor. Such evidence (and there is more along the same lines) runs counter to the idea that it is sufficient to summate such components of the model in terms of "strain." But the more important general point is that theoretical development concerning aetiological processes may well require that we make an effort to conceive of factors as *conceptually* non-equivalent. This has pushed recent work towards a cognitive-emotional view of the origins of depression that involves low self-esteem and the development of a general feeling of hopelessness following an event, rather than the somewhat lame notion of amount of background strain.

A further point is raised by the example. Log-linear analysis because of its built-in assumptions is less likely than more traditional approaches to find statistical interaction, and it was this that arguably pushed Tennant and Bebbington to their particular interpretation (Brown, 1986). But it is up to the would-be user to decide whether the assumptions about the world implicit in statistical procedures are appropriate. This cannot usually be settled in statistical terms alone.

This last point can be used to illustrate another critical boundary issue—how to draw the line between relevant and non-relevant depression. Work with multiple regression (probably currently the most popular method of multivariate analysis) encourages the use of a continuous measure of depression. This gains credence from the obvious fact that depression appears to be continuous. But it does not follow that this is the most effective way to proceed. A common design has been to use clinical and social measures at time 1 to predict depression at time 2. Let us assume that continuous clinical measures have been utilized on both occasions, and the standardized beta weights have been used to assess the relative importance of the time 1 measures. Under these circumstances time 1 depression will typically greatly outweigh that of the time 1 social factors. Now the use of multiple regression with a continuous measure pretty well guarantees this result. (I leave aside technical questions concerning the appropriateness of using beta weights—Achen, 1982.) The argument is as follows. Such a measure will reflect degrees of psychological well-being rather than clinically relevant depression since the latter is relatively rare in the general population. Because of this, measures of association (based on variance explained) will largely reflect the ability to predict *well being* at time 2 from well being at time 1. This will explain a good deal of the relevant variance and tend to dwarf the contribution of any non-clinical factors known to be relevant to clinical outcome at the other end of the dimension (Brown, et al., 1989). The unthinking acceptance of a built-in perspective of a particular statistical method can therefore lead us astray. In this instance there is a great deal to be said for the use of a categorical measure with an arbitrary boundary reflecting depression—but, of course, one which makes clinical sense.

It is possible to make a more general point by drawing an analogy between my earlier point about the importance of interplay in the research interview along conversational lines. The need is now for eye contact with data to encourage ideas about possible causal processes. And here the notion of the story may again not be inappropriate. The investigator has to converse with the data in order to elaborate and test emerging ideas. A task traditionally met by the hundreds of cross-tabulations required by an analysis carried out in the Lazarsfeldian tradition (Rosenberg, 1968). Instead of this kind of exploratory interplay, the microcomputer (and its complex statistical packages) has increasingly kept investigators that much more distant from their data. They are no longer likely to know them in quite the same intimate way. This can be hazardous on several grounds.

First, a Lazarsfeldian interplay is an excellent way of picking up errors in computer material. (I have in mind particularly worrisome ones that can so easily emerge when combining variables.) Second, working with cross-tabulations encourages questions about the membership of certain critical cells and is an important impetus to return to original descriptive material. It is also an unrivalled way of gaining ideas of what may be going on, as well as acting as a check on simplistic assumptions about the meaning of a measure. However good a rating scale in terms of reliability and validity, it is still possible to have erroneous ideas about a measure *when thinking about it*. In a recent analysis, for example, I got carried away with the implications of a complex index ("negative elements in core relationships") and into equating a positive score with a highly uncomfortable and unpleasant set of circumstances. It was only eventually by reading the detailed descriptive accounts of the women with high scores that I realized that this was far from so. Many had, at most, a pedestrian relationship with perhaps some potential for deterioration under stress. Boundary problems therefore can still arise even when the more formal measurement tasks have been reasonably well-accomplished. It is still useful to *think* about measures appropriately.

Two Broader Issues

The apparent lack of the kind of interplay just outlined between computer printouts and basic material in many research reports may go some way to explain fairly widespread disenchantment with much current enquiry in social psychiatry. In *The Future of Psychiatry,* Kleinman (1988) is particularly critical. He argues, for example, that stress and support are not separable, discrete categories of social variables (i.e., yet another boundary issue): "Instead there is a mutually determining relationship between stressor and support. . . . The psychologists and sociologists who divide them into neatly dichotomized predictor variables quantified on different scales are creating artifacts of measurement that lack validity in the patient's life world" (Kleinman, 1988, p. 64). It should, of course, be part of the job of the social scientist to help his reader to interpret his findings in human form. (What does an average one-point difference on a 14-point scale of support represent?) But having said this, all measurement is artifactual and, as with contextual ratings, there is a case to be made at times for deliberately exaggerating their contrivance. The basic purpose of model-building is not to represent the world as seen by those we study but to help our search for critical processes and mechanisms.

One way of interpreting Kleinman's argument is that it is largely a matter of at what point in our research the world is "neatly dichotomized." If an index is created from a jumble of items reflecting support received from different individuals and this is then arbitrarily divided along its length, then there is much to be said for Kleinman's unease. How, even if the scale should predict risk, are we to relate it to an individual's experience? But the dichotomy of "adequate" versus "inadequate support" of the Islington study is not of this kind. Ratings were developed to reflect characteristics of particular relationships. A long winnowing process was necessary to establish that only certain kinds of relationships and only certain kinds of "support" were relevant. (Fortunately these results broadly reflected what had been expected from prior cross-sectional studies.) Only at this point was it established that under some conditions certain relationships were substitutable while under other conditions they were not. For example, support in a crisis from a sister or from a woman friend named as very close was as effective in reducing risk of depression as long as the woman had not been "let down" in terms of the support expected from her husband. If she had been let down in this way, no other support appeared helpful (Brown et al., 1986).

Another problem of measurement concerns an even broader issue. Whether a research program flourishes in the longer term cannot be entirely divorced from political considerations. Supporters have to be mustered if critical financial backing is to be obtained. Assuming the research is promising, any sign that findings appear to be incapable of replication by others is bound to be a serious threat to such support. One means of coping with this is to insist that any user of an instrument stick closely to prescribed procedures. It is doubtful whether research such as that with EE and schizophrenia could have sustained its steady momentum without such an insistence. The strategy has the advantage that it is impeccable scientifically (even though motives may be less elevated). But while it is also justified by the real danger of the collapse of a research program in its early years, there is the alternative danger that the need for replicability will stultify new insights.

The solution is to seek measures that can serve both a conservative and innovative function. The intensive tradition is well-placed to do this as it does not depend on the kind of standardization that can be easily upset by the introduction of new features.

One way is to seek to keep constant only the definition of the basic unit of study—say what is to be included as a life event. But then to allow the addition of any more "qualities" that are thought necessary to define the unit—say the degree of danger, loss, goal frustration, challenge involved in a severely threatening event. This can give all the flexibility likely to be required, as long as the basic units were well enough designed not to require change. The objective, of course, is to be able to recreate the earlier measures exactly, whatever the subsequent innovations. Given this, it is possible with a leap-frogging strategy to give up earlier measures only when the new ones are fully established. It follows that development at work should be enough to establish effective units of study. Once this is done the theoretically more important insights likely to be embodied in the measurement of qualities can be spread over the life of a program.

Finally, what about the models themselves? What in particular are the implications for the question of boundaries of the fact that aetiological variables can be surprisingly highly correlated?

An Aetiological Model of Depression—Putting Things Together

The role of loss, disappointment, and rejection in depression can be seen as a brutal thrusting of disorder on a person, more or less out of the blue. Such a catastrophic view was made more plausible by the development of the brought-forward time coefficient (BFT) which indicated that the depression following a severe event would typically not have occurred for several years, if at all, without the occurrence of the event (Brown, et al., 1973). The subsequent identification of the important role for a woman of "matching severe events" underlines the plausibility of this conclusion. However, this is likely to require amendment to the degree to which it can be shown that the depression develops among a quite small group of women and that there is a tight interrelationship among the causal components of the model.

A recent model centers on measures made at the time of first contact with women in Islington before any onset of depression in the follow-up year. A Conjoint Index incorporating both external and internal features of their lives is used to represent their situation at this time. The components of the Index were brought together because there is no fully convincing way of giving any single element temporal priority. The external component, *"negative elements in core relationships,"* combines various "objective" measures of quality of relationships, mostly involving husband and children (Brown, in press(b)). The internal component reflects the presence of either *low self-esteem* or *chronic subclinical symptoms* (typically involving depression or anxiety). The Conjoint Index itself is defined by a positive score on the external component *and* at least one of the two internal components. It has two interesting properties. First, the external component is quite unrelated to subsequent onset without the presence of one of the internal components. This also holds in reverse: the presence of the external is also required for the internal to predict onset. Secondly, only a quarter of the inner-city population of Islington, once women with depression had been excluded, are positive on the Index. And it was from this relatively small group of women that almost all of those who became depressed in the follow-up period were drawn (25/32).

The two key aetiological processes are *"event production,"* related to the increased chance of a severe event occurring, and *"vulnerability,"* already discussed. The two processes lie behind the considerable predictive power of the Conjoint Index. It is powerfully related to the subsequent occurrence of an important sub-group of severe events likely to lead to onset, that is, those that match an ongoing difficulty or role conflict (Brown et al., 1987). It also acts as a powerful vulnerability factor for those experiencing any type of severe event. Of women with a positive Index who experience such a matching severe event approximately half became depressed (Brown, in press(b)).

But it needs to be added that much of the power of the Index can be explained by its correlation with inadequate support in the aftermath of a severe event (either because of not receiving crisis support or being "let down" - see table 3.2). This, of course, confirms the emerging picture of depression as being grounded in the quality of core relationships. We have therefore:

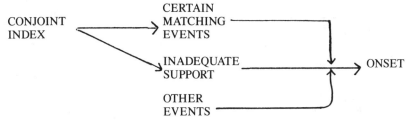

It is possible that middle-class women will show a different, looser, picture, with their depression occurring more often "out of the blue." But for working-class women in Islington, some half of the onsets appeared to be largely foreordained by the situation faced at the time we first saw them; and for the remainder developing depression, the odds against a number must have been formidable. What are the chances of a sexual affair going well for a working-class single mother living in an inner-city area?

But while this *combining* of the internal and external is good practice in the sense that we cannot be sure of the time order between the two, it is unsatisfactory theoretically since very different features are brought together. There is much to be said for imposing some time order and assuming that the greater part of any causal effect runs from the environment represented by the "negative elements in core relationships" index to the two "internal" states (although there will certainly be some interplay).

It follows from this realignment of boundaries that it is the two internal states (low self-esteem and chronic sub-clinical conditions) that are the vulnerability factors, and not negative elements in core relationships; the latter are critical because they are highly predictive of these two internal states as well as certain matching severe events and inadequacy of support. It still follows that a combination of factors is required for high risk—but now it is one of the internal states plus at least one of the subsequent risk factors.

Of course, this simplifying assumption about time order can be criticized, and it can also with justice be pointed out that notions like being "let down" may overlap with the depressive reaction we wish to explain. But while these are significant issues (to which I will return), it is necessary to keep in mind the very high order of prediction achieved by the Conjoint Index which *only* utilizes material collected at first contact. In this sense, there is clearly something to explain in real terms and the second, more

FIGURE 3.1
Schematic Aetiological Model of Depression

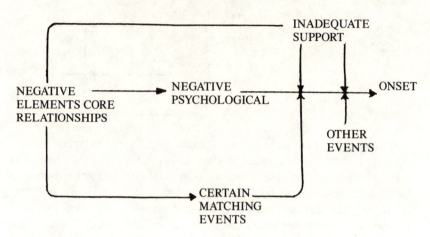

articulate, version of the model has the merit of highlighting a theoretically plausible possibility.

Extending the Model

It is doubtful whether such models can be developed outside an intensive measurement tradition. It is fortunate, therefore, that they have other benefits, not least that they are an excellent basis for exploring the past.

The original version of the model just outlined included loss of mother before eleven as a vulnerability factor (Brown, et al., 1977). While there has been a good deal of controversy about the role of loss of parent (Brown and Harris, 1986b; Harris and Brown, 1985; Crook and Eliot, 1980; Tennant, et al., 1980; Harris, et al., 1986), the basic effect has now been replicated in two further studies (Brown, et al., 1986; Harris, et al., 1986, 1987; Bifulco, et al., 1987).

Recent research also suggests that more fundamental than early loss is the quality of replacement parental care. If this is inadequate (in terms of an index of parental indifference and lax control, termed *lack of care*), the risk of current depression is doubled, irrespective of loss of mother. The presence of such inadequate care related to an increased overall risk of depression of about one third—that is, in Islington three women instead of two developed depression in the year.

Current research indicates that intervening experiences between past and present can serve to reduce as well as increase such risk (Quinton and

Rutter, 1984a and b; Rutter et al., 1983; Rutter, 1988), and that certain experiences in adolescence and early adulthood can lead to depressogenic situations in the present (Harris et al., 1987). In a study of another inner-city population, premarital pregnancy, for instance, appears to have played a particularly critical mediating role between early lack of care and subsequent depression (Brown, 1988b). What seems to have been crucial is that such pregnancies trapped women in relationships which they might well not otherwise have chosen, and which ultimately became a source of provoking agents. In interpreting this, a conveyor belt of adversities was outlined, on which some were moved from one crisis to another, starting with lack of care in childhood and passing via premarital pregnancy to current working-class status, lack of social support, and high rates of provoking agents. These experiences were certainly also often parallelled by feelings of helplessness and low self-esteem, capable of influencing how the external environment was interpreted and dealt with.

In the present model, an index of inadequate parenting is quite highly related to the Conjoint Index; and the past is entirely unassociated with the occurrence of a severe event unless the relevant event-producing life structure is also current (Brown, 1989). Such results suggest that the present environment by and large provides the essential intervening link between inadequate parenting and later depression.

However, this is probably not the whole story. There was a hint in the Islington material of a link between early adverse parenting and inadequate support that was independent of the Conjoint Index and that a personality characteristic stemming from early experience might be involved. Women with inadequate parental care were more likely than others to turn to unsuitable or inappropriate persons for support once a crisis had occurred (Andrews and Brown, 1988). Such women also tended to romanticize close relationships and to deny any incipient problems with them. It often seemed that they wanted to believe, in spite of clear contrary evidence, that those they had named as closest to them were reliable, helpful, and supportive. Personality factors should therefore not be seen as necessarily outside the confines of the model. Indeed, it is possible that their importance for depression will be largely found to stem from their role in helping to produce experiences such as inadequate support important in the model.

Perhaps the greatest need in pursuing such clues is to deal with the intricacies of temporal order over the life course. Prospective studies on their own are unlikely to prove sufficient as contacts can never be frequent enough to settle all questions about time order, and intensive measurement will be necessary to fill in details experiences occurring in the lengthy periods between contacts. Work on the recall of life events over a ten-year period suggests that the technical problems are not insuperable (Neilson et al., 1989). There is also a need to pursue issues of time order when we turn to the situation that provides the immediate background for a depressive disorder, although here more minute documentation is likely to be necessary, together with attention to the fact that components of the model may serve both to produce and perpetuate each other. We may have a break-up of a marriage (aetiological agent) which does not at once provoke clinical depression (outcome). However, the resulting isolation and lack of support may lead in a matter of weeks to feelings of low self-worth (vulnerability). These feelings may increase the risk of further crises (aetiological agents) because of the risky sexual adventures embarked upon in an effort to deal with these feelings (coping); and one such crisis, combined with ongoing vulnerability, may eventually provoke depression within a year of the original event. Fortunately, in terms of the question of boundaries, such effects will typically take place over a period—that is, in this instance, low self-worth played a role in event-production and then, once an event has occurred, acted as a vulnerability factor. It will also be necessary to establish, in some detail, what happens between provoking event and onset, a demanding task given that in many instances clinical depression appears to follow a crisis within a matter of weeks.

Other Questions

We have just seen how aetiological models encourage the exploration of a host of substantive questions. To the degree significant aetiological processes are identified, questions about intervention are bound to arise. Recent work arising in the context of schizophrenia and EE illustrates how such intervention can both test and elaborate theory derived from non-experimental research. So far this has not occurred with depression, despite the obvious need to relate the apparent beneficial (and sadly often non-persistent) effects of anti-depressant drugs and cognitive therapy to possible parallel changes in social milieu. How far do such treatments, for example, have an influence via their facilitation of "fresh start" events (Brown, et al., 1988), an influence that is only transient due to the fact that the milieu does not change? It is also possible—as with schizophrenia—that drugs will be shown to interact with psychosocial factors. An obvious candidate for an experimental approach is the apparent beneficial impact of a "volunteer" befriending service for women who are either at high-risk or already chronically depressed (Mills and Pound, 1985).

Such substantive issues are many. There is also a need to relate the current model to factors influencing who receives psychiatric care (Goldberg and Huxley, 1980). With current pressure on services, particularly in inner-city areas, psychiatrists probably see a highly selected group of depressive conditions. "Acting out" behavior among women, often linked to an early experience of separation from mother, appears to be a powerful determinant of who is referred to psychiatric services (Brown, et al., 1985). Factors influencing who receives care are likely to overlap, at least in part, with those of aetiological importance, and there may even be a possibility that those increasing risk may, once depression has developed, reduce the chance of a woman receiving any form of treatment (Brown and Harris, 1978). Here it is necessary to face the shocking indifference of many studies to issues of sampling and selection—yet another boundary problem. How often are patients not considered in a treatment evaluation because they have discontinued contact (many out-patients attend only once)? How far does enthusiasm for a treatment determine inclusion? How far are "mixed" conditions (say of alcoholism and depression) considered?

The question of "co-morbidity" is important in its own right, and there is increasing recognition of the inhibiting effect on research of hierarchical diagnostic schemes. Intensive research has made a contribution by suggesting that severely threatening events reflecting specific types of meaning are involved in the onset of different conditions—loss, disappointment and rejection relating to depression and danger to anxiety (Finlay-Jones and Brown, 1981; Miller and Ingham, 1983). Where recovery is concerned there may well also be equally specific effects, where events reflecting hope and renewal are important for depression and increased predictability and security for anxiety (Brown et al., 1988; Brown et al., 1989).

The recent upsurge of biological research in psychiatry has so far remained distant from such models and has concentrated on biological changes during a depressive episode and on the likely mode of drug effects. However, it is possible that biological markers of predictive importance are at present being revealed that are not simply reflections of current clinical state. The need to foster collaborative research, as in the area of treatment, hardly need emphasis.

Equally important is the area of comparative research. Already there is evidence for the relevance of such models for other cultures (Leff, 1989); the one outlined has been shown to hold, for example, in Spain (Uria and Gaminde, 1988) and Italy (Lora, and Fava, 1990). However, these same two studies have also failed to replicate certain findings. There is no evidence in either that (as in London) women with a child at home are particularly at risk (Brown and Harris, 1978; Bebbington et al., 1984). The paradoxical feature of such failures is that they may prove to be strict replications at a conceptual level. In this particular example, we may well be seeing an influence of the relative weight placed by the different cultures on the importance of women's work in the home, and the greater difficulties faced by women in the kind of non-traditional setting found in London.

The most intriguing possibilities concern the study of different protective social arrangements (say, the key importance of same-sex peers in some cultures). There is also the possibility that subtle differences in the events and difficulties found to be capable of provoking and perpetuating depression (and anxiety for that matter) will tell us a good deal about the nature of the societies themselves.

Another area worth mentioning is the increasing awareness of the way case and borderline conditions of affective disorder can intervene between stressor and onset of physical disorder (e.g., menorrhagia—Harris, 1989, and onset of gastrointestinal disorder—Craig, 1989) or fail to act in this way (e.g., coronary heart disease—Neilson et al., 1989). It is particularly important here to consider the intervening role of non-depressive reactions. The onset of secondary amenorrhea, for example, appears to be associated with prior tension rather than depression or anxiety (Harris, 1989).

But these must be by way of illustration; there are too many questions for me to be comprehensive. One of the fascinations of depression is its universal nature and the way it links with basic questions in most, if not all, the social, psychological, and biological disciplines.

None of the issues just sketched are incompatible with the aetiological model I outlined; nearly all, indeed, promise to elaborate it in some significant way. Biological markers, for instance, may act independently of the basic psychosocial processes, interact with them or run parallel, and there should be no problem in principle in incorporating all three possibilities. There is reason to hope that research on depression during the next decade will begin to break out of the somewhat narrow disciplinary boundaries that have developed. In so far as cross-disciplinary collaboration does take place, existing psychosocial models should provide one initial basis for integrating findings, and the intensive approach to measurement should give a sufficiently sensitive and flexible set of methods to meet any new demands for accuracy and theoretical relevance. The danger (and it is a big one) is that, under increasing financial pressure and the need to develop methods acceptable to all participants, we will settle for measures that are merely expedient, and are insufficient for the kind of boundary marking I have discussed.

I should like to thank Tirril Harris and Elizabeth Davies for their helpful criticism of an earlier draft of this chapter.

References

Achen, C. (1982) *Interpreting and Using Regression.* Beverly Hills: Sage Publications.

Adam, K.C., Bouckoms, A. and Streiner, D. (1982) Parental loss and family stability in attempted suicide. *Archives of General Psychiatry, 39,* 1081–1085.

Ainsworth, M.D., Blehar, M.C., Waters, E. and Wall, S. (1978) *Patterns of Attachment: assessed in the Strange Situation and At Home.* Hillsdale, New Jersey: Lawrence Erlbaum.

Alloway, R. and Bebbington, P. (1987) The buffer theory of social support—a review of the literature. *Psychological Medicine, 17,,* 91–108.

Andrews, B. and Brown, G.W. (1988) Social support, onset of depression and personality: an exploratory analysis. *Social Psychiatry, 23,* 99–108.

Bebbington, P. (1986) Establishing causal links—recent controversies. In: Katschnig, H. (Ed.) *Life Events and Psychiatric Disorders: Controversial Issues.* Cambridge: Cambridge University Press.

Bebbington, P.E., Sturt, E., Tennant, C. and Hurry, J. (1984) Misfortune and resilience: a community study of women. *Psychological Medicine, 14,* 347–364.

Blalock, H.M. (1968) The measurement problem: a gap between the language of theory and research. In: Blalock, H.M. (Ed.) *Methodology in Social Research.* New York: McGraw Hill.

Brown, G.W. (1986) Statistical interaction and the role of social factors in the aetiology of clinical depression. *Sociology, 20,* 601–606.

Brown, G.W. (1989a) Life events and measurement. In: Brown, G.W. and Harris, T.O. (Eds.) *Life Events and Illness.* New York: Guilford.

Brown, G.W. (in press) Epidemiological studies of depression: definition and case finding. In: Becker, J. Kleinman, A. (Eds.) *Affective Disorders: Theory and Research: Psychosocial Aspects, I.* (In press).

Brown, G.W. (in press). A psychosocial view of depression. In: Bennett, D. and Freeman, H. (Eds.) *Community Psychiatry.* Churchill Livingstone (in press).

Brown, G.W., Adler, Z. and Bifulco, A. (1988) Life events, difficulties and recovery from chronic depression. *British Journal of Psychiatry, 152,* 487–498.

Brown, G.W., Bifulco, A. and Harris, T.O. (1987) Life events vulnerability and onset of depression: some refinements. *British Journal of Psychiatry, 150:* 30–42.

Brown, G.W., Bifulco, A., Harris, T.O. and Bridge, L. (1986) Life stress, chronic psychiatric symptoms and vulnerability to clinical depression. *Journal of Affective Disorders, 11:* 1–19.

Brown, G.W., Bifulco, A. and Lemyre, L. (1988) Recovery from anxiety and depression. Paper presented at University of London Seminar in Epidemiological Psychiatry, 12th October 1988.

Brown, G.W., Birley, J.L.T. and Wing, J.K. (1972) The influence of family life on the course of schizophrenic illness: a replication. *British Journal of Psychiatry, 121:* 241–258.

Brown, G.W. and Harris, T.O. (1978) *Social Origins of Depression: a Study of Psychiatric Disorder in Women.* London: Tavistock.

Brown, G.W., Craig, T.K.J. and Harris, T.O. (1985) Depression: disease or distress? Some epidemiological considerations. *British Journal of Psychiatry, 147:* 612–622.

Brown, G.W. and Harris, T.O. (1986) Stressor, vulnerability and depression: a question of replication. *Psychological Medicine, 16:* 739–744.

Brown, G.W. and Harris, T.O. (1986a) Establishing causal links: the Bedford College studies of depression. In: Katschnig, H. (Eds.) *Life Events and Psychiatric Disorders: Controversial Issues.* Cambridge: Cambridge University Press.

Brown, G.W., Harris, T.O., Bifulco, A. (1986) Long-term effect of early loss of parent. In: Rutter, M., Izard, C. and Read, P. (Eds.) *Depression in Childhood: Developmental Perspectives*. New York: Guilford Press.

Brown, G.W., Harris, T.O., Copeland, J.R. (1977) Depression and loss. *British Journal of Psychiatry, 130:* 1–18.

Brown, G.W., Harris, T.O. and Lemyre, L. (in press). Now you see it, now you don't—same considerations on multiple regression. In: Magnusson, D., Bergman, L.R., Rudinga, G. and Torested, B. (eds). *Problems and Methods in Longitudinal Research: Stability and Change*. Cambridge: Cambridge University Press.

Brown, G.W., Harris, T.O., and Peto, J. (1973) Life events and psychiatric disorders: 2. Nature of causal link. *Psychological Medicine, 3:* 159–176.

Brown, G.W. and Rutter, M. (1966) The measurement of family activities and relationships: a methodological study. *Human Relations, 19,* 241–263.

Brown, G.W. and Harris, T.O. (1989) *Life Events and Illness*. New York: Guilford.

Brown, G.W., Andrews, B., Harris, T.O., Adler, Z. and Bridge, L. (1986) Social support, self-esteem and depression. *Psychological Medicine, 16,* 813–831.

Craig, T.K.J. (1989) Abdominal pain. In: Brown, G.W. and Harris, T.O. (Eds.) *Life Events and Illness*. New York: Guilford.

Creed, F. (1981) Life events and appendicectomy. *The Lancet, i, 1381–1385.*

Dohrenowend, B.P., Link, B.G., Kern, R., Shrout, P.E. and Markowitz, J. (1987) In: Cooper, B. (Ed.) *Psychiatric Epidemiology: Progress and Prospects*. London: Croom Helm.

Finlay-Jones, R. and Brown, G.W. (1981) Types of stressful life events and the onset of anxiety and depressive disorders. *Psychological Medicine, 11:* 803–815.

Friedman, M. and Rosenman, R.H. (1974) *Type A Behavior and Your Heart*. New York: Alfred Knopf.

Frijda, N.H. (1986) *The Emotions*. Cambridge: Cambridge University Press.

Gellner, E. (1985) *Relativism and the Social Sciences*. Cambridge: Cambridge University Press.

Gilbert, P. (1988) Psychobiological interaction in depression. In: Fisher, S. & Reason, J. (Eds.) *Handbook of Life Stress, Cognition and Health*. New York: John Wiley & Sons.

Goldberg, D. and Huxley, P. (1980) *Mental Illness in the Community: the Pathway to Psychiatric Care*. London: Tavistock.

Harris, T.O. (1989) Disorders or menstruation. In: Brown, G.W. and Harris, T.O. (Eds.) *Life Events and Illness*. New York: Guilford Press.

Harris, T.O. and Brown, G.W. (1985). Interpreting data in aetiological studies: pitfalls and ambiguities. *British Journal of Psychiatry, 147,* 5–15.

Harris, T.O., Brown, G.W., Bifulco, A. (1986) Loss of parents in childhood and adult psychiatric disorder: the Walthamstow Study, 1. The role of lack of adequate parental care. *Psychological Medicine, 16,* 641–659.

Harris, T.O., Brown, G.W., Bifulco, A. (1987) Loss of parent in childhood and adult psychiatric disorder: the Walthamstow Study, 2. The role of inadequate substitute care. *Psychological Medicine, 17,* 163–183.

Henderson, A.S., and Brown, G.W. (1988) Social support: the hypothesis and the evidence. In: Henderson, A.S. and Burrows, G.D. (Eds.) *Handbook of Social Psychiatry*. Amsterdam: Elsevier.

Henderson, A.A., Byrne, D.G. and Duncan-Jones, P. (1981) *Neurosis and the Social Environment*. Academic Press: Sydney.

Hinde, R. (1987) *Individuals, Relationships and Culture: Links Between Ethology and the Social Sciences.* Cambridge: Cambridge University Press.

Jaspers, K. (1963) *Allegemeine Psychopathologie.* Translated by Hoenig, J. and Hamilton, M.W. Manchester: Manchester University Press.

Kaplan, A. (1964) *The Conduct of Inquiring.* California: Chandler Publishing Company.

Kleinman, A. (1988) *The Future of Psychiatry.* New Jersey: Erlbaum.

Lazarus, R. (1966) *Psychological Stress and the Coping Process.* New York: McGraw-Hill.

Leff, J. (1988) *Psychiatry Around the Globe: A Transcultural View.* London: Gaskell.

Leff, J. and Vaughn, C. (1985) *Expressed Emotion in Families.* New York: Guilford Press.

Lora, A. and Fava, E. (1990) Provoking agents, vulnerability factors and depression in an Italian Setting: a replication of Brown and Harris's model. (Manuscript).

McKee, D. and Vilhjalmsson, R. (1986) Life stress, vulnerability and depression: a methodological critique of Brown et al. *Sociology, 20,* 601–606.

Miller, P. McC. and Ingham, J.G. (1983) Dimensions of experience. *Psychological Medicine, 13,* 417–449.

Neilson, E., Brown, G.W., Marmot, M. (1989) Life events and myocardial infarction. In: Brown, G.W., Harris, T.O. (Eds.) *Life Events and Illness.* New York: Guilford Press.

O'Connor, P. and Brown, G.W. (1984) Supportive relationships: fact or fancy? *Journal of Social and Personal Relationships, 1:* 159–175.

Quinton, D. and Rutter, M. (1984a) Parents with children in care: 1. current circumstances and parenting skills. *Journal of Child Psychology and Psychiatry, 25,* 211–229.

Quinton, D. and Rutter, M. (1984b) Parents with children in care: 2. Intergenerational continuities. *Journal of Child Psychology and Psychiatry, 25,* 231–250.

Roth, J.A. (1966) Hired hand research. *American Sociologist, 1,* 190–196.

Rutter, M. (1981) Stress, coping and development: some issues and questions. *Journal of Child Psychology and Psychiatry, 22:* 323–354.

Rutter, M. and Quinton, D. and Liddle, C. (1983) Parenting in two generations: looking backwards and looking forwards. In: Madge, N. (Ed.) *Families at Risk.* London: Heinemann Educational.

Rutter, M. and Brown, G.W. (1966) The reliabillity of family life and relationships in families containing a psychiatric patient. *Social Psychiatry, 1:* 38–53.

Surtees, P. (1980) Social support, residual adversity and depressive outcome. *Social Psychiatry, 15:* 71–80.

Tennant, C. and Bebbington, P. (1978) The social causation of depression: a critique of the work of Brown and his colleagues. *Psychological Medicine, 8:* 565–575.

Uria, M. and Gaminde, I. (1988) Desordenes afectivos y factores sociales en la comunidad autonoma vasca - 3: Comarca de tolosa. Ms.

Vaughn, D. (1986) *Uncoupling: How Relationships Come Apart.* Oxford: Oxford University Press.

4

Elective Affinities in Schizophrenia and Childhood Autism

Christopher D. Frith and Uta Frith

Do Childhood Autism and Schizophrenia Show a Hidden Relationship?

"Let me anticipate," said Charlotte, "to see if I understand what you are aiming at. Just as everything is related to its own kind so it must be related to other things" . . . "Quite so" replied the Captain, . . . "We talk of affinities when things meet together and interact with each other. Take alkalis and acids. Despite their antagonism, or perhaps because of it, they seek each other most determinedly. They modify each other and form something new. Here is affinity." . . . "I must confess," said Charlotte, "when you mention these strange examples they don't make me think of blood relations, but of relationships of the mind . . ."

In Goethe's *Elective Affinities* (*Die Wahlverwandtschaften,* 1809), from which this extract is taken, the characters go along with the idea that there is greater merit in bringing together elements, opposites even, than there is in separating them. We follow their example by bringing together some very different concepts which can yet reveal surprising compatibilities. Clearly the two psychotic disorders that we have chosen to relate to each other, schizophrenia and autism, each belong to a different category of onset, one late, one early. Delusions and hallucinations commonly occur in schizophrenia, but are an exclusion criterion for the diagnosis of autism. There are major differences in epidemiological statistics, such as sex ratio, family history, and incidence of mental retardation. Nevertheless the term "autism" was originally coined by Bleuler in 1911 in order to characterize a type of social impairment that seemed characteristic of schizophrenia.

Profound and intransigent social impairments are indeed a feature of both disorders, and it is no coincidence that both Kanner (1943) and Asperger (1944) independently of each other chose the label "autistic" to name the disorder that we now call childhood autism.

In some respects it is easy to see similarities in different psychiatric disorders. Impaired performance on cognitive tests or impaired emotional responses are examples of very common deficits. Such commonalities are not the areas where we would like to discover a hidden relationship. We wish to know whether there are similarities of a specific rather than a general nature, features that hold uniquely and universally true for both disorders. Our first problem is therefore to decide which features are, in fact, fundamental to both. Once chosen, we would like to explain them in terms of a similar underlying dysfunction in the processing of information and, underlying this, a similar neurophysiological dysfunction.

The Key Features of Autism

When identifying key features, the picture is clearer in many ways for early childhood autism. Autism research benefited from methodological advances that were made in the study of mental retardation (e.g., Ellis, 1979; Hermelin and O'Connor, 1970). The most important advance was the strategy of comparing retarded children with mental age-matched autistic children. The problem of misidentifying chronological age-inappropriate behavior as abnormal when it is, in fact, mental age-appropriate is therefore avoided. Abnormalities can be specifically attributed to autism rather than to mental retardation when this strategy is followed. Wing and Gould (1979) used this insight in order to clarify the key symptoms of autism. In an important epidemiological study, they contrasted children with and without severe social impairment. As a result of this study a cluster of signs were identified which sharply divide children with and without persistent social impairments. These signs are largely independent of other additional handicaps such as sensory or motor handicap, and of accompanying mental retardation. The three signs are: 1) impaired social relations including aloofness, passivity, and oddness, 2) impaired communication, verbal and non-verbal, and 3) impaired imaginative activity with the substitution of stereotyped behavior. This triad applies to all individuals who are diagnosed as autistic according to various diagnostic schemes (Wing, 1988a,b). It includes "pure" cases as well as cases with additional handicaps, and degree of severity can vary. For all affected individuals the triad is the common denominator. It thus defines a whole spectrum of autistic disorders.

The triad is frequently, but not necessarily, associated with general mental retardation (Wing and Gould, 1979). Thus it is possible to study cases in which the three key signs are unconfounded by general intellectual impairment. With different levels of development and different degrees of ability, the signs show different behavioral manifestations, but they are always distinctly recognizable. The able and verbally articulate individual may show a communication impairment by engaging in lengthy accounts of a favorite topic without any consideration of the listener's wish to be told. This is just as much a failure of communication as can be observed in a mute child who persists in repetitive action without regard to the teacher's efforts towards a more constructive activity. It is sometimes hard to spot impairments at the extreme ends of the spectrum. At one extreme, difficulty arises because very young or very retarded children have too limited a repertoire to allow the key behavior to be observed. At the other extreme, the difficulty is that older, well taught and able autistic individuals can show remarkable compensation, and their well-rehearsed and often wide behavioral repertoire can deceive the non-expert observer. It is therefore not surprising that the middle range of the autistic spectrum includes the most typical cases.

The Key Features of Schizophrenia

For schizophrenia, the question of comparison groups is not so clear. As long as schizophrenia was considered not to be associated with organic damage, it was appropriate to compare schizophrenia with the other "functional" psychoses, and even the neuroses. However, such a view is now untenable. It is generally accepted that there is an organic basis to schizophrenia (e.g., Cutting, 1985), and in the majority of cases there is evidence of significant intellectual impairment (Aylward et al., 1987). It therefore might be more appropriate to compare schizophrenia with neurodegenerative disorders. Studies of this kind on a large scale in the manner of Wing and Gould's study of social impairment in children have yet to be done. In the absence of such definitive studies, there continues to be argument about which should be considered the key features of schizophrenia. The at present undisputed contenders are the positive symptoms (particularly Schneider's first rank symptoms, i.e., specific forms of abnormal experience underlying some hallucinations and delusions). In most of the leading standardised diagnostic schemes (e.g., PSE, Wing et al., 1974; DSM IIIR; American Psychiatric Association, 1987) these symptoms are necessary, but not always sufficient for the patient to be classified as suffering from schizophrenia. On the other hand, there are also the negative signs of psychomotor slowness, affective blunting, and intellectual deficit. These often precede as well as follow the first onset of the positive symptoms which attract attention both in the early stages and in acute phases of relapse. In the later stages of the illness, only one or the other type may be shown. Crow (1980) even suggested that these symptom clusters belong to discrete syndromes with different aetiologies.

In terms of the quality of life that the patient can lead, and in terms of long-term adaptation, there is little doubt that it is the negative signs that are most important (Owens and Johnstone, 1980). This is true, too, in terms of association with neurological signs (Owens et al., 1985). However, recent speculations about the psychological abnormalities that underlie schizophrenia have largely been concerned with the striking positive symptoms and have ignored the less visible negative ones. An example is the theory that positive symptoms are caused by a disorder of selective attention. The idea is that the patient cannot help but attend to irrelevant events in his environment. It is then suggested that the negative signs are merely consequences of a strategy that is deliberately adopted to overcome this failure of selective attention (Hemsley, 1977). For instance, the patient would avoid complex situations in which many competing stimuli are likely to occur and in which any attention failure would be particularly serious. In this sort of theory, social withdrawal and lack of communication are explained simply by the fact that social situations are examples of complex situations. Unfortunately, this explanation begs the question of what situations count as complex and why. A more serious problem for the theory is the finding that there are patients who show negative signs (e.g., poverty of speech), in the absence of any significant cognitive decline (Frith and Done, 1983). Presumably, their social impairment is not due to non-specific problems concerning complex information processing. Rather, their problem is in dealing specifically with *social* situations, and in particular, communication (Wing and Freudenberg, 1961).

As Bleuler (1911) originally suggested, we ourselves believe that social withdrawal and lack of communication do not reflect a coping strategy for some other cognitive impairment. Instead, they are themselves primary features and in need of explanation by a psychological theory. If we add to these a third feature, namely lack of spontaneous, creative behaviour with increased stereotyped activity (Frith and Done, 1983; Lyon et al., 1986; Frith and Done, in press), then we have an exact parallel to Wing's triad of impairments. The negative signs of schizophrenia can therefore be seen as a distinctive cluster of social, communicative, and imaginative impairments. Because these impairments together most clearly predict long-term outcome and brain pathology (Johnstone et al., 1986; Owens and Johnstone, 1980; Owens et al., 1985), it seems justified to consider them as key features of chronic schizophrenia over and above the definitive positive features.

As in the examples elaborated in Goethe's *Elective Affinities,* there are both attractions and risks in the attempt to relate separate or opposite entities. The attraction of our attempts to relate Wing's triad of impairments to the negative symptoms of schizophrenia is that we can build on cognitive theories that have already been proposed for both autism and schizophrenia. We are therefore in a position to put together a tentative model that can link related symptoms to underlying cognitive processes and can attempt to link these cognitive processes to brain function.

What then are the risks in our search for hidden similarities? Of course, when we suggest that certain key features of autism and chronic schizophrenia are related, we do not mean to imply that the two disorders are the same. This is plainly not the case, and on no account should differences be obscured (Wing and Attwood, 1987). The single most important difference is in the age of onset. Thus, the social-cognitive impairment that is associated with autism is manifest in early childhood, while that associated with schizophrenia may not appear until middle age. It follows that social knowledge and abilities in the adult autistic person are an outcome of abnormal development, while the schizophrenic individual even in his illness can draw on a store of normally acquired skills. Epidemiological and genetic studies point to a difference in aetiology. However, given the large variety of biological causes that are likely to exist for both disorders, we do not wish to speculate here about them.

Wing's Triad and Second-Order Representations.

The theory that can explain Wing's triad of impairments as the consequence of a specific cognitive dysfunction has been presented elsewhere (e.g., Baron-Cohen et al., 1985, 1986; Leslie, 1987; Leslie and Frith, 1988; Frith, 1989), and we shall therefore consider it only briefly. Crucial to the theory is Leslie's (1987; 1988a; 1988b) distinction between two kinds of knowledge. First, there is knowledge about objects in the world, such as bananas and telephones. This knowledge concerns the properties of the objects (color, texture) and the appropriate responses to be made to them (eating, dialing). It provides a more or less "true" representation of the world, and stored knowledge of this type is referred to as a *first-order representation*. It is the mind's window to the world. Second-order representations are what the mind makes of first-order representations. These are not like a window, but are "once removed" from reality as we perceive it. By cutting themselves off from a direct view (via a decoupling mechanism, in Leslie's terminology), these representations become the basis for a different kind of knowledge from which new inferences can be drawn. This knowledge knows about knowing. The ability to form second-order representations is a quantum leap in development. According to Leslie, one of the first unequivocal manifestations is the ability to pretend, which emerges around 18 months. From now on, the child is capable of taking into account that something is the case (a real state of affairs and a first-order representation), and yet can playfully ignore or contradict this knowledge (a "pretend" state and a second-order representation). An empty cup can be treated as if full, without the child being mistaken about the real state of affairs.

A later, highly important spin-off of the ability to handle second-order representations is the development of a "theory of mind." Of course, a well developed "theory of mind" depends on a great number of other things as well, not least learning and experience (Astington et al., 1988). It is a theory because we are talking of systematic social knowledge as opposed to mere social-emotional responding. This systematic knowledge is precisely what enables fast learning of social rules, and flexible, sophisticated use of the rules. Without such a theory, learning would be a slow process.

Having a "theory of mind" crucially depends on being aware that there are mental states (thoughts, desires, beliefs) which people have *about something,* and that other people have minds with different contents to our own. It is this aspect of "theory of mind" that depends on the ability to form second-order representations. Having a "theory of mind" enables us to mind-read, in a manner of speaking. We can work out what somebody is thinking by using inferences because we know mental states have causes and effects (e.g., we know something not by magic, but because someone told us). Furthermore, being able to mind-read implies that we are aware that actions, words and expressions produced by other people are not necessarily true reflections of their state of mind. By elaborating on this discrepancy we can deceive, lie and bluff. One could mention many more aspects of sophisticated social know-how and manipulation but here we are concerned only with that aspect that critically enables this sophistication to develop at all, namely second-order representation.

Impairment of pretend play and imaginative activity is one of the components of Wing's triad which can be seen as a consequence of a failure with second-order representations. This could itself be due to a variety of problems in mechanisms that underlie our handling of second-order representations. The impairment of two-way social interaction is a more indirect consequence due to a lack of a 'theory of mind.' Autistic aloneness is not so much a lack of first-order social responsiveness (this seems to be a non-specific feature of mental retardation) but a lack of second-order social know-how. Autistic aloneness is a kind of mind-reading blindness (Frith, 1989). It implies that thinking about people is

similar to thinking about very complex and unpredictable objects. However, it does not imply avoidance of people. In fact, autistic children prefer
to be in the company of others rather than alone, and show attachment to
particular individuals (Sigman and Ungerer, 1984; Sigman et al., 1986;
Mundy et al., 1986), suggesting that primary social responsiveness is not
impaired. Mind-reading blindness can accommodate also the fact that the
social impairment in autism comprises the aloof, the passive, and odd. All
three forms can be explained as manifestations of the inability to conceive
of people as having mental states.

What of the impairment of communication? Here too we must distinguish two levels. Certainly, straightforward *instrumental* communication
is possible for autistic children (Attwood et al., 1988; Landry and Loveland, 1988). On the other hand, two-way *intentional* communication depends upon making inferences about the minds of others. This requirement
has been discussed in detail by Sperber and Wilson (1986). Thus, the lack
of a "theory of mind" will leave communication very impoverished. For
example, the appropriate response to the query "Can you get out of bed?"
depends upon inferring something about the context and the speaker's
intentions. In the case of the mother speaking to her adolescent son, she
intends him to get up, and if he simply said "yes" without moving, this
would make her angry. On the other hand, if the question was asked by a
doctor of a Parkinson's patient, the answer "yes" would be noted as
satisfactory, even without an accompanying demonstration. Typically, in
pure autism, unconfounded by mental retardation, we find that the individual takes no account of the speaker's likely wishes and merely decodes
the messages literally. "Can you get out of bed?" would be decoded as a
request for information about mobility. In this way, we can explain the
elusive quality of the able autistic individuals comprehension failure which
includes lack of humor, irony, and make-believe. At the same time we can
allow for the fact that a great deal of social competence exists in such
individuals.

Difficulty with second-order representations explains Wing's triad of
autistic features in terms of a single cognitive deficit. This theory also
enables predictions to be made about aspects of autistic behavior that were
not previously investigated. In particular, it was predicted that autistic
children should have difficulty in understanding false beliefs. This prediction has been tested in a number of experiments (Baron-Cohen et al., 1985;
1986; Leslie and Frith, 1988). In one of these (Perner et al., 1989), the child
is disappointed to discover that a "smarties" tube contains, not Smarties,
but a small, blunt pencil. The child is then asked "What will your friend
say/think is in the tube when she comes into the room?". In order to give
the correct answer (Smarties), the child must recognize that, although

there is really a pencil in the tube, his friend does not know this and will falsely believe that there are Smarties in the tube. Unlike normal 4-year olds, the majority of autistic children (with a mental age well above 4) incorrectly answered, "a pencil." They behaved as if they believed that when they know something, everyone else knows it too. In this sense, they do not know what causes their own knowledge (they *saw* what was in the tube) or somebody else's ignorance (they did *not see*). Many of the anecdotes about communication failure in autistic children can be understood in terms of this kind of mind-reading blindness.

The cognitive deficit we envisage is very specific: it is a difficulty in forming and applying second-order representations, not first-order representations. When there is mental retardation (with or without autism) the efficiency of both systems would be impaired, but in autism without mental retardation, only the second order system is affected. This need not be a serious deficit for adapting oneself to the physical world, but it is when it comes to adapting oneself to the social world. Here it is necessary to be able to represent and continually update the mental states of others. This must be kept separate from updating information about the true state of the world. Hence, we are aware that others can have different beliefs from us, and this drives our wish to communicate. Second-order representation is just as necessary to represent one's own mental states as it is for that of others, and thus the ability is a necessary component of self-consciousness.

Schizophrenic Symptoms and Second-Order Representations.

Having identified a triad of social and communicative impairments with stereotypes in schizophrenia, we propose that here too is a problem with second-order representations. We also propose that the cognitive dysfunction giving rise to this problem would manifest itself very differently in the two disorders. The major difference between the schizophrenic and the autistic person is that the autistic individual shows cognitive impairment from early in life, whereas the schizophrenic patient manifests the impairment long after the various cognitive abilities and language are fully developed. Thus we expect to see differences between those two groups, just as we do when comparing people who are congenitally deaf with those who acquired deafness in later life (Myklebust, 1964; Bloom and Lahey, 1978).

For the first decade or so of his life, the future schizophrenic patient will have had plenty of experience inferring the mental states of others and acknowledging (and no doubt taking advantage of) their false beliefs. Thus it is plausible that he will be able to draw on this experience when the psychosis first manifests itself, and that he will continue to take account of the fact that other people have different mental states, knowledge, and beliefs. He would still also systematically take account of possible causes and effects of mental states, his own as well as others. We propose, that as his illness progresses the schizophrenic patient will have increasing difficulty in using a theory of mind in the normal way, and will often fail to interpret mental states correctly. This difficulty will result in major problems with social interaction and communication. However, there is no reason to doubt that a well established self-awareness persists, as well as an ingrained knowledge about routine social roles and relationships.

We would expect differences too in the type of imaginative impairment that would result from problems with second-order representations, because the patient prior to his illness has fully developed normal imagination. As this becomes difficult to handle, stereotyped activites take over.

Communication Impairment in Schizophrenia

There have been extensive studies of language in schizophrenia but far fewer of communication. The results of these studies suggest that schizophrenic language is remarkably intact, that is in terms of phonology, syntax, and semantics (see review by Frith and Allen, 1988). Nevertheless problems always emerge, but these have proved difficult to characterize. The problems include lack of cohesion (Rochester and Martin, 1979), failures of discourse planning (Hoffman, 1986), failure to make inferences (Allen, 1984), use of simplified syntax (Morice and Ingram, 1982) and, above all, poverty of ideas and production. All these problems can readily be interpreted in terms of failures of communication rather than of language. To reiterate, in order to communicate intentionally, it is necessary to infer the mental state of the partner. This is because we cannot understand what the point of a remark is unless we take into account what the partner intends and what he already knows and expects. These inferences determine whether to reply to a message at all, as well as the precise form of the reply. There is some evidence of a failure in schizophrenic patients to make inferences of mental states (Allen, 1984).

The problem with the use of referents and with discourse can largely be understood as a consequence of not taking into account the needs of the listener (in terms of his current knowledge). For example, we use complex rather than simple syntax only if the needs of the listener make such complexity necessary for communication. If varying needs are not taken into account then either the simplest syntax will always do, or else pedantic language is used at all times. Just such strategies are found in schizophrenic language as in the signs "poverty of speech" and "stilted speech.'' In the extreme, if the needs of the listener are not inferred and thus not recognized, then there is no need for communication at all and muteness results. Poverty of speech is a common sign in chronic schizophrenic patients, and is also observed in autistic patients when adults (Rumsey, et al., 1986). Thus many of the ''language'' problems associated with schizophrenia can be explained in terms of a failure to infer continuously the relevant mental states of others.

The expression of affect is also largely to do with communication of inner states and one's awareness of the effect this has on other people's inner feelings. Thus flattening of affect can be seen as a direct consequence of the same problem, namely a difficulty in forming and using second-order representations. At this deeper level of analysis—but not necessarily in surface behavior—similarities of autistic and schizophrenic communication failure are striking.

Self-Monitoring and Willed Intentions

Many of the negative and some of the positive symptoms of schizophrenia have been explained in terms of defects in the initiation and monitoring of willed actions (Frith, 1987; Frith and Done, 1988). Briefly, this refers to a fault in the ability to know whether or not an action was one's own. Certain types of symptoms, such as delusions of control by outside agencies were said to arise because the patient was not aware of his own willed intentions. A precise prediction made on the basis of this hypothesis was that patients showing these symptoms should have difficulty correcting their own errors in a reaction time task (Frith and Done, 1989). This prediction was confirmed experimentally. Negative symptoms according to this theory occur when the patient fails to form willed intentions. This account had almost nothing to say about communication problems in schizophrenia. In contrast, the triad of impairments in autism and its explanation has almost entirely been concerned with communication, and not with action and self monitoring. How will these different accounts fare when we relate them together? What are the hidden affinities?

Communication is a special kind of action. Therefore, it can be understood in the same way as other actions. Initiation and monitoring of actions play an important role in communication. Otherwise, one would not know what one said and meant as opposed to what someone else said and meant. Second-order representation is necessary for this type of monitoring, and must therefore be necessary for certain kinds of action as well. In fact, it applies whenever one needs to consider whether one did or did not do something, and also when one forms willed intentions.

Figure 4.1 is taken from Leslie (1988a) and illustrates his model for

FIGURE 4.1
First and Second Order Representations (after Leslie, 1988)

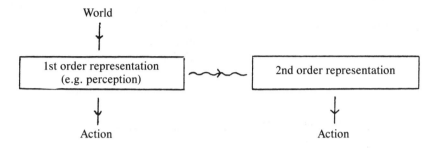

FIGURE 4.2
Two Routes to Action (after Frith and Done, 1988)

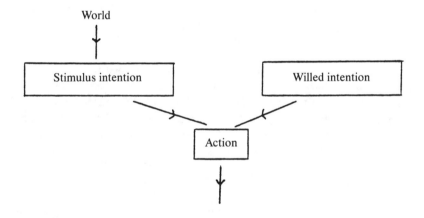

pretend play. Two sources of action are shown. The first depends on first-order representations and enables us to respond appropriately to objects (e.g., answering the telephone). The second depends on second-order representations and enables us to pretend (e.g., answering the banana). There is a striking similarity between this figure and that concerning the two routes to action discussed by Frith (1987), and by Frith and Done (1988) (Figure 4.2). This similarity suggests that stimulus elicited action depends upon first-order representation, while spontaneous or willed action depends on second-order representation. We propose therefore that both intentional communication and willed action depend upon second-order representation. The difference between these systems is that communication depends especially on representing the mental states of others, while willed action depends on representing the mental states of the actor himself, in particular his wishes and intentions. We therefore can postulate one single fault in the underlying processes that would explain the social failure as well as the poverty of ideas and actions.

Sperber and Wilson (1986) analyze in some detail the series of processes involved in a successful two-way communication. Essentially the relevance of the message has to be understood. First, the subject must recognize that there is an intent to communicate. Sperber and Wilson call an indication of an attempt to communicate an ostensive stimulus. This often takes the form of speech (as in "Oy, Jimmy"), but can also be a subtle and non-verbal stimulus (as in a raised eyebrow). Having recognized that there is an attempt to communicate, the subject must decode the message that is presented (e.g., from sound to phonology to semantics). However, decoding the message is not enough. The subject must also make inferences about the mental state of the communicator in order to extract the relevance of the message. The subject's representations of the mental state (e.g., wishes) of the communicator must be kept distant from his own wishes and also distinct from his representations of the real state of the world.

The development of a willed action can be described in a very similar way. First, the subject must recognize that one of his goals is achievable. He must then infer the series of states of the world that has to be produced in order to achieve that goal. These desired states of the world (second-order representation) must be kept distinct from the actual states of the world (first-order representations).

Negative and Positive Symptoms in Communication

In Table 4.1 we suggest some of the problems that might arise if there was a fault in the processes that compute relevance in communication. A fault can result in two kinds of error, false positives and false negatives. If there is something wrong with the subject's ability to recognize an attempt to communicate (an ostensive stimulus) he might either see an attempt to communicate when there wasn't one (false positive), or he might fail to see an attempt to communicate which was in fact genuine (false negative). In both cases, there is misinterpretation and faulty communication of relevance. In the first case, too much relevance is attributed, in the second case, too little.

The false positive error in this case corresponds to a *delusion of reference,* where the subject erroneously believes that people are communicating with him. The false negative error would result in a lack of social responsiveness which is one aspect of *social withdrawal.* In general, we

TABLE 4.1
The Normal Processes Underlying Communication and Possible Abnormalities

False Negative (negative symptoms)	Normal Process	False Positives (positive symptoms)
Failure to respond to ostensive stimuli	Recognition that communication is intended by other	Delusions of reference
No inference about mental states of other	Inferences about mental states of other	Paranoid delusions
Unable to represent mental states of others	Distinction between mental states of self and others	Incoherent speech, auditory hallucinations (3rd person)

suggest that false positive errors lead to so-called "positive" symptoms, while false negative errors lead to "negative" symptoms.

Paranoid delusions can arise if the subject makes false but coherent inferences about the mental state of others.

If the subject confuses the mental states he might attribute to himself and to others, then it would follow that he apparently takes no account of the fact that he knows things that his hearers do not know. This could lead to certain kinds of *incoherence of speech* in which the subject fails to provide referents and introduces apparently unrelated topics without explanation (Rochester and Martin, 1979; Hoffman, 1986).

In extreme cases, the subject confuses his representations of the mental states of others with first-order representations of the real world. This could lead to certain auditory *hallucinations*. Auditory hallucinations have been explained as arising when the patient perceives his own thoughts as coming from an external source (e.g., Frith, 1987). However, it has always been difficult to explain why the "voices" are reported by patients to talk about them in the 3rd person, and why for the same patient there can be several different voices, male as well as female. It seems likely that what is most important to us in the beliefs of others is what they think about us. This content of their beliefs would be particularly important in determining the precise form of our communications. Therefore representations about the beliefs of others might take the form of 3rd person commentaries, for example, "he's not going to speak to me, he's too arrogant." Thus the common first rank symptom of hearing voices discussing the patient might be seen as a result of faulty interpretation of second-order representations. The mental states of others are still internally represented but misperceived as first-order representations of the real world. Hence the experience of hallucinations is created.

The false negative errors of the communication system all lead to varying degrees of *social withdrawal* and *lack of communication*. It is clear that all the examples of negative symptoms given in this column of the table apply very straightforwardly to autism.

Negative and Positive Symptoms in Willed Action

Table 4.2 suggests the problems that might arise in the system for willed action. They would arise from the same fault in relevance computing processes. Hence, the arguments relating symptoms to abnormal processes are essentially the same as those we have outlined for Table 4.1 The failure to infer the appropriate actions leading to goals might lead to *incoherent speech* of a different kind from that associated with failures in the communication system. The patient meanders through a series of topics without ever reaching the point. Auditory hallucinations associated with failures in the action system would occur because the subject failed to distinguish between his own mental states and states in the real world. The patient might hear his thoughts as if they were coming from an external source. Likewise, the patient's own intentions might be perceived as having an external source, thus leading to *delusions of control*.

The false negative errors associated with the action system would lead to a general *lack of volition* and inability to achieve goals. In addition *flattening of affect* might occur if the subject was unable to represent his own mental states. For all three negative symptoms there are examples in relation to autistic individuals, most clearly documented in biographical accounts (e.g., Park, 1987).

The relations between symptoms and processing failures outlined in

TABLE 4.2
The Normal Processes Underlying Action and Possible Abnormalities

False Negatives (negatives symptoms)	Normal Process	False Positives (positive symptoms)
Lack of volition	Recognition that a goal is achievable	Grandiose delusions
Unable to infer actions appropriate to goals	Inference of actions appropriate to goals	Delusions of causality, incoherent speech and acts
Unable to represent own mental states (flattening of affect)	Distinction between mental states and states of the world	Delusions of control, auditory hallucinations (thought broadcast)

tables 4.1 and 4.2 are very tentative, but the tables imply interesting possibilities for classifying psychotic symptoms in terms of type and severity. First, there is the obvious distinction between symptoms associated with communication and those associated with action. If these systems are to some extent independent then we might expect the associated types of symptoms to be independent also.

Since the communication system is more complex, requiring the distinction between mental states of ourselves and others, we might expect this system to be more vulnerable, and thus symptoms associated with communication should reflect an earlier stage or a less severe form of the illness than those associated with action. Within both systems, the underlying processes are hierarchical. Thus if no distinction can be made between the mental states of the self and of others, the ability to infer the mental states of others is irrelevant. Likewise, if second-order representations cannot be formed at all, there are no mental states of self and others to be confused. Such a hierarchy indicates which symptoms are more or less severe. In this way, the present approach to the understanding of psychosis suggests the beginning of a rational and theoretically based scheme for classifying and relating symptoms.

For both tables the division into negative and positive symptoms reflects two types of processing error. For theoretical reasons, faults in the decision process have to allow for both false positives and false negatives. In practice, however, we see only false negatives in the case of autism, and only false positives in the case of acute phases of schizophrenia. Only some schizophrenic patients experience both positive and negative symptoms, while many chronic patients experience only negative symptoms.

How is this pattern to be explained? The key is the distinction between first- and second-order representations. Only if second-order representations are available and used can false positives occur. If second-order representations are not available at all, then false negatives are bound to occur, and only those. This would be the case in severe cases of autism, and might be the case in certain severe and late stages of schizophrenia where all vestiges of the formerly acquired second-order representation systems have disappeared.

It remains to be seen whether in mild cases of autism the ability to use second-order representation can be developed and practiced with time. If so, symptoms due to false positives would also occur. However, this has not been shown. Indeed, it might be very difficult to show, because the subjective experience of positive symptoms will depend on the patient's past experience. This past experience will be different for a person whose whole development took an abnormal course.

Differences Between Schizophrenia and Autism.

Having drawn out the affinities between the two disorders, we must again turn to the vast differences between them. We have repeatedly stated that although similar cognitive dysfunction may underlie both schizophrenia and autism, this will not automatically mean that the signs and symptoms are similar. Nor does it exclude the possibility of additional cognitive deficits, which might well result in totally different additional impairments. To identify critical underlying cognitive differences is not an easy task. One initially striking difference, namely, the absence of positive symptoms in autistic individuals and their presence in schizophrenic patients, is less impressive now, because we can explain both presence and absence by the malfunctioning of one and the same cognitive process. We therefore think it could be misleading to stress the absence of delusions and hallucinations in autistic children. This absence might be of no greater significance than the absence of reading and spelling abnormalities in someone who has never been literate in the first place.

From their past experience schizophrenic patients know that people have mental states and what causes or changes them. We suggest, however, that when they are ill, these patients have great difficulty in inferring what these mental states are and how they are caused. Symptoms such as delusions of reference and delusions of persecution are a result of making incorrect inferences about the mental states of others. Autistic people do not make such attributions. They simply would not make the attempt to interpret the mental states of others, since they have never been sufficiently aware of their existence.

In addition to differences that might be explained by different age of onset, there are other differences that might be due to different causes. For instance, there is the characteristically uneven profile of abilities of autistic people of all levels of intelligence (Lincoln et al., 1988), and there are the peculiarly narrow interests, the occasional savant capabilities, the odd preoccupations and elaborate routines that are unique to classically autistic children. There are also characteristic odd movements, speech intonations, and sensory responses that are a frequent feature in autism, but rare in schizophrenia. None of these particular symptoms is universally present throughout the spectrum of autistic disorders, none is part of Wing's triad, and none can be explained by communication or monitoring of action failure. It remains to be seen whether these and other additional impairments can be explained as consequences of the early age of onset, or whether they are of separate origin.

How Can One Study the Neurophysiological Basis of First- and Second-order Representations?

An entirely independent line of thinking leads us to believe that underlying the psychological deficit that we postulated for both autism and schizophrenia is some fairly specific damage to the brain. The existence of well adapted and able autistic and schizophrenic people suggests that the structures necessary for second-order representation can be damaged while leaving other cognitive structures intact. One would therefore assume that there are brain structures specifically concerned with the mechanisms necessary for second-order representation. In any case, we need to ask what these hypothetical structures are, and where they are located. We would also like to know what happens if these structures are damaged in the immature organism on the one hand, and the mature organism on the other. However, if we are properly to understand brain and behavior relationships we need to consider work with animals, since only here can true experiments be conducted.

The brain structures needed for second-order representation cannot have suddenly come into existence. They must have evolved, and thus animals must at least possess the precursors of such an ability. Before we can relate second-order representations to brain structures, we must attempt to delineate what this ability implies and what ability in animals might resemble it.

Leslie and Frith (1990) suggest that there are at least three components necessary for handling second-order representations: a decoupling mechanism, an inference mechanism, and a specific mechanism for relating first- and second-order representations. The decoupling mechanism is one component where one might look for a fault. According to Leslie (1987), the decoupling mechanism is designed to release a representation from its primary aim, namely to represent a real state of affairs. The primary representation is decoupled from this purpose and is now suspended from considerations of truth. There are three important consequences. First there is the detachment of the representation from its normal semantic associations. This means that other associations which we know to be incorrect can nevertheless be temporarily attached. The second feature is that it is not our perception that changes with decoupling. When pretending a banana is a telephone we still see that it is a banana, just as we still "know" it is a banana. Rather it is our responses that change. In other words, we behave as if the banana was a telephone (we put it to our ear, talk into it, etc.). Thus, while pretending we detach the responses appropriate to one object (which in some sense are the meaning of that object) and arbitrarily attach these responses to another object. The third feature of decoupling is that any rearrangement of stimuli and responses is temporary. When we have finished pretending we easily revert to our "normal" responses, eating bananas and not eating telephones.

It is these three consequences of decoupling that we can relate to phenomena reported in the literature on animal learning. In an extensive review of the kinds of tasks used to study learning and memory in monkeys, Ridley and Baker (submitted) suggest that there is a fundamental distinction between two kinds of learning. To us these two kinds of learning are reminiscent of the two types of knowledge. In one type the animal learns about the nature of the objects involved (i.e., their permanent properties). In particular it learns which objects to approach and which objects to avoid. For example food is placed always under the ballerina and never under the soldier. The monkey has to learn to approach the ballerina and avoid the soldier. Essentially, what is learned is the meaning of the object (e.g., the ballerina means food), and this is learned in terms of the appropriate response to be made to that object. This corresponds to first-order representations.

In contrast, according to Ridley and Baker, there is another type of learning where the animal learns to use the object as a sign. For example, if both food wells are covered by *green* plaques the food is in the left well, but if both are covered by *red* plaques then the food is in the right well. Here the animal has to learn to attach an arbitrary response to objects while the objects themselves remain neutral, neither to be generally approached nor avoided. Many more trials are needed to learn this task than are required to learn the ballerina vs. soldier task.

We suggest that the result of this type of learning is an analogue of the forming of second-order representations. In principle, the color plaques could be replaced by objects well known to the aninmal which, in the context of this particular task, would not represent their familiar meaning, but act as signs for something else. In an experiment reported by Gaffan and Bolton (1983; Experiment II, Stage 2) a monkey learned that a carrot meant "choose the black penny" and a sultana meant "choose the white penny." The black penny led to a food reward only when the carrot was there, but not the white penny, and vice versa. The cognitive requirements in this situation show certain similarities to those required for pretence. The representation of the object has to be detached from the representation of its normal meaning (e.g., eat) and has to be responded to in a new arbitrarily decided way (e.g., select a color). These responses apply only in the context of the experiment, and are thus temporary. Outside this context, carrot and sultana retain their semantic meaning and are eaten immediately.

Thus Ridley and Baker's distinction between two types of learning can be mapped readily onto Leslie's model of pretence (Figure 4.1). The first type of learning could be thought of as akin to forming first-order representations by which the permanent and real properties of objects are represented. The second and much more effortful type of learning might be akin to forming second-order representations, insofar as it is the context which determines which responses are to be (briefly and arbitrarily) attached to objects. Given that such a distinction can be made in animal learning, experiments could be conducted to find out which brain systems are involved. This is as far as we can go at present in suggesting ways of exploring the brain functions that underly the critical processes that we discussed in the main part of this essay.

The next step is to think about the kind of brain dysfunction that we might expect to give rise to a dysfunction in the formation of second-order representations. The justification for the distinction between the two kinds of learning in animals derives from studies of the effects of brain lesions. A great many experiments, reviewed by Ridley and Baker, have shown that "stimulus-reward association" (first-order) learning is impaired by lesions of the amygdala, while "arbitrary rule" (second-order) learning is impaired by lesions of the hippocampus. Here then a structural basis for the two types of processing is suggested. However, the results do not imply that the equivalent of first- and second-order representations in animals are stored respectively in the amygdala and hippocampus. Indeed, it has been shown that the hippocampus and amygdala are only necessary for the learning, not for the retention of the two types of tasks (Ridley et al., submitted; Jones and Mishkin, 1972). It remains quite open what other brain structures might be involved.

Some Ideas from Neuropsychology

In current mainstream neuropsychology (Warrington and Weiskrantz, 1982), it is assumed that long term semantic memory is critically subserved by structures in the temporal lobe. This would be equivalent to first-order representations of the world. On the other hand, the central executive component of working memory is believed to be subserved by the frontal cortex (Goldman-Rakic, 1987). We would like to suggest that this component is responsible not only for temporary representations, but also for the arbitrary context-dependent meanings of objects. This demands second-order representations. Of course second-order representations do not exist on their own. In Leslie's (1987) model, a second-order representation is a "decoupled" first-order representation as indicated in his diagram (Figure

4.1). Warrington and Weiskrantz (1982) propose that there is a "cognitive mediational memory system" by which long term information from the posterior association cortex (i.e., temporal and parietal lobes) is additionally represented in a frontal system. We can therefore hypothesize that for second-order presentations both the frontal lobes and the connection from these to the temporal lobes need to be intact.

Bringing together these various ideas, we suggest that the processing of second-order representations is the job of the frontal cortex and its connections with various posterior structures. As yet, there is insufficient evidence for even the most tentative suggestions about which brain structures are involved in decoupling, and in keeping first-order and second-order representations distinct. However, a beginning is already made by elaborating the concepts of first- and second-order representations. On this basis, tasks can be designed that will permit the study of these issues in animals and in patients with known circumscribed lesions.

So far, neuropsychological tests have not been designed within the framework we are using in this chapter. All too often they are not designed within a cognitive framework at all, but rather in terms of brain areas (i.e., frontal tests, temporal tests, etc.). In these terms, we would expect that schizophrenic and autistic patients would be impaired on frontal tests rather than those concerned with more posterior regions. This need not mean, however, that the "lesion" is actually in the frontal cortex. In terms of our formulation, any difficulties with second-order representations might arise from malfunctioning connections between posterior regions and the frontal cortex.

There is currently considerable interest in the frontal lobes as a source of schizophrenic impairments (e.g., Weinberger, 1988). However, while many studies find that schizophrenic patients perform badly on frontal tests, they frequently perform badly on tests associated with other areas as well (e.g., Kolb and Wishaw, 1983). This is perhaps not surprising, since many patients show evidence of a general cognitive decline.

Since most neuropsychological tests presuppose a near normal general intellectual level, it is necessary to study autistic and schizophrenic patients of higher ability. A recent study adopted this strategy (Rumsey and Hamburger, 1988), and found that high IQ autistic patients are impaired only on frontal tests. As far as we are aware, this strategy has not yet been applied to schizophrenic patients. Tests derived specifically to examine the ability to form and use second-order representations should be used not only to study autistic and schizophrenic patients, but also neurological patients with various developmental or acquired disorders.

Summary and Conclusions

In this paper, we have put together the separate disorders of autism and schizophrenia and have drawn out the striking affinity between the negative signs of schizophrenia and the signs implied by Wing's triad. The affinity prompted us to propose that there is one and the same key abnormality that underlies the distinctive and profound communication failure in autism and the negative features of schizophrenia. This abnormality can be seen as a failure in the use of second-order representations. This failure leads to specific abnormalities of verbal and non-verbal communication, and of social interaction. It also leads to difficulties with the initiation of spontaneous willed action.

The positive symptoms of schizophrenia occur when erroneous representations of mental states are formed (through faulty inference), or when mental states and real states of the world are not properly distinguished. Such symptoms are not observed in autism because the awareness of mental states has never been fully developed. Hence misinterpretations do not arise.

The key abnormalities affect two systems: that concerned with communication (requiring representation of the mental states of others) and that concerning willed action (requiring representation of mental states of self). The representation of mental states as well as the representation of willed intentions require the ability to form second-order representation.

In order to look for a biological basis for the hypothesized cognitive processes, it is necessary to search for analogues in animal learning. Primates may have a capacity that is a precursor of the capacity to form second-order representations, and this could provide a useful tool for future investigations. Studies with animals and neurological patients suggest that while first-order representations (knowledge about the world) are processed in the posterior regions of the brain, especially the temporal lobes, objects may be "re-represented" in the frontal lobes. We can hypothesize that second-order representations depend on both the frontal lobes and connections from these to the temporal lobes.

In this brief account, we have done little more than to relate together psychotic symptoms, animal learning and brain function in terms of one cognitive process, namely the capacity to form and use second-order representation. The next step must be to develop techniques for studying this process in adults, children and animals.

References

Allen, H.A. (1984) Positive and negative symptoms and the thematic organisation of schizophrenic speech. *British Journal of Psychiatry,* 144: 611–617.

American Psychiatric Association (1987) *Diagnostic and Statistical Manual for Mental Disorders.* Revised edition (DSM-III-R). American Psychiatric Association: Washington, D.C.

Asperger, H. (1944) Die "Autistischen Psychopathen" im Kindesalter. Archiv für Psychiatrie und Nervenkrankheiten, 117: 76–136.

Astington, J.W., Harris, P.L. and Olson, D.R. (eds.) (1988) *Developing Theories of Mind.* Cambridge: Cambridge University Press.

Attwood, A.H., Frith, U. and Hermelin, B. (1988) The understanding and use of interpersonal gestures by autistic and Down's syndrome children. *Journal of Autism and Developmental Disorders,* 18: 241–257.

Aylwood, E., Walker, E. and Bettes, B. (1984) Intelligence in schizophrenia: Meta-analysis of the research. *Schizophrenia Bulletin,* 10: 430–459.

Baron-Cohen, S., Leslie, A.M. and Frith, U. (1985) Does the autistic child have a "theory of mind"? *Cognition,* 21: 37–46.

Baron-Cohen, S., Leslie, A.M. and Frith, U. (1986) Mechanical, behavioural and intentional understanding of picture stories in autistic children. *British Journal of Development Psychology,* 4: 113–125.

Bleuler, E. (1911) Dementia praecox oder Gruppe der Schizophrenien. V. Aschaffenburg (ed.): *Handbuch der Psychiatrie,* Vol. 4., Chap. 1. Deuticke, Leipzig/Wien.

Bloom, L. and Lahey, M. (1978) *Language Development and Language Disorders.* New York: Wiley.

Crow, T.J. (1980) Molecular pathology of schizophrenia. More than one dimension of pathology? *British Medical Journal,* 280: 66–68.

Cutting, J. (1985) *The Psychology of Schizophrenia.* (Chapter 5) Churchill-Livingstone: Edinburgh.

Ellis, N.R. (1979) *Handbook of Mental Deficiency.* Hillsdale N.Y.: Erlbaum.

Frith, C.D. and Done, D.J. (1983) Stereotyped responding by schizophrenic patients in a two-choice guessing task. *Psychological Medicine,* 13: 779–786.

Frith, C.D. (1987) The positive and negative symptoms of schizophrenia reflect impairments in the perception and initiation of action. *Psychological Medicine,* 17: 631–648.

Frith, C.D. and Allen, H.A. (1988) Language disorders in schizophrenia and their implications for neuropsychology. In: P. Bebbington and P. McGuffin (Eds.) *Schizophrenia: The Major Issues .* Oxford: Heineman.

Frith, C.D. and Done, D.J. (1988) Towards a neuropsychology of schizophrenia. *British Journal of Psychiatry,* 153: 437–443.

Frith, C.D. and Done, D.J. (1989) Experience of alien control in schizophrenia reflect a disorder in the central monitoring of action. *Psychological Medicine,* 19, 359–364.

Frith, C.D. and Done, D.J. (In press) Stereotyped behavior in madness and in health. In: S.F. Cooper and C.T. Parish (Eds.) *The Neurobiology of Behavioural Stereotype.* Oxford: Oxford University Press.

Frith, U. (1989) *Autism: Explaining the Enigma.* Oxford: Blackwell.

Gaffan, D. and Bolton, J. (1983) Learning object—object associations by monkeys. *Quarterly Journal of Experimental Psychology,* 35B: 149–156.

Goldman-Rakic, P.S. (1987) Circuitry of primate prefrontal cortex and regulation of behaviour by representational memory. In: *Handbook of Physiology: The Nervous System.* Vol. 5 (Eds. F. Plum and V. Mountcastle) American Physiological Society, Bethesda, pp. 373–417.

Hemsley, D.R. (1977) What have cognitive deficits to do with schizophrenic symptoms? *British Journal of Psychiatry,* 130: 167–173.

Hermelin, B. and O'Connor, N. (1970) *Psychological Experiments with Autistic Children.* Oxford: Pergamon Press.

Hoffman, R.E. (1986) Verbal hallucinating and language production processes in schizophrenia. *The Behavioural and Brain Sciences,* 4: 503–548.

Johnstone, E.C., Owens, D.G.C., Frith, C.D. and Crow, T.J. (1986) The relative stability of positive and negative features in chronic schizophrenia. *British Journal of Psychiatry,* 150: 60–64.

Jones, B. and Mishkin, M. (1972) Limbic lesions and the problem of stimulus reinforcement associations. *Experimental Neurology,* 36: 362–377.

Kanner, L. (1943) Autistic disturbances of affective contact. *Nervous Child,* 2: 217–250.

Landry, S.H. and Loveland, K.A. (1988) Communication behaviours in autism and developmental language delay. *Journal of Child Psychology and Psychiatry,* 29: 621–634.

Leslie, A.M. (1987) Pretence and representation: the origins of 'theory of mind'. *Psychol. Review,* 94: 412–426.

Leslie, A.M. (1988a) Some implications of pretense for mechanisms underlying the child's theory of mind. In: Astington, J., Harris, P. and Olson, D. (eds.) *Developing Theories of Mind.* Cambridge: Cambridge University Press.

Leslie, A.M. (1988b) The necessity of illusion: perception and thought in infancy. In: Weiskrantz, L. (ed.) *Thought Without Language.* Oxford: Oxford University Press.

Leslie, A.M. and Frith, U. (1988) Autistic children's understanding of seeing, knowing and believing. *British Journal of Developmental Psychology,* 4: 315–324.

Leslie, A.M. and Frith, U. (1990) Prospects for a cognitive neuropsychology of autism: Hobson's choice. *Psychology Review 97,* 122–131.

Lincoln, A.J., Courchesne, E., Kilman, B.A., Elmasian, R. and Allen, M. (1988) A study of intellectual abilities in high-functioning people with autism. *Journal of Autism and Developmental Disorders,* 18: 505–524.

Lyon, N., Mejsholm, B. and Lyon, M. (1986) Stereotyped responding by schizophrenic out-patients. *Journal of Psychiatric Research,* 20: 137–150.

Kolb, B. and Wishaw, I.Q. (1983) Performance of schizophrenic patients in tests sensitive to left or right frontal, temporal or parietal function in neurological patients. *Journal of Nervous and Mental Disease,* 171: 435–443.

Morice, R.D. and Ingram, J.C.L. (1983) Language complexity and age of onset in schizophrenia. *Psychiatry Research,* 9: 233–242.

Mundy, P., Sigman, M., Ungerer, J. and Sherman, T. (1986) Defining the social deficit of autism: the contribution of non-verbal communication measures. *Journal of Child Psychology and Psychiatry,* 27: 657–669.

Myklebust, H. (1964) *The Psychology of Deafness: Sensory Deprivation, Learning, and Adjustment.* N.Y.: Grune and Stratton.

Owens, D.G.C. and Johnstone, E.C. (1980) The disabilities of chronic schizophrenia: their nature and the factors contributing to their development. *British Journal of Psychiatry,* 136: 384–395.

Owens, D.G.C., Johnstone, E.C., Crow, T.J., Frith, C.D., Jagoe, J.R. and Kreel, L. (1985) Lateral ventricular size in schizophrenia: relationship to the disease process and its clinical manifestations. *Psychological Medicine,* 15: 27–41.

Park, C.C. (1987) *The Seige: The First Eight Years of an Autistic Child.* 2nd Edition with epilogue "Fifteen Years After". Boston, Massachusetts: Atlantic-Little Brown.

Perner, J., Frith, U., Leslie, A., Leekham, S. (1989) Exploration of the autistic child's theory of mind: knowledge, belief and communication. *Child Development, 60,* 689–700.

Ridley, R.M., Aitken, D.M. and Baker, H.F. (1989) Learning about rules, but not about reward is impaired following lesions of the cholinergic projection to the hippocampus. *Brain Research 502,* 306–318.

Ridley, R.M. and Baker, H.F. A critical evaluation of primate models of amnesia and dementia. (Submitted to *Brain Research Reviews*).

Rochester, S.R. and Martin, J.R. (1979) *Crazy Talk: A Study of the Discourse of Schizophrenic Speakers.* New York, Plenum.

Rumsey, J.M., Andreasen, N.C. and Rapoport, J.L. (1986) Thought, language, communication and affective flattening in autistic adults. Archives of General Psychiatry, 43: 771–777.

Rumsey, J.M. and Hamburger, S.D. (1988) Neurophysiological findings in high functioning men with infantile autism, residual state. *Journal of Clinical and Experimental Neuropsychology,* 10: 201–221.

Sigman, M., Mundy, P., Sherman, T. and Ungerer, J. (1986) Social interactions of autistic mentally retarded and normal children and their caregivers. *Journal of Child Psychology and Psychiatry,* 27: 647–656.

Sigman, M. and Ungerer, J.A. (1984) Attachment behaviours in autistic children. *Journal of Autism and Developmental Disorders,* 14: 231–244.

Sperber, D. and Wilson, D. (1986) *Relevance: Communication and Cognition.* Oxford: Blackwell.

Venables, P.H. (1964) Input dysfunction in schizophrenia. In: B.A. Maher (Ed.) *Contributions to the Psychopathology of Schizophrenia.* New York, Academic Press.

Warrington, E.K. and Weiskrantz, L. (1982) Amnesia: a disconnection syndrome. *Neuropsychological,* 20: 233–248.

Weinberger, D.R. (1988) Schizophrenia and the frontal lobe. *Trends in the Neurosciences,* 11: 367–370.

Wing, J.K. and Freudenberg, R.K. (1961) The response of severely ill chronic schizophrenic patients to social stimulation. *American Journal of Psychiatry,* 118: 311.

Wing, J.K., Cooper, J.E. and Sartorius, N. (1974) *The Description and Classification of Psychiatric Symptoms: An Instruction Manual for the PSE and CATEGO Systems.* Cambridge University Press, Cambridge.

Wing, L. and Gould, J. (1979) Severe impairments of social interaction and associated abnormalities in children: epidemiology and classification. *Journal of Autism and Developmental Disorders,* 9: 11–79.

Wing, L. and Attwood, A. (1987) Syndromes of autism and atypical development. In: Cohen, D.J., Donnellan, A. and Paul, R. (eds.) *Handbook of Autism and Pervasive Developmental Disorders.* New York: Wiley.

Wing, L. (1988a) The continuum of autistic characteristics. In: Schopler, E. and Mesibov, E.B. (eds.) *Diagnosis and Assessment.* New York: Plenum.

Wing, L. (1988b) The autistic continuum. In: L. Wing (ed.) *Autism: Biological Aspects* London: Gaskill and Royal College of Psychiatrists.

5

Cognitive Perspectives on Social Psychiatry

Chris R. Brewin

Introduction

Research in social psychiatry has established the important influence of environmental factors on the onset and course of psychiatric disorder. Such factors as life events, chronic difficulties, social support, and the emotions expressed by patients' families, have all emerged as significant determinants of outcome. These findings have still, however, to be explained at the psychological level if they are to be effectively translated into strategies for prevention and treatment. We need to know how and why social events such as these can evoke strong individual reactions. Why, for example, do some people have poorer social support and smaller social networks than others, and why do the emotional attitudes of families differ? Why, even when faced with severe environmental stressors, do people differ so greatly in the nature and intensity of their reaction and in their ability to cope? These are precisely the sort of questions addressed by theories drawn from experimental and social cognitive psychology, and many of their principles have now been incorporated into effective therapeutic interventions.

Cognitive perspectives are certainly not without precedent in social psychiatry. In his writings on schizophrenia, Wing (e.g., 1978) has distinguished for many years between intrinsic impairments and secondary adverse reactions such as low self-confidence arising from the individual's attitudes towards self and symptoms. Yarrow et al. (1956) graphically described the difficulties faced by relatives in coming to an understanding of the unusual behavior exhibited by patients displaying for the first time the symptoms of schizophrenia. Cognitive perspectives have also been influential in depression research (Bebbington, 1985). For example, Brown and Harris (1978) speculated that events and difficulties provoke depression because they create a state of hopelessness and that the influence of vulnerability factors is mediated by levels of self-esteem. It is fair to say, though, that cognitive perspectives have not been systematically applied in social psychiatry, and where they have they have tended not to draw upon available psychological theory.

In the context of psychiatric and other conditions cognitive factors may have a wide range of potential effects. They may precipitate or increase vulnerability to illness, or may be involved in hastening or retarding recovery processes. In addition, they are likely to be major determinants of emotional responses on the part of patients, relatives, and care-givers (Brewin, 1988). In this chapter I shall briefly describe some of the cognitive influences and processes that have been the subject of research, and then give examples of how they may further our understanding of issues of concern to social psychiatry.

Cognitive Approaches in Psychology

The main distinguishing feature of a cognitive approach to psychological investigation lies in the emphasis given to mental processes that intervene between an environmental event and a person's behavior. The vast majority of environmental events impinging on a person are thought to be mentally evaluated in various ways, including being compared to prior experiences stored in memory before being acted on. Experimental cognitive psychology is largely concerned with explaining how people perceive, attend to, classify, store, and remember information, and how they then use this information to make decisions. Typically the aim has been to develop general models of these processes, and little account has been taken of individual differences or motivational variables. Because the processes of interest are usually unavailable to introspection, inferences about their nature are often derived from measures such as reaction time or speed of recall on experimental tasks.

The idea that there are mental processes that intervene between stimulus and response is historically associated with the Gestalt school of psychology. Their theories were not only influential in explaining how objects in the physical world are perceived but were soon extended to the perception of social objects and hence influenced the course of social psychology as well as the study of perception and thinking. Throughout the period when Behaviorism was in the ascendant, social psychologists such as Lewin, Heider, and Festinger continued to emphasize the importance of conscious perceptions and evaluations in determining human behavior. These theories invoked such mentalist concepts as expectancy, level of aspiration, balance, consistency, causal attribution, and cognitive dissonance, which did not correspond to directly observable behavior but rather to hypothetical processes designed to account for behavior. Unlike the theories stemming from experimental cognitive psychology, they were very much concerned with motivational processes, individual differences, and with the specific content of the information available to the person. Many current theories in clinical psychology, such as social learning theory (Bandura, 1977a) and learned helplessness theory (Abramson, Seligman and Teasdale, 1978; Seligman, 1975), have their roots in this work.

In practice, the knowledge people require consciously to evaluate stressful situations properly and decide on the appropriate course of action is often missing, or forgotten. Simply telling people relevant facts about the frequency of the problem or its most likely outcome may be extremely helpful to them. Even if relevant knowledge is available, the inferences that people are called upon to make about themselves and their circumstances are often complex and difficult, and human judgment is known in many cases to be all too fallible. For example, parents trying to explain why their child is truanting may have to integrate a huge amount of information about school circumstances, the behavior of peers, current sources of stress, their own attitudes towards school and disciplinary styles, and so on. There is now a great deal of evidence that even in simple situations people's ability to recognize the interdependence of events, identify causes, estimate the degree of control they have, and draw valid conclusions from a set of data are quite limited, and prone to be influenced by a variety of factors (e.g., Nisbett and Ross, 1980). It is known that people are strongly affected by prior expectations, that they are subject to various errors and biases, and that they tend to rely on simple rules or heuristics when faced with large quantities of information. Under these circumstances erroneous and premature judgments, made either by the patient or by the clinician, are likely to flourish, sometimes with the most unfortunate consequences.

Clinicians themselves have come up with influential cognitive theories to account for the wide individual differences they meet in their work. For example, Kelly (1955) proposed that people have unique systems of personal constructs with which they categorize the objects in their world, interpret the events that happen to them, and predict the future. One of the main purposes of therapy, he suggested, is to help people free themselves from the restrictions imposed by their own construct systems. Ellis (1962) and Beck (1967) have also argued that dysfunctional emotions such as anxiety and depression follow from people's perceptions and evaluations of the events in their lives rather than from the events themselves. Ellis' Rational-Emotive Therapy and Beck's Cognitive Therapy are both designed to alter these perceptions by a number of techniques, including challenging faulty underlying assumptions such as "I cannot live without this person" or "Nobody will ever speak to me again if I make a fool of myself."

The important point to bear in mind is that, although all cognitive theories emphasize the importance of intervening mental processes, there is no one "cognitive approach." Theories may deal with processes such as selective attention, or with structures such as "schemata" or "associative networks" that describe the organization of material in memory. They may be concerned with specific kinds of content, such as ideas, images, expectations, and attitudes, and this content may be accessible or inaccessible to consciousness. They may assert different kinds of causal relations between mental processes, emotions, and behavior. This diversity means that the potential contribution of cognitive theories is considerable.

Cognitions as Precipitating Factors

The major factor associated with the onset of a wide range of physical and psychiatric disorders is life stress (e.g., Brown and Harris, 1978; Dohrenwend and Dohrenwend, 1974; Totman, 1979). The most stressful events involve fear of pain or other punishment, frustration of goal-directed behavior, conflict between equally attractive or equally unattractive goals, approach-avoidance conflict, helplessness, and loss of or separation from significant others. But simply counting the number of events, commonly regarded as stressful, that a person has experienced does not allow one to predict with any great accuracy whether he or she will become ill. Even responses to very serious stressors such as earthquakes or being interned in a concentration camp show enormous individual variation. Many authors have concluded that this is because the stressfulness of events depends, at least in part, on how they are evaluated or appraised by the individual (e.g., Lazarus, 1966).

The role of individual appraisal is particularly marked in the case of experiences which are ambiguous. For example, it is often difficult for patients with physical sensations such as chest pain to distinguish between alternative explanations, one of which may have an extremely threatening label whereas the other is not at all threatening. Illness presents many attributional problems, with patients trying to decide whether the cause is internal or external to themselves and whether an organic or psychological explanation is most appropriate (Watts, 1982). Experiences are explained in the light of the knowledge that people have available, knowledge that may be thought of as consisting of a set of categories plus rules for assigning events to categories. Each category will be associated with its own set of information concerning the frequency of the problem, the likely outcome, and so on, information which may be accurate, inaccurate, or simply missing. For example, it has often been noted that the effects of overbreathing or hyperventilation are similiar to the experience of a panic attack. In both conditions the person has an intense feeling of apprehension or impending doom accompanied by distressing physical sensations such as vertigo, blurred vision, palpitations, numbness, tingling in the hands and feet, and breathlessness.

According to a recent model of panic attacks (Clark, Salkovskis, and Chalkley 1985; Salkovskis and Clark, 1986) some individuals increase their respiratory ventilation and overbreathe when under stress, which produces a range of these unpleasant sensations. These are then consciously labelled by the patient as symptoms of a heart attack or other medical emergency, or as indications that the patient is going mad. The frightening consequences of these labels lead to further apprehension, to further increases in ventilation, and so on in a vicious cycle. Subsequent conditioning processes may lead to these feelings being associated with particular situations, and to the development of agoraphobia (Franklin, 1987). Cognitive treatment based on this analysis consists of helping patients to relabel their sensations as symptoms of hyperventilation rather than of some more catastrophic condition. Patients first practice voluntary overbreathing, then introspect on their sensations and compare them to those experienced during panic attacks. The therapist then trains them in a pattern of slow breathing which is incompatible with hyperventilation. Although cognitive treatment for panic attacks contains a number of disparate elements, so that improvement need not be the result of relabelling, Salkovskis and Clark argue that the extremely rapid initial reduction in panic attack frequency and self-reported anxiety points to be importance of the cognitive element.

Similar processes may account for different reactions to less ambiguous but equally stressful experiences. Recent research by Brown, Bifulco, and Harris (1988) has described the kind of life events that tend to precede depression in female community residents. They point out that whereas on average four-fifths of depressed women have experienced a major stressor, only about one in five women experiencing such a stressor go on to become depressed. This association can be strengthened by considering only severe events that correspond either to ongoing difficulties (D-events), to particular areas of strong commitment (C-events), or to areas where role conflict exists (R-events). Although presented as a classification of events, their account explicitly recognizes the role of cognitive evaluations. The significance of D-events is presumed to lie in the high levels of helplessness that accompany them, while C-events and R-events can be readily understood in terms of goal frustration and conflict. The authors conclude: "The role of matching difficulties and commitments indicates the importance of the loss of something upon which one has heavily staked a part of oneself. . . . The findings of course underline the importance of social environment and cognitive factors in the aetiology of depression" (p. 41).

Cognitions as Vulnerability Factors

The wide variability in people's response to stressful life events has also led to the suggestion that events only have severe consequences for individuals who are in some way permanently vulnerable. This vulnerability has traditionally been expressed as an aspect of personality, with neuroticism, a personality dimension that reflects differences in the strength and reactivity of emotional responses, being most often considered a vulnerability factor for psychological disorder. Neuroticism (N) scores have been found to be elevated in many groups of psychiatric patients (Eysenck, 1967). The notion that people have stable, highly consistent personality traits that influence their behavior across many situations has, however, come under increasing criticism in recent years. One reason is that, in general, people do not behave with a high degree of consistency in different situations, and it appears more useful to think of behavior as the product of complex person-environment interactions (Mischel, 1973). Mischel's solution was to integrate personality research with the approach of cognitive and social learning theory, shifting the unit of study from global traits inferred from behavioral signs to the individual's cognitive activities and behavior patterns, studied in relation to particular circumstances. The variables he identified as likely to be important in predicting behavior, including abnormal behavior, were competencies, encoding and categorization of events, expectancies, subjective values, and self-regulatory systems and plans.

In the case of depression, several psychological factors have been consistently considered as vulnerability factors. They fall roughly into two groups, one concerned with individual personality characteristics (e.g., self-esteem and neuroticism), and one concerned with interpersonal characteristics (e.g., dependency and attachment style). Currently such psychological characteristics tend to be viewed in cognitive terms, by relating them to individuals' conscious and nonconscious mental representations of themselves and other people (Brewin, 1988). Thus neuroticism has been interpreted as a particular style of processing emotional material, in which there is faster and more frequent recall of negative self-related information, and slower and less frequent recall of positive self-related information (Martin, 1985). Bowlby (1982) has for many years proposed that mental representations of early attachments mediate the formation of affectional bonds in later life.

The cognitive perspective has suggested important commonalities between concepts previously thought to be disparate, such as self-esteem, neuroticism, and memory biases. Other proposed cognitive precursors of depression include attributional style (Brewin, 1985; Peterson and Seligman, 1984), hardiness (Kobasa et al., 1981), and locus of control (Nelson and Cohen, 1983). It should be noted, however, that cognitive and personality characteristics have been variously defined and have been thought of as operating in a number of quite distinct ways, including: (a) being permanently observable or measurable factors that directly increase the risk of depression, (b) being permanently observable factors that interact with life stress to increase risk, (c) being latent factors that are only measurable in the context of life stress and that then interact with stress to increase risk. In addition it has been proposed that personality variables have a causal influence on other risk factors for depression, such as the propensity to experience life events or the ability/willingness to utilize social support.

Studies of self-reported attributions, attitudes, and beliefs in acutely ill and recovered patient samples have in general found that dysfunctional cognitions are only present in the acute phase. With recovery, patients' scores return to normal levels and are comparable to those of non-psychiatric controls (Teasdale, 1988). Consistent with these findings, attitudinal measures taken when people are well have generally failed to predict the onset of clinical depression (e.g., Ingham et al., 1987; Lewin-sohn et al., 1981). This suggests that cognitive vulnerability is not a permanently observable characteristic that directly increases the risk of depression.

It is possible, however, that different kinds of cognitive measure might reveal evidence for such vulnerability. The existence of memory biases in depression is well-established, with the depressed tending to recall more negative material and less positive material than the nondepressed (Blaney, 1986). It has been suggested that the existence of such biases is not specific to the depressive episode but may also predate and predispose individuals to become depressed. This hypothesis has received some support from a study by Teasdale and Dent (1987) which compared memory for positive and negative self-descriptive material in women who had recovered from depression and women who had never been depressed. Teasdale and Dent reported that the recovered depressed revealed a poorer memory for positive material than did the never depressed. However, Bradley and Mathews (1988) failed to replicate this result, finding that currently depressed subjects remembered more negative than positive self-referent adjectives, whereas both recovered depressed and controls recalled a similar preponderance of positive rather than negative self-referent adjectives. Thus, in contrast to Teasdale and Dent, there was no evidence for a memory bias existing independently of the current episode of depression.

Other researchers have looked specifically for an interaction of cognitive vulnerability with life stress, and several studies with mildly depressed student samples have found that such an interaction predicts subsequent depression, even when the initial levels of symptoms are controlled for (Brewin, 1989). One of the few comparable prospective studies to have been carried out using standardized diagnostic procedures investigated whether the interaction of low self-esteem and high life stress would predict the onset of depression in a sample of working-class women. Brown et al. (1986) confirmed that it was this combination of variables that was most highly related to onset, whereas low self-esteem on its own was not so related. Interestingly, however, this interaction was particularly predictive for single mothers who had not received adequate crisis support, whereas it was not so predictive for similarly unsupported married women. These more detailed findings underscore the complex relations between cognitive and social variables.

Other studies employing strict diagnostic procedures, but using different measures, have not produced similar findings. Hammen et al. (1988) tested the notion that a vulnerable attributional style, in conjunction with life stress, would be a risk factor for depression in children. This vulnerable style consisted of the tendency to attribute failures and other negative outcomes to causal factors that were internal to the child, long-lasting, and with wide-ranging effects. Children who consistently blamed their problems on lack of intelligence, or personality defects, would be demonstrating such an attributional style. Hammen et al.'s sample of children included offspring of women with affective disorders and hence presumed to be at high risk for depression. Hierarchical multiple regression analyses failed to support the main hypothesis: over a 6-month period depression was best predicted by initial symptoms and by life stress but not by attributions and life events. However, when coupled with high stress, a negative attribution style was found to increase a child's likelihood of a non-affective diagnosis.

Parry and Brewin (1988) investigated the plausibility of a similar cognition x stressful event model in accounting for depression in a sample of working-class mothers. However, they used a cross-sectional rather than a longitudinal design. They divided their sample into four groups, according to whether women were cases of depression or non-cases, and had or had not recently experienced a major stressor. Following the diathesis-stress model, they expected that the most dysfunctional cognitions, involving self-attributions of blame and self-depreciation, should be found in the group of women who had become depressed following a major stressor. In fact the data showed quite a different pattern. There was some evidence that depression itself produced more dysfunctional cognitions, but the data were also consistent with a model in which stressors and dysfunctional cognitions produced depression independently, rather than in combination.

To date, then, the evidence that cognitive vulnerability is a permanently observable factor that interacts with life stress to produce depression is at best inconclusive, with studies using questionnaire and interview methods yielding different results. One possible explanation for this is that cognitive vulnerability is latent and not readily measured by questionnaire and interview. Rather, this vulnerability only becomes apparent when it is elicited by an appropriate stressful event (e.g., Beck et al., 1979). The disadvantage of this theory is that it is very difficult to test. It either requires subjects to be assessed after a stressful event and before the onset of symptoms, or it requires the development of new measures to tap the hypothesized vulnerability directly. Initial attempts at using information-processing measures such as speed of recall for this purpose have not been uniformly successful, but this research is in a very early stage.

Cognitions and the Course of Illness

Although social psychiatric research on depression has been predominantly concerned with understanding its onset, a number of studies have also investigated the influence that environmental factors have on its course. A slower recovery has been related to persistent ongoing major difficulties (Brown and Harris, 1978), and a faster recovery to the occurrence of events that "neutralize" the effects of prior events and difficulties (Parker, Tennant, and Blignault, 1985; Tennant, Bebbington, and Hurry, 1981). Most recently Brown, Adler, and Bifulco (1988) confirmed that reductions in ongoing difficulties often preceded recovery from chronic depression. They also identified a category of "fresh start" events that also appeared to lead to clinical improvement.

The effects of environmental events on recovery may or may not be mediated by similar mechanisms to those that mediate the effects of events and difficulties on onset. One possibility is that events can influence how patients perceive, respond to, and try to control their symptoms, a process in which cognitions are likely to play an important role. The analysis of people's choice of coping strategy, and what determines the persistence with which they pursue it, comes within the scope of research on motivation. The important factors here are people's views about the cause of the problem, their knowledge and beliefs about the range of appropriate strategies, their estimate of the resources, both personal and environmental, that they think are available to carry out these strategies, and the existence of values and goals that are in opposition to particular coping strategies or coping efforts in general (Brewin, 1988). Faulty analysis of the cause of a problem, ignorance of an effective strategy, and overestimation of the difficulty involved, could all lead to giving up coping attempts prematurely.

In support of this cognitive perspective there is evidence that the anxious and depressed do generally feel they have less control over their lives when they are ill than when they recover (Strickland, 1978). Firth-Cozens and Brewin (1988) found that current life events and symptoms were perceived as less controllable by patients when they were anxious and depressed than after a course of psychotherapy. Positive changes in perceptions of controllability were also correlated with improvements in symptoms. These findings confirm earlier research indicating that the more control depressed women perceived themselves to have over their symptoms and life events, the less depressed they were six weeks later (Firth and Brewin, 1982). In one of the few studies to have investigated the cognitive appraisal of symptoms in a severely handicapped psychiatric sample, MacCarthy, Benson, and Brewin (1986) interviewed 39 patients attempting to control chronic symptoms. Half the sample were diagnosed as suffering from schizophrenia, and the majority had a psychiatric history stretching back at least 10 years. Despite this, patients gave reliable and consistent accounts of their problems, described their coping strategies and appraised the effectiveness of these strategies.

The major contribution of a cognitive approach to explaining recovery is at present, however, a largely theoretical one. I shall describe two types of theory, one concerned with motivation and one concerned with vulnerability. Cognitive theories of motivation have been dominated by a very simple idea, namely that the intensity or persistence of behavior is determined by a combination of the value of the goal the person is trying to achieve and the expectancy that the behavior will be effective in attaining that goal. Little effort will be expended when the goal is unimportant or when the behavior is seen as unlikely to achieve the desired ends. Sometimes the goal is very attractive, such as overcoming life long shyness, but the expectancy that one will change is too small to encourage social experimentation. At other times, one might be confident of eliminating a tic or nervous habit but be unwilling to be referred to a psychologist or psychiatrist.

The above ideas, which are usually referred to as expectancy-value theories, underpin such influential approaches to psychopathology as Bandura's (1977a) social learning theory, and Seligman's (1975) learned helplessness theory. While not ignoring the value component, both theories have placed particular emphasis on the importance of expectancies. Bandura has emphasized the distinction between outcome expectancies, people's beliefs about the likely success of a treatment or other course of action, and efficacy expectancies, their beliefs about their own ability actually to carry out those actions. Thus it is possible to imagine a person who believes flooding to be an effective form of treatment for his phobia (high outcome expectancy) but does not believe himself capable of exposing himself to his most feared situation (low efficacy expectancy). Seligman has similarly placed the expectation of uncontrollability at the heart of his explanation of motivational deficits in behavior.

There has as yet been little research that attempts to measure helplessness directly, but Bandura (1977b, 1982) has developed measures of efficacy expectancies or "self-efficacy" beliefs. His thesis is that people vary greatly in the confidence which they feel when coping with difficult situations, particularly ones which produce unpleasant emotional arousal. The more confident they feel about responding skillfully to the varying demands of the situation or, in his terms, the greater their self-efficacy, the harder they will try to overcome the problem and the longer they will persist at it. From this Bandura deduces that successful psychological therapies are those which are most effective at increasing self-efficacy: it is a mechanism which accounts for why some therapies are generally better than others and why some people do better than others at the same therapy. There is now a great deal of evidence for Bandura's claim that self-efficacy predicts avoidance behavior. Furthermore, although most research has been concerned with the treatment of fear, self-efficacy appears to be a motivational construct that is applicable to a wide variety of situations.

Cognitive mechanisms may be related to recovery in quite separate ways, however. Various authors (e.g., Ingram, 1984; Teasdale, 1988) have proposed that the cognitive vulnerability factors described in the previous section are related to the persistence of depression rather than to its onset. They suggest that the presence of depressive mood is likely to elicit negative memories and dysfunctional patterns of thinking to differing extents in different people, depending on their prior experience (the "differential activation" hypothesis). These negative memories are, in turn, likely to be recycled through consciousness, promoting rumination, increasing sensitivity to new setbacks, and undermining coping efforts. Depressive thinking may, then, be a symptom as well as a cause of depression, but one that has important consequences for how long the person takes to recover. Much of the available data on cognitions as vulnerability factors for depression are consistent with this view (Brewin, 1985; Teasdale, 1988).

Cognition and Interpersonal Emotion

A consistent theme in social psychiatry is the significance of personal relationships to the onset and course of illness. In a study of the rehabilitation of patients with chronic schizophrenia, Wing (1961) noted that positive attitudes on the part of Industrial Rehabilitation Unit staff were related to greater helpfulness towards patients and were likely to aid clinical improvement. Conversely, in life event research, the lack of an intimate relationship has frequently been found to be a vulnerability factor for women, increasing the likelihood of depression in the presence of a provoking agent (Brown and Harris, 1986). Another well-replicated finding concerns the effect of relatives' levels of Expressed Emotion (EE) on patients' probability of relapse. Depressed and schizophrenic patients are more likely to relapse when living with a high EE relative (Hooley, Orley, and Teasdale, 1986; Karno et al., 1987; Nuechterlein et al., 1986; Vaughn and Leff, 1976; Vaughn et al., 1984). It seems likely that the adverse effects of high EE are not confined to psychiatric patients, however, and may include patients who are simply trying to lose weight (Fischmann-Havstad and Marston, 1984).

These findings suggest the importance of interventions aimed at caregivers and at patients' relatives, as well as at patients themselves. Although little researched, marital therapy appears to be a promising treatment for depression (Jacobson, 1984; O'Leary and Beach, 1990). Interventions with the families of schizophrenic patients have shown that it is possible to lower relatives' levels of Expressed Emotion with beneficial effects on patients' relapse rates (Leff et al., 1982). The psychological processes underlying positive and negative interpersonal emotions are as yet, however, poorly understood. This would appear to be a key area for future research, in order to develop more effective and precisely-targeted interventions.

Attribution theory suggests several ways in which cognitive appraisal might affect marital, family, therapeutic, and other close relationships (Brewin, 1988). Jones and Nisbett (1972) proposed that the divergent perspective of actors and observers would lead a person explaining their own behavior to place relatively greater weight on situational causes, whereas a person observing it would emphasize internal, dispositional causes. This is known as the "actor-observer bias." In a marital context, it would mean that a couple should differ in their explanation of negative behavior such as arriving home later than promised: the one arriving late should see the cause as primarily related to the situation ("I had too much work to do"), whereas the partner should locate the cause in that person's negative personality characteristics ("You're selfish and unreliable"). The actor-observer bias is an example of the pervasive "fundamental attribution error" (Nisbett and Ross, 1980), the tendency to underrate situational influences on behavior. They both indicate cognitive mechanisms that may underlie divergent beliefs and attributional conflict between individuals.

Weiner (1985) has identified several specific emotional consequences of attributing outcomes to internal vs. external and to controllable vs. uncontrollable causes. His theory proposes that when a person experiences a positive outcome, an attribution to the controllable (intentional) actions of another person elicits the emotion of gratitude. A negative outcome attributed to the controllable actions of another produces anger. When the negative outcome has been experienced by another person, on the other hand, attributions to causes external to and uncontrollable by that person elicit the emotion of pity. Interpersonal emotions such as gratitude, anger, and pity are important in understanding the tension and distress that arises in families and the willingness of family members to tolerate difficult behavior and support each other at stressful times. There is now a considerable amount of research supporting the view that positive and negative emotions are based, at least in part, on specific patterns of causal belief (e.g., Butler, Brewin, and Forsythe, 1986).

Marital Conflict

The role of actor-observer biases in marital conflict was investigated by Orvis, Kelley, and Butler (1976), who got each member of a couple to write down their own explanation of areas of conflict as well as what they thought would be their partner's explanation. They found that actors more often explained their behavior in terms of such causes as environmental circumstances, temporary internal states, and judgments of what was preferable or necessary, whereas the partner's explanation was more likely to be in terms of the actor's characteristics (lazy, forgetful, irresponsible, violent), and the actor's negative attitude toward the partner. These findings are consistent with the idea of an actor-observer bias, although actors also appear to emphasize reasons and justifications for their actions as well as situational constraints. A subsequent study by Harvey, Wells, and Alvarez (1978) obtained independent explanations for the same events from each member of a couple, as well as predictions about the partner's explanations. They found that even highly satisfied couples with relatively long-term relationships had inaccurate perceptions of each other's understanding of areas of conflict. Each member of the couple tended to think that the other's causal analysis would agree with their own, and both tended to be unaware of the existence of divergent explanations.

The clinical significance of actor-partner differences was further investigated in a comparison of nondistressed couples with distressed couples seeking counselling (Fincham, Beach, and Baucom, 1987). Distressed spouses saw their own actions as more positively motivated and more deserving of praise than positive partner behavior, whereas the causes of their own negative actions were rated as being more external, less stable, and less global than the causes of partners' negative actions. In contrast, nondistressed spouses made more benign attributions for their partner's behavior than for their own behavior. As Fincham et al. comment, "It is precisely this pattern of attributions that is likely to maximize the impact of negative partner behavior for distressed spouses and positive partner behavior for nondistressed spouses . . . distressed spouses may discredit positive spouse behavior, because they do not believe it matches the motivation that characterizes their own behavior, and instead focus on negative partner behavior . . . this may account in part for the long chains of negative interchanges that distinguish distressed from nondistressed spouses" (p. 746).

The general conclusion from a large number of studies is that distressed spouses are more likely to see their partner and their relationship as the source of their difficulties. They also tend to see these causes as more global, i.e., affecting many areas of the marriage, as more blameworthy, and as more reflective of their spouse's negative attitude toward them. Recent evidence (Fincham and Bradbury, 1988) builds on these correlational findings and suggests that causal and responsibility attributions are predictive of future marital satisfaction (at least for wives). There are also promising indications that the experimental manipulation of attributions for one's partner's behavior can lead to changes in behavior, suggesting that this line of research is highly relevant to the practice of marital and family therapy.

Expressed Emotion

The key components of EE are criticism, hostility, and emotional overinvolvement. Attribution theory, however, suggests that the origins of these components in relatives are quite different. From an attributional perspective, hostility and criticism on the part of a relative stem from causal beliefs emphasizing the patient's control over and responsibility for their symptoms and negative behaviors. Overinvolvement, on the other hand, may be linked to pity (and seeing the patient as not responsible and not in control) or to guilt (and seeing oneself as in some way responsible).

These ideas have been investigated in a recent study of relatives of patients with schizophrenia (Brewin et al., in press). Camberwell Family Interview tapes originally used to classify relatives as high or low EE were listened to, and the causal attributions that relatives spontaneously made for patients' symptoms or negative behaviors were extracted. The range of individual causal factors mentioned was very wide, so attributions were rated on seven general dimensions, using the Leeds Attribution Coding System (LACS: Stratton et al., 1986). On the whole, relatives tended to attribute behaviors to unstable factors that were internal to the patient and uncontrollable by either the patient or themselves. Their explanations differed significantly, however, according to whether the outcome was the illness itself, antisocial behavior, interpersonal problems, or the negative symptoms of schizophrenia. In a test of the main hypothesis, critical comments and hostility were found to be associated with attributions to causal factors idiosyncratic to and controllable by the patient, whereas the attributions of overinvolved relatives did not differ from those of relatives low in expressed emotion.

As in the studies of marital distress, Brewin et al. (in press) found clear evidence that family members did spontaneously make attributions for each other's behavior, and that these attributions were enormously varied. In part this reflected low levels of education about the nature of schizophrenia, and difficulties in interpreting the nature of unusual behavior (cf. Yarrow et al., 1956). The study also revealed attributional conflict between family members, who sometimes made different explanations for the same behavior. Some important theoretical links between EE and different explanations received support, although the direction of causality was not interpretable from a study of this nature. Future research, however, will examine the relation between change in EE status and change in relatives' attributions.

Cognition, Social Interaction, and Social Support

Social support from other people appears to be very important in protecting physical and mental health during stressful periods of one's life (e.g., Berkman and Syme, 1979; Brown et al., 1986; Cohen and Wills, 1985; Parry and Shapiro, 1986), although the evidence for this buffering role is not always consistent (Alloway and Bebbington, 1987). Yet many psychiatric patients who would appear to be particularly in need of such support have smaller social networks and interact less with others than do nonpsychiatric controls (Brugha, 1984; Brugha et al., 1982). Some depressed women in the community additionally show a pattern of "nonoptimal confiding," in which they confide in critical or otherwise unsuitable others (Andrews and Brown, 1988). Even in the general population, shyness, loneliness, and anxiety in social situations is very common, and in some cases social anxiety is so intense that the mere presence of other people becomes highly aversive and leads to social withdrawal. Two main types of cognitive explanation have been offered for social anxiety and withdrawal, one to do with beliefs about social competence, and one that emphasizes the role of social comparison processes. The various theories of social anxiety and withdrawal are not mutually exclusive, and all may be helpful in analyzing the problems of a particular individual. Their different causal focus does, however, point to different kinds of intervention strategy for improving social performance.

Shy and lonely people tend to attribute interpersonal failures (but not necessarily other kinds of failure) to internal, stable, and uncontrollable factors such as lack of social ability (Anderson, Horowitz, and French, 1983; Teglasi and Hoffman, 1982). As we have already noted, these kinds of attribution lead to low self-esteem and to low expectations of success or, in Bandura's (1977b) terms, to low self-efficacy. This in turn would be expected to reduce the amount of effort expended to initiate and persist at social encounters. Leary et al. (1986) have also investigated attributions for subjective feelings of nervousness, one of the factors claimed by Bandura to contribute to estimates of self-efficacy. In support of this model, Leary et al. showed that people who attribute their feelings of social anxiety to stable characteristics of themselves are more likely to avoid social encounters than people who attribute them to unstable characteristics of themselves or to situational factors.

Theories based on beliefs about social competence are particularly relevant to those individuals who desire social interaction but have low expectations of being able to perform adequately. Other individuals may be socially competent, and know it, but actively avoid interaction because they have other attributes or experiences which they consider to be abnormal and of which they are embarrassed or ashamed. Goffman (1968) has described the many social difficulties experienced by stigmatized individuals who belong to a despised race or religion, or who have physical deformities or character blemishes. The adverse reactions of others may lead to a self-imposed isolation from society. In many cases, however, a process of self-stigmatization may produce similar effects in a person who does not fall into one of Goffman's socially despised categories, and who may not have experienced actual societal rejection. Örner (1987) described these reactions in a group of British servicemen who had fought in the Falklands war five years previously and continued to experience the after-effects in the form of vivid memories or nightmares (post-traumatic stress disorder). According to Örner, they felt marked out by their experiences and different from other people in an important way. In the absence of other servicemen with similar experiences, they felt unable to talk to others and chose rather to isolate themselves from society.

Social comparison theory suggests that people with a "problem" they are uncertain or fearful about should avoid "normal" (i.e., dissimilar) people and seek out similar others, sharing their problem with selected friends or perhaps joining self-help groups composed of people in related situations. Receiving information that others share their problems should increase their self-esteem and reduce self-stigmatization. But many factors may interfere with this process of gaining consensus information via direct social comparison. The individual may be unable to identify a group of similar others, and may be prevented from mixing with their peers because of excessive shame and embarrassment and lack of social skills.

A great deal may depend on people's initial estimate of the frequency of their "problem". The more unusual they think themselves, the more likely they are to doubt the availability of similar others, and on this basis fear social interactions in which their "secret" might be unmasked. This process may account for the fact that depressed patients have smaller social networks than the nondepressed. The depressed believe that they are dissimilar to others and that negative experiences are more likely to happen to them than to other people (e.g., Brewin and Furnham, 1986; MacCarthy and Furnham, 1986). Brewin and Furnham suggested that these beliefs should lead the depressed to avoid others, thus restricting their access to normative or consensus information. In this way inaccurate consensus judgments would tend to persist through lack of disconfirmatory evidence, and social interaction would continue to be aversive. According to this approach, the reduced network size and relative lack of intimacy enjoyed by those prone to depression is explained by specific consensus beliefs that influence the attractiveness, and hence the probability, of social interaction. Consistent with this model, Brewin, MacCarthy, and Furnham (1989) found that the seeking of support following a stressful experience was associated with consensus beliefs independently of level of depression.

There is, therefore, a case to be made that the frequency of different kinds of social interaction, including the seeking and utilization of social support, is linked to social comparison processes. But the relation between social comparison, social interaction, and negative emotions such as anxiety, depression, or embarrassment is a complex one. It does seem likely that inaccurate consensus beliefs are related to negative emotions and that these in turn are related to social withdrawal. For some patients the opportunity to gain consensus information, either in written form or by actually mixing with similar others, may therefore be extremely valuable. But mixing with similar others is less likely to appeal to those who do not wish to evaluate their feelings and experiences, either because they have access to adequate expert advice or because their coping strategies depend on attending to certain kinds of information and not others. For example, patients who use the "downward comparison" strategy to maintain their self-esteem may find it upsetting to meet others who are managing better than they are and who make them feel like a failure. Patients who use the "upward comparison" strategy, on the other hand, may be uncomfortable mixing with others they perceive as worse off than themselves, since this may bring home the reality of their problem or disability.

Conclusion

In this chapter, I have tried to show that cognitive theories are extremely relevant to social psychiatry. Factors in the social environment precede and modify psychiatric disorder because they have the power to create certain states of mind, such as fear, helplessness, or self-blame, in significant numbers of individuals. The psychological characteristics that interact with social factors to give rise to these states of mind may consist of attitudes, beliefs, and attributions, and be susceptible to self-report, or they may consist of aspects of individuals' information-processing system that are less accessible to the investigator. For example, suicide attemptors may be distinguished from controls by their latency to retrieve certain sorts of autobiographical memory (Williams and Broadbent, 1986), and patients with generalized anxiety are characterized by a greater sensitivity to threatening stimuli, even when these are presented beneath the threshold of awareness (Mathews and MacLeod, 1986).

Ultimately, the mutual influence of cognitive and social factors can be traced back through an individual's life history. For example, cognitions such as self-blame for current experiences of victimization may be related to preceding social factors such as repeated abuse in childhood (Andrews and Brewin, 1990). Like the clay that records the passing of the long-dead dinosaur, cognitions are the substratum that bears the impress of previous social events. At present, research into the influence of this substratum on psychiatric disorder is in an early stage, and few conclusions can be drawn about causal relationships and their direction. Most studies with patients have been concerned with the acutely ill, and have helped to illuminate the cognitive processes underlying symptoms such as hypervigilance and "automatic" negative thoughts. No cognitive vulnerability factors that precede illness or relapse have yet been clearly established, although there are a number of promising candidates. Studies with relatives and care-givers are of even more recent origin but point to the importance of cognition and emotion in determining the course of illness. For the future, the cognitive perspective holds out the promise of providing a link between established research findings in social psychiatry and the development of more sophisticated clinical interventions with both patients and relatives.

References

Abramson, L.Y., Seligman, M.E.P., and Teasdale, J.D. (1978). Learned helpless-ness in humans: Critique and reformulation. *Journal of Abnormal Psychology*, *87*, 49–74.

Alloway, R., and Bebbington, P.E. (1987). The buffer theory of social support—a review of the literature. *Psychological Medicine*, *17*, 91–108.

Anderson, C.A., Horowitz, L.M., and French, R. (1983). Attributional style of lonely and depressed people. *Journal of Personality and Social Psychology*, *45*, 127–136.

Andrews, B., and Brewin, C.R. (1990). Attributions of blame in the victims of marital violence: A study of antecedents and consequences. *Journal of Marriage and the Family*, *52*, 757–767.

Andrews, B., and Brown, G.W. (1988). Social support, onset of depression, and personality: An exploratory analysis. *Social Psychiatry and Psychiatric Epide-miology*, *23*, 99–108.

Bandura, A. (1977a). *Social Learning Theory*. Englewood Cliffs, N.J.: Prentice-Hall.

Bandura, A. (1977b). Self-efficacy: Toward a unifying theory of behavioral change. *Psychological Review*, *84*, 191–215.

Bandura, A. (1982). The self and mechanisms of agency. In J.Suls (Ed.), *Psycho-logical Perspectives on the Self. Vol. 1*. Hillsdale, N.J.: Lawrence Erlbaum.

Bebbington, P.E. (1985). Three cognitive theories of depression. *Psychological Medicine*, *15*, 759–769.

Beck, A.T. (1967). *Depression: Clinical, Experimental, and Theoretical Aspects*. New York: Hoeber.

Beck, A.T., Rush, A.J., Shaw, B.F., and Emery, G. (1979). *Cognitive Therapy of Depression*. New York: Wiley.

Berkman, L.F., and Syme, S.L. (1979). Social networks, host resistance, and mortality: A nine-year follow-up study of Alameda County residents. *American Journal of Epidemiology*, *109*, 186–204.

Blaney, P.H. (1986). Affect and memory: A review. *Psychological Bulletin*, *99*, 229–246.

Bowlby, J. (1982). *Attachment and Loss: Vol. 1. Attachment*. (2nd Ed.). London: Hogarth Press.

Bradley, B.P., and Mathews, A. (1988). Memory bias in recovered clinical depres-sives. *Cognition and Emotion*, *2*, 235–245.

Brewin, C.R. (1985). Depression and causal attributions: What is their relation? *Psychological Bulletin*, *98*, 297–309.

Brewin, C.R. (1988). *Cognitive foundations of clinical psychology*. London: Lawrence Erlbaum.

Brewin, C.R. (1989). Psychological factors in the aetiology of depression. *Current Opinion in Psychiatry, 2*, 213–216.

Brewin, C.R., and Furnham, A. (1986). Attributional versus pre-attributional variables in self-esteem and depression: A comparison and test of learned helplessness theory. *Journal of Personality and Social Psychology, 50*, 1013–1020.

Brewin, C.R., MacCarthy, B., Duda, K., and Vaughn, C.E. (in press). Attribution and expressed emotion in the relatives of patients with schizophrenia. *Journal of Abnormal Psychology*.

Brewin, C.R., MacCarthy, B., and Furnham, A. (1989). Social support in the face of adversity: The role of cognitive appraisal. *Journal of Research in Personality, 23*, 354–372.

Brown, G.W., Adler, Z., and Bifulco, A. (1988). Life events, difficulties, and recovery from chronic depression. *British Journal of Psychiatry, 152*, 487–498.

Brown, G.W., Andrews, B., Harris, T.O., Adler, Z., and Bridge, L. (1986). Social support, self-esteem and depression. *Psychological Medicine, 16*, 813–831.

Brown, G.W., Bifulco, A., and Harris, T.O. (1988). Life events, vulnerability and onset of depression: Some refinements. *British Journal of Psychiatry, 150*, 30–42.

Brown, G.W., and Harris, T.O. (1978). *The Social Origins of Depression*. London: Tavistock.

Brown, G.W., and Harris, T.O. (1986). Stressor, vulnerability and depression: a question of replication. *Psychological Medicine, 16*, 739–744.

Brugha, T.S. (1984). Personal losses and deficiencies in social networks. *Social Psychiatry, 19*, 69–74.

Brugha, T.S., Conroy, R., Walsh, N., Delaney, W., O'Hanlon, J., Dondero, E., Daly, L., Hickey, N., and Bourke, G. (1982). Social networks, attachment and support in minor affective disorders: A replication. *British Journal of Psychiatry, 141*, 249–255.

Butler, R.J., Brewin, C.R., and Forsythe, W.I. (1986). Maternal attributions and tolerance for nocturnal enuresis. *Behaviour Research and Therapy, 24*, 307–312.

Clark, D.M., Salkovskis, P.M., and Chalkley, A.J. (1985). Respiratory control as a treatment for panic attacks. *Journal of Behavior Therapy and Experimental Psychiatry, 16*, 23–30.

Cohen, S., and Wills, T.A. (1985). Stress, social support, and the buffering hypothesis. *Psychological Bulletin, 98*, 310–357.

Dohrenwend, B.S., and Dohrenwend, B.P. (Eds.) (1974). *Stressful Life Events: Their nature and effects*. New York: Wiley.

Ellis, A. (1962). *Reason and Emotion in Psychotherapy*. New York: Lyle Stuart.

Eysenck, H.J. (1967). *The Biological Basis of Personality*. Springfield, Illinois: C.C. Thomas.

Fincham, F.D., Beach, S., and Baucom, D. (1987). Attribution processes in distressed and nondistressed couples: 4. Self-partner attribution differences. *Journal of Personality and Social Psychology, 52*, 739–748.

Fincham, F.D., and Bradbury, T.N. (1988). The impact of attributions in marriage: Empirical and conceptual foundations. *British Journal of Clinical Psychology, 27*, 77–90.

Firth, J., and Brewin, C.R. (1982). Attributions and recovery from depression: A preliminary study using cross-lagged correlation analysis. *British Journal of Clinical Psychology, 21,* 229–230.

Firth-Cozens, J., and Brewin, C.R. (1988). Attributional change during psychotherapy. *British Journal of Clinical Psychology, 27,* 47–54.

Fischmann-Havstad, L., and Marston, A.R. (1984). Weight loss maintenance as an aspect of family emotion and process. *British Journal of Clinical Psychology, 23,* 265–272.

Franklin, J.A. (1987). The changing nature of agoraphobic fears. *British Journal of Clinical Psychology, 26,* 127–133.

Goffman, E. (1968). *Stigma: Notes on the Management of Spoiled Identity.* Harmondsworth, Middx.: Penguin Books.

Hammen, C., Adrian, C., and Hiroto, D. (1988). A longitudinal test of the attributional vulnerability model in children at risk for depression. *British Journal of Clinical Psychology, 27,* 37–46.

Harvey, J.H., Wells, G.L., and Alvarez, M.D. (1978). Attribution in the context of conflict and separation in close relationships. In J.H. Harvey, W.J. Ickes, and R.F.Kidd (Eds.), *New Directions in Attribution Research* (Vol. 2). Hillsdale, N.J.: Lawrence Erlbaum.

Hooley, J.M., Orley, J., and Teasdale, J.D. (1986). Levels of expressed emotion and relapse in depressed patients. *British Journal of Psychiatry, 148,* 642–647.

Ingham, J.G., Kreitman, N.B., Miller, P. McC., Sashidharan, S.P., and Surtees, P.G. (1987). Self-appraisal, anxiety and depression in women: A prospective enquiry. *British Journal of Psychiatry, 151,* 643–651.

Ingram, R.E. (1984). Toward an information-processing analysis of depression. *Cognitive Therapy and Research, 8,* 443–478.

Jacobson, N.S. (1984). Marital therapy and the cognitive-behavioral treatment of depression. *Behavior Therapist, 7,* 143–147.

Jones, E.E., and Nisbett, R.E. (1972). The actor and the observer. In E.E. Jones, D.E. Kanouse, H.H. Kelley, R.E. Nisbett, S. Valins, and B. Weiner (Eds.), *Attribution: Perceiving the Causes of Behavior.* New Jersey: General Learning Press.

Karno, M., Jenkins, J.H., de la Selva, A., Santana, F., Telles, C., Lopez, S., and Mintz, J. (1987). Expressed emotion and schizophrenic outcome among Mexican-American families. *Journal of Nervous and Mental Disease, 175,* 143–151.

Kelly, G.A. (1955). *The Psychology of Personal Constructs. Vols. 1 & 2.* New York: W.W. Norton.

Kobasa, S., Maddi, S., and Courington, S. (1981). Personality and constitution as mediators in the stress-illness relationship. *Journal of Health and Social Behavior, 22,* 368–378.

Lazarus, R.S. (1966). *Psychological Stress and the Coping Process.* New York: McGraw-Hill.

Leary, M.R., Atherton, S.C., Hill, S., and Hur, C. (1986). Attributional mediators of social avoidance and inhibition. *Journal of Personality, 54,* 704–716.

Leff, J., Kuipers, L., Berkowitz, R., Eberlein-Vries, R., and Sturgeon, D. (1982). A controlled trial of social intervention in the families of schizophrenic patients. *British Journal of Psychiatry, 141,* 121–134.

Lewinsohn, P.M., Steinmetz, J.L., Larson, D.W., and Franklin, J. (1981). Depression-related cognitions: antecedent or consequence? *Journal of Abnormal Psychology, 90,* 213–219.

MacCarthy, B., Benson, J., and Brewin, C.R. (1986). Task motivation and problem appraisal in long-term psychiatric patients. *Psychological Medicine, 16*, 431–438.

MacCarthy, B., and Furnham, A. (1986). Patients' conceptions of psychological adjustment in the normal population. *British Journal of Clinical Psychology, 25*, 43–50.

Martin, M. (1985). Neuroticism as predisposition toward depression: A cognitive mechanism. *Personality and Individual Differences, 6*, 353–365.

Mathews, A., and MacLeod, C. (1986). Discrimination of threat cues without awareness in anxiety states. *Journal of Abnormal Psychology, 95*, 131–138.

Metalsky, G.I., Halberstadt, L.J., and Abramson, L.Y. (1987). Vulnerability to depressive mood reactions: Toward a more powerful test of the diathesis-stress and causal mediation components of the reformulated theory of depression. *Journal of Personality and Social Psychology, 52*, 386–393.

Mischel, W. (1973). Toward a cognitive social learning reconceptualization of personality. *Psychological Review, 80*, 252–283.

Nelson, D., and Cohen, L. (1983). Locus of control and control perceptions and the relationship between life stress and psychological disorder. *American Journal of Community Psychology, 11*, 705–722.

Nisbett, R.E., and Ross, L. (1980). *Human Inference: Strategies and Shortcomings of Social Judgment.* Englewood Cliffs, N.J.: Prentice-Hall.

Nuechterlein, K.H., Snyder, K.S., Dawson, M.E., Rappe, S., Gitlin, M., and Fogelson, D. (1986). Expressed emotion, fixed dose fluphenazine decanoate maintenance, and relapse in recent-onset schizophrenia. *Psychopharmacology Bulletin, 22*, 633–639.

Oatley, K., and Bolton, W. (1985). A social-cognitive theory of depression in reaction to life events. *Psychological Review, 92*, 372–388.

O'Leary, K.D., and Beach, S.R.H. (1990). Marital therapy: A viable treatment for depression and marital discord. *American Journal of Psychiatry, 147*, 183–186.

Örner, R.J. (1987). *Post-traumatic stress disorders in victims of the Falklands war: Syndrome and treatment.* Paper delivered at the British Psychological Society Annual Conference, Brighton.

Orvis, B.R., Kelley, H.H., and Butler, D. (1976). Attributional conflict in young couples. In J.H. Harvey, W.J. Ickes, and R.F. Kidd (Eds.), *New Directions in Attribution Research* (Vol 1). Hillsdale, N.J.: Lawrence Erlbaum.

Parker, G., Tennant, C., and Blignault, I. (1985). Predicting improvement in patients with non-endogenous depression. *British Journal of Psychiatry, 146*, 132–139.

Parry, G., and Brewin, C.R. (1988). Cognitive style and depression: Symptom-related, event-related, or independent provoking factor? *British Journal of Clinical Psychology, 27*, 23–35.

Parry, G., and Shapiro, D.A. (1986). Social support and life events in working class women: Stress-buffering or independent effects? *Archives of General Psychiatry, 43*, 315–323.

Peterson, C., and Seligman, M.E.P. (1984). Causal explanations as a risk factor for depression: Theory and evidence. *Psychological Review, 91*, 347–374.

Salkovskis, P.M., and Clark, D.M. (1986). Cognitive and physiological approaches in the maintenance and treatment of panic attacks. In I. Hand and H-U. Wittchen (Eds.), *Panic and Phobias.* Berlin: Springer-Verlag.

Seligman, M.E.P. (1975). *Helplessness: On Depression, Development, and Death.* San Francisco: Freeman.

Stratton, P., Heard, D., Hanks, H.G.I., Munton, A.G., Brewin, C.R., and Davidson, C. (1986). Coding causal beliefs in natural discourse. *British Journal of
Social Psychology, 25,* 299–314.

Strickland, B.R. (1978). Internal-external expectancies and health-related behaviors. *Journal of Consulting and Clinical Psychology, 46,* 1192–1211.

Teasdale, J.D. (1988). Cognitive vulnerability to persistent depression. *Cognition
and Emotion, 2,* 247–274.

Teasdale, J.D., and Dent, J. (1987). Cognitive vulnerability to depression: An
investigation of two hypotheses. *British Journal of Clinical Psychology, 26,*
113–126.

Teglasi, H., and Hoffman, M.A. (1982). Causal attributions of shy subjects. *Journal
of Research in Personality, 16,* 376–385.

Tennant, C., Bebbington, P., and Hurry, J. (1981). The short-term outcome of
neurotic disorders in the community: the relation of remission to clinical factors
and to "neutralising" life events. *British Journal of Psychiatry, 139,* 213–220.

Totman, R.G. (1979). *Social Causes of Illness.* London: Souvenir Press.

Vaughn, C.E., and Leff, J.P. (1976). The influence of family and social factors on
the course of psychiatric illness. *British Journal of Psychiatry, 129,* 125–137.

Vaughn, C.E., Snyder, K.S., Jones, S., Freeman, W.B., and Falloon, I.R.H. (1984).
Family factors in schizophrenic relapse: Replication in California of British
research on expressed emotion. *Archives of General Psychiatry, 41,* 1169–1177.

Watts, F.N. (1982). Attributional aspects of medicine. In C. Antaki and C.R.
Brewin (Eds.), *Attributions and Psychological Change.* London: Academic
Press.

Weiner, B. (1985). An attributional theory of achievement motivation and emotion.
Psychological Review, 92, 548–573.

Williams, J.M.G., and Broadbent, K. (1986). Autobiographical memory in suicide
attempters. *Journal of Abnormal Psychology, 95,* 144–149.

Wing, J.K. (1961). Attitudes to the employability of chronic schizophrenic patients.
Occupational Psychology, 35, 58–64.

Wing, J.K. (1978). *Reasoning about madness.* Oxford: Oxford University Press.

Yarrow, M.R., Schwartz, C.G., Murphy, H.S., and Deasy, L.C. (1956). The
psychological meaning of mental illness in the family. *Journal of Social Issues,
11,* 12–24.

6

Mental Retardation and the
Autistic Continuum

Lorna Wing

Introduction

The subjects of mental retardation and childhood autism, originally investigated separately, are now considered to be closely connected. The MRC Social Psychiatry Unit has had a long tradition of research in these fields. As in all Unit work, three inter-related themes have predominated, namely, exploration of basic psychological impairments, epidemiology, and evaluation of services. The story of the sequence of studies over the course of time illustrates the gradual evolution from the initial broad, general view to the present detailed analysis of the nature of these developmental disorders.

Early Unit Work on Mental Retardation

Interest in mental retardation preceded that in autism. In the early days of the MRC Social Psychiatry Unit (then called the Unit for Research in Occupational Adaptation) O'Connor and Tizard (1956) examined the prevalence of mental retardation, the services available at the time, and methods of training mildly retarded people from institutions for gainful employment in the community. The authors measured the levels of ability of the subjects and assessed in various ways their degree of emotional instability, which they referred to as "neurosis." They mentioned that psychotic symptoms could be seen in some severely retarded people. At this period in the Unit's investigations, concepts of behavior disorder were derived from adult psychiatry. Ideas linking behavior patterns to underlying cognitive dysfunctions were still in the embryonic stage.

Tizard (1964, 1966), in the introduction to his book on the prevalence of mental retardation and research into the development of better services, briefly discussed the problem of classifying by clinical types or syndromes. He pointed out that (at the time he was writing) a definite cause could be found in only a minority of cases and that, in any case, aetiology was not related to level of disability or service needs. He concluded that the primary disability was best described in terms of "grade of defect." However, in desribing his study of a small unit run on family lines that provided a new lifestyle for children taken from an institution, Tizard noted that "psychotic" children were excluded.

The classification system based on the degree of retardation was in line with attitudes prevalent at the time, although a few workers, such as Gellner (1959) were attempting to sub-group on patterns of impairments and to link these with specific sites of brain dysfunction.

The present author (Wing, 1971) carried out a prevalence study of severe mental retardation (IQ below 50) among children in the Camberwell area of London. A schedule designed by Kushlick, Blunden and Cox (1973) was completed for each child, and some additional medical information was also collected. From the results, the children could be classified on aetiology into those with Down's syndrome and the rest due to other causes, and also, independently, according to their social and physical incapacities, that is, inability to walk, incontinence, and severe behavior disorder. Each of these problems was defined on operational criteria based on ratings from the schedule. This latter system of sub-grouping, while still comparatively crude, was more helpful for service planning than that based solely on level of IQ.

The Origins of the Unit's Interest in Autism

In the late fifties and early sixties, O'Connor and Hermelin (1962), while members of the Social Psychiatry Unit, carried out a series of experiments to investigate speech and thought in severe mental retardation, using subjects with IQ scores between 25 and 50 who were living in institutions. The observations they made during this study led them to conclude that severe mental retardation could not be regarded as unitary in its functional deficits. They had, for example, found significant differences in task performance between those with and without Down's syndrome. Following this series of studies, O'Connor and Hermelin became interested in the possibility of identifying other diagnostic sub-groups that might also show some specific patternss of cognitive dysfunction.

Their attention was drawn to a group of children they saw in mental handicap hospitals who were suffering from untreated phenylketonuria. These children stood out as having a peculiar pattern of behavior characterized by severe impairment of social interaction and communication and repetitive, stereotyped movements. O'Connor and Hermelin noted that Kanner's (1943) description of the cluster of features he named "early infantile autism" had much in common with the behavior of the children with phenylketonuria.

The literature on autism tended to emphasize the presence of isolated skills contrasting with retardation in other areas. From their own observations and published clinical accounts, it seemed to O'Connor and Hermelin that autistic children might show qualitative differences from other types of retarded children in their strategies for processing information. Despite doubts expressed to them by Professor Sir Aubrey Lewis concerning the validity and reliability of the diagnosis, they went ahead with a series of experiments that have taken their place in the classical literature on autism (Hermelin and O'Connor, 1970; O'Connor and Hermelin, 1978). Nevertheless, the cautious attitude of Lewis was reasonable, in that a diagnosis of autism had a much less secure basis than that of Down's syndrome, as will be discussed later in this chapter.

Autism: the Historical Background

The story of the development of ideas concerning autism and related conditions has been told elsewhere (Cantor, 1988; J. K. Wing, 1976), and only a brief summary will be given here.

In the historical literature, the most famous example of a child who would now be called autistic is that of Victor, the boy found wandering wild in the woods of Aveyron in France (Itard, 1801;1807). In the nineteenth century, various writers described cases of "insanity" in children, characterized by abnormalities of social interaction, language, and behavior some of which are also recognizable as fitting present day definitions of autism and related conditions (e.g., Connolly, 1862; Haslam, 1809; Maudsley, 1867). None of their suggestions for sub-grouping such conditions have withstood the test of time.

During the present century, a number of writers have attempted to define specific syndromes among the many patterns of strange behavior generally grouped under the heading of childhood psychosis. These include De Sanctis (1906;1908), Heller and Weygandt (see Hulse, 1954), Earl (1934), and Mahler (1953), but the author whose ideas became most widely known and accepted was Leo Kanner (1943), perhaps because his descriptions of the children he observed were so clear. He described a group of children, abnormal from birth or within 2½ years of age, with social aloofness and indifference to others, mutism or characteristic deviance of language development (echolalia, repetitive speech, reversal of pronouns, idiosyncratic use of words and phrases), poor or no interpresonal communication, fascination with and dexterity in manipulating objects, and marked resistance to change in their stereotyped pattern of activities. He considered that they were of potentially normal intelligence because of their bright, alert, attractive faces, good visuo-spatial skills and excellent rote memories. He excluded children who were known to have organic brain disorders. Boys were affected three or four times more often than girls. He believed this to be a unique and separate syndrome and named it "early infantile autism." He also thought it was caused by a genetic trait inherited from intelligent but cold, detached parents, or because of abnormal upbringing by such parents, or a combination of both (Kanner 1949).

In 1944, one year after Kanner's original publication on the subject, Asperger produced a paper on a pattern of behavior he termed "autistic psychopathy." The characteristics were an odd, naive style of social interaction, good grammar and vocabulary, but a pedantic long-winded style of speech, impairment of non-verbal aspects of communication, poor motor co-ordination, circumscribed interests in special subjects, a very god rote memory but rather poor comprehension of the meaning of the facts remembered, a marked lack of common sense, and egocentricity related to lack of understanding of other people's needs and feelings. Asperger considered that many of those with his syndrome were of normal or high intelligence, but there were also some who were mildly mentally retarded. He did not exclude from the group those with known organic brain dysfunction. He wrote in German, during the Second World War, and it was many years before his ideas were discussed in the English language literature (Gilberg and Gilberg, 1989; Tantam, 1988a, b; Van Krevelen, 1961; Wing, 1981).

While some workers were engaged in trying to define and name subgroups, others wrote about childhood psychosis as a unitary condition (the "splitters" and the "lumpers"). A number of authors used the term "childhood schizophrenia" as a general label (for example, Bradley, 1967; Bender, 1947; Creak, 1963; Despert, 1938; Goldfarb, 1961; Potter, 1963) apparently including all the so-called syndromes described by the writers mentioned above. Difficulties in comparing results of studies were compounded by the tendency for the terms childhood autism, psychosis, and schizophrenia to be used interchangeably or to be defined in different ways by different authors (Rutter, 1968).

The scientific as opposed to the anecdotal approach gained momentum from the sixties onwards. A working party, chaired by Creak (1961; 1964), made the first attempt to produce a set of diagnostic criteria for the group of conditions they referred to as the "schizophrenic syndromes of childhood" but which evidently covered autism and autistic-like clinical pictures. The "nine points" that resulted from the working party's deliberations were heavily criticized for the imprecision of the definitions allowing for a wide range of interpretations, and the lack of guidance as to the relative importance of the different items. Nevertheless, the exercise was useful in highlighting the existing diagnostic confusion and in promoting debate on the nature of the problems being defined. To quote from DeMyer, Hingtgen, and Jackson's (1981) extensive review of research into infantile autism, "Perhaps no condition in the past has carried more different terms or more different names for sub-categories than early childhood psychosis. The use of these multiple terms—considering that no clear difference among them has been demonstrated—causes confusion, not only in literature reviews and among professionals, but also in parents trying to understand the import of their child's diagnosis."

Three major problems had to be solved before some order could emerge from chaos. These were, first, the relationships among the various clinical pictures loosely grouped together as "childhood psychoses," especially that between childhood schizophrenia and the rest; second, the relationship with organic brain dysfunction; and, third, the relationship with mental retardation.

The Relationship of Autism and Schizophrenia

The solution of the first problem was adumbrated by Anthony (1958a, b; 1962) who pointed out that different clinical pictures were associated with different ages of onset. Kolvin and his colleagues (Kolvin, 1971) carried out a series of studies of "psychotic" children and found that a very small group had a clinical picture like that in typical adult schizophrenia narrowly defined as in the PSE-ID-CATEGO system (Wing et al., 1974), with the characteristic experiences of interference with thoughts, auditory hallucinations and delusions. The onset in these cases was after 5 years of age, being very rare in middle childhood but becoming more common with increasing age. This group could be differentiated on clinical grounds (family history, symptoms, course, prognosis) from those with some or all of the features of Kanner's autism in whom the onset was, in most cases, before three years of age. Kolvin and his colleagues found a very few children who regressed in skills and behavior between three and five years of age in whom the final picture was more like that of the early onset group, not schizophrenia.

This work helped to clarify one aspect of terminology, at least for workers prepared to accept a narrow definition of schizophrenia. There are still some who, like Cantor (1988), Bender (1947), and Fish (1977), use a definition broad enough to encompass some, if not all, cases of autism and autistic-like conditions. However, the use of the term childhood schizophrenia has markedly decreased in papers published in the later seventies and the eighties. Follow-up studies into adult life have shown that autistic and autistic-like children do not develop adult schizophrenia (Rutter, 1970; DeMyer et al., 1973; Wing, 1988a).

The Relationship of Autism and Brain Dysfunction

The relationship of autism and autistic-like conditions to organic brain dysfunction has also been clarified by a wide range of studies carried out from the sixties onwards. DeMyer, Hingtgen, and Jackson, in 1981, reviewed the work published up to that time, which clearly demonstrated the involvement of neurobiological factors. Since then, improvements in techniques of examination have provided more evidence of associated neurological, biochemical, genetic and chromosomal abnormalities (Coleman and Gillberg, 1985; Folstein and Rutter, 1988; Schopler and Mesibov, 1987; Wing, 1988b, c).

Kanner (1943) created future diagnostic problems by excluding children with known brain dysfunctions from his autistic group. What Kanner did not know in 1943 was that there would be advances in medical technology, which, had they been available then, might have revealed organic abnormalities in the children he diagnosed as classically autistic, nor that such abnormalities tend to become more obvious with increasing age (Rutter, 1970). Writers before and after Kanner have described typically autistic behavior, in some cases indistinguishable from Kanner's classic accounts, occurring much more often than chance would allow in association with certain conditions causing brain dysfunction. These include, among others, untreated phenylketonuria (Jervis, 1963), maternal rubella (Chess, 1971; 1977), tuberose sclerosis (Critchley and Earl, 1932, Hunt and Dennis, 1987), Rett's syndrome (Hagberg et al., 1983), a history of infantile spasms (Taft and Cohen, 1971), and peri-natal trauma (DeMyer, 1979).

The occurrence of epileptic fits in one third or more of people with autism or autistic-like conditions is additional support for organic as opposed to emotional causes (Rutter, 1970; Wing, 1988b). In recent years, evidence has been reported for the presence of a genetic trait in some cases of autism (Folstein and Rutter, 1988), and an association with the fragile x chromosome (Hagerman, 1987). Over the course of time, the number of possible causes that have been identified has steadily increased. There is still much work to be done before it will be possible to assign a definite cause, genetic, or pre-, peri-, or post-natal, for each individual case, but there is no doubt that major advances have been made. In parallel with increases in understanding of the neurobiology of autism, a number of studies have demonstrated that parents of autistic and autistic-like children are no more likely to have abnormal methods of child rearing than are parents of other children with chronic handicaps (Pitfield and Oppenheim, 1964; Cox et al, 1975; DeMyer, 1979).

The Relationship of Autism and Mental Retardation

The other diagnostic problem created by Kanner resulted from his belief in the potentially normal or superior intelligence of his autistic group, based on their isolated skills in visuo-spatial tasks or rote memory. Poor performance overall on intelligence tests was explained by refusal to co-operate.

Workers who have tested large groups of autistic and autistic-like children have found overall IQ scores that covered the whole range from severe retardation to normal or superior intelligence, but the majority were below 50 and only around ten to twenty per cent scored IQ 70 or above (DeMyer, 1976; Lotter, 1966; Rutter, 1970; Wing and Gould, 1979). Despite the consistency of such results, it could still be argued that the apparently retarded children were not co-operating. DeMyer, Barton, and Norton (1972) helped to dispose of this hypothesis. They selected items from intelligence tests for infants and children and used them to test autistic children, beginning with the easiest items designed for the lowest mental ages and using rewards to reinforce performance. They found that, if they began low enough on the mental age scale, virtually every child was testable. Within the domains of language, motor, and visuo-spatial skills, the children completed the tasks consistently without any evidence of refusal until they reached an age level at which they failed. There were discrepancies between, but not within domains. The authors argued that autistic children were unlikely to decide not to co-operate with tests above a certain age level. The most convincing hypothesis was that they failed tasks because of genuine inability to perform. The proper technique of testing is to begin at a low enough level. Most autistic children are genuinely mental retarded. Follow-up studies have added further indirect evidence to this view in that they have shown the close association between intelligence level in childhood and prognosis in adult life (DeMyer et al., 1973; Rutter, 1970; Wing, 1988a).

Investigations of Cognitive Function

O'Connor and Hermelin, when they left the Social Psychiatry Unit, set up the MRC Developmental Psychology Unit and continued their studies on autistic children (Hermelin and O'Connor, 1970; O'Connor and Hermmelin, 1978) together with Frith (1970a,b; 1971). They confirmed the generally uneven profile of skills and concluded that autistic children showed both delays and deviance in their cognitive and language development. The details of their findings are complex and vary with the children's levels of ability, but of particular interest are the authors' observations that autistic children, on experimental tests, resembled deaf children in some aspects and blind children in others. Although they could perceive all forms of sensory stimulation, they seemed unable to derive internal representations from them. When presented with either random or patterned sensory stimuli, they tended to impose their own simple repetitive patterning with little relation to the observable features of the input (Frith, 1970a,b; 1971). This defect tended to affect auditory-vocal more than visual or motor modalities, but, nevertheless, was a general tendency that the authors considered to be a basic impairment in autism.

Shah (1988), while a member of the Social Psychiatry Unit, investigated the cognitive processes underlying the tendency for autistic people to have better scores on visuo-spatial than on other types of tasks. She selected autistic subjects aged sixteen to twenty-five with a non-verbal IQ of above 50. (Those chosen ranged in non-verbal IQ from 57 to 108). Three different control groups variously matched for age and IQ were used.

One of the findings of particular interest was the superior "segmentation" ability, compared with controls, of all the autistic subjects in the study. This is the ability to focus on the separate elements making up a whole task. such as the block design test from the Wechsler Intelligence Scales (Wechsler, 1949; 1974), and to resist being distracted by the meaning of the whole display. This ability is of advantage in certain kinds of visuo-spatial tasks, but would be a disadvantage in situations where attention to meaning was of paramount importance, such as in complex social interactions.

O'Connor and Hermelin (1984; 1988; O'Connor, 1989) have extended the exploration of unusual patterns of cognitive abilities and deficits. They are currently examining the remarkable skills, contrasting with retardation in other areas, that can be found in so-called "idiot-savants," many of whom have autism or autistic-like conditions.

Epidemiology

Another area in which there were few facts available before the 1960s was the prevalence of autism and autistic-like conditions. Kanner (1943) suggested that his syndrome was rare, but made no estimates of rates. The first geographically based population study was carried out by Lotter (1966; 1967) who was at the time a member of the staff of the MRC Social Psychiatry Unit. He chose to study children aged eight, nine, and ten years living in the former county of Middlesex who had the behavioral features described by Kanner as characteristic of early infantile autism. He screened the total population in a series of steps, each more detailed than the last. Lotter collected information on a range of behavioral abnormalities in the children he identified as possibly autistic, covering the features described by Kanner and other workers, but, in making his final diagnosis, he placed emphasis on two items that Kanner and Eisenberg (1956) had decided were of primary importance for the diagnosis of Kanner's syndrome—namely, profound lack of affective contact (aloofness and indifference to others) and insistence on maintaining sameness in elaborate repetitive activities. An elaborate activity required some evidence of a capacity to organize the environment, such as making lines or patterns of objects, insisting upon a particular pre-bedtime routine, or complicated whole body movements. Simple stereotypes, such as rocking or finger flicking, were not accepted as sufficiently complex.

Lotter found 2.1 per 10,000 children with the classic syndrome described by Kanner, and 2.4 per 10,000 with most of the features, making a total of 4.5 per 10,000. It is important to note that Lotter identified children solely on their behavior. He did not exclude any on grounds of mental retardation, possible organic causation, or age of onset after 30 months. He found that 56 percent had IQs below 50, 25 percent were between 50 and 69 and 19 percent had IQs of 70 or above. Nearly one third had evidence suggestive of neurological abnormalities (by the standards of investigation available at that time). Three children had an onset between 3 and 4½ years, but had autistic behavior like the rest when seen by Lotter. He corroborated the excess of boys reported by Kanner (1943). This was around 2.5 to 1 for the whole group, but all 10 of those with IQs above 55 were boys. He also found a tendency for higher socioeconomic class in the parents, especially in those with children with most typical autism, but this was less marked than in Kanner's reports.

Lotter's study confirmed the fact that autistic behavior, as described by Kanner, could occur in association with mild or severe mental retardation as defined by overall IQ level. However, testing by psychologists experienced in this field demonstrated that the profiles of sub-tests tended to be different in autistic children from those in non-autistic mental retarded children of a similar IQ level. Lockyer and Rutter (1969) reported that autistic and autistic-like children more often showed extreme variability among sub-test scores. The most usual pattern was a higher score on tests depending upon simple visuo-spatial skills and rote memory, and a much lower score on language and related tasks. A minority had higher scores on certain language related tests, and were poor on visuo-spatial and motor tasks, but even this group did poorly on abstract comprehension as opposed to verbal production.

Gould (1977), while a member of the Social Psychiatry Unit, tested fifty-six severely mental retarded children selected from among those taking part in an epidemiological study by Wing and Gould (1979) described later in this chapter. She found that those with autistic or autistic-like behavior differed from the non-autistic retarded children in having a lower mean score on the Vineland Social Maturity scale (Doll, 1953) and a very much lower score on the Reynell Language Comprehension scale (Reynell, 1969), but a score similar to the non-autistic children on the visuo-spatial items of the Merrill-Palmer scale (Stutsman, 1931).

A New Approach to Classification

Returning to the questions of diagnosis and classification, by the middle of the seventies solid evidence had been produced that early childhood psychoses were often associated with mental retardation, but were different from schizophrenia, narrowly defined, occurring in childhood. However, the relationship between Kanner's autism and other forms of early childhood psychoses had not been elucidated. Furthermore, the present author (Wing, 1969) had compared small groups of autistic, expressive "aphasic," receptive "aphasic," partially deaf plus partially blind, severely retarded Down's syndrome, and normal children on ratings obtained from a schedule completed by the parents. The conclusions were that autistic children appeared to have multiple handicaps, combining various problems that occurred in other syndromes. From this preliminary study, it was evident that further examination was also needed of the relationship of autism to other developmental disorders.

An Epidemiological Study in Camberwell

Consideration of these unsolved problems led Gould and the present author (Wing and Gould, 1979) to undertake an epidemiological study of children under fifteen years on a specified day (December 31st, 1970) whose parents lived in the former London borough of Camberwell. The aim was to find all children with autism or any other form of early childhood psychosis by collecting information from parents and teachers, using the MRC Handicaps, Behavior, and Skills (HBS) schedule described in Chapter 9, psychological testing of the children and examination of all available case notes. The diagnoses were made by the authors, not from existing case records. Those children who were still alive were later followed up in adolescence or early adult life (Wing, 1988a).

Definition of "Childhood Psychosis"

The first difficulty was that of defining what was meant by "childhood psychosis." Autism had been vividly described by Kanner (1943, 1973), but descriptions of other so-called syndromes, or "childhood psychosis" in general, were like the Creak committee's "nine points," that is, couched in general terms capable of any interpretation (for example, "unawareness of personal identity," "loose associations," "fragmentation of speech"), or else comprised lists of items of behavior including some that could be seen in a variety of general or specific developmental disorders (such as poverty of speech, perseveration, oppositional behavior, anxiety).

In the event, we decided to make the parameters as wide as possible by searching for any child who had one or more of the features described by Kanner, plus any other child whom teachers or other professional workers in direct contact considered to be peculiar, odd, strange for any reason, taking into account the child's level of development. Children of this kind were to be included regardless of their level of intelligence. In addition, we included all children who functioned as severely mentally retarded regardless of their behavior. Thus, in effect, we defined "childhood psychosis" as behavior that was strange in the light of the child's mental age, which made more sense to us than many of the definitions we found in the literature. Children who were severely retarded but not strange in behavior provided a comparison group.

The Triad of Social Impairments

Applying the criteria used by Lotter (1966) it was possible to identify children who had the classic autistic behavior pattern and those who had most of the features (Wing and Gould, 1979). But it was very evident, as Lotter himself found, that there were no clear cut-off points, and although there were some very typical children at the center of the group, the boundaries were difficult to define. What did strike us very forcibly was that the 166 children who were alive at the time of the initial study (out of total of 173 who had originally been eligible for inclusion) could be divided into two groups. The first were those who derived interest and pleasure from social interaction at a level that was appropriate in the light of their mental age. (It should be remembered that normal babies respond to other people virtually from birth). The second group comprised those whose social interactions were inappropriate for any mental age. Once again, some children were on the boundary line between these two groups, but most could be classified easily. Inappropriate social interaction could be shown as aloofness or indifference to others, or as passive acceptance of approaches with little or no spontaneous social activity, or as active but odd, one sided, repetitive, basically egocentric approaches to others. These categories were abbreviated to the aloof, the passive, and the active but odd.

Inappropriate social interaction, referred to for brevity as "social impairment" was virtually always associated with impairment of two way social communication, affecting non-verbal as much or more than verbal aspects and the so-called "pragmatic" skills (Baltaxe, 1977), as distinct from formal language structure, and with impairment of social aspects of imaginative development, which was replaced by repetitive, stereotyped activities. This cluster was named "the triad of social impairments." Each aspect could occur in varying degrees of severity. At one end of the scale were children who were aloof and indifferent to others, who communicated only to obtain simple needs, and whose only activities were flicking their hands or objects. At the other end were children who approached everybody, friend or stranger, to ask the same series of questions over and over again, and who had a kind of pseudo-pretend play comprising, for example, enacting repetitively a scene from a television program, such as *Batman* or *Bionic Man*. It should be noted that the triad was seen in some children who were unable to walk independently. Most of these were profoundly retarded in all areas of function and the social impairment was just one more problem among many. It might be argued that it is irrelevant to diagnose the presence of the triad in such cases, but a non-mobile person's level of social responsiveness is of great importance to those giving care. Furthermore, for research into the nature of social impairment, it is necessary to observe all the conditions under which it can occur.

Prevalence Rates

By definition, all children with Kanner's autism had the triad, the prevalence of this group being 4.9 per 10,000 children (2.0 classic and 2.9 nearly classic), close to the rates found by Lotter (1966). But there were, in addition, 17.6 mobile and 4.6 non-mobile children per 10,000 who also had the triad but did not fit the autistic picture. The total prevalence of all with the triad was 27.1 per 10,000 including the non-mobile group, and 22.5 for the mobile children only. Mobile children of first generation immigrants from third world countries had a prevalence of the triad of 51.4

per 10,000, compared with 13.6 for children of native British parents (Wing, 1979). The figures for classic autism were 7.1 and 4.3 respectively (Wing, 1980). Similar findings of higher prevalence of the triad among children of immigrants have reported by Akinsola and Fryers (1986) and Gillberg et al. (1987). Pre-, peri-, or post-natal exposure to unfamiliar viruses is one possible explanation of this phenomenon.

Abnormalities of Behavior

Behavior problems such as temper tantrums, screaming, random aggression, and destructiveness, self injury, wandering, and creating chaos aimlessly were seen significantly more often in those with the triad. It was the children with the triad whose behavior was described by those who knew them as strange, different, unpredictable, and inexplicable.

The majority of the sociable, severely retarded children had behavior that was more or less appropriate in the light of their mental ages. A minority had behavior problems, such as cheekiness, bullying, and minor delinquency, but these tended to occur within a social context. These problems did not appear strange, unlike the behavior of the socially impaired children. A few socially impaired children in the higher ranges of ability broke the law, but, in their case, they did so in pursuit of some circumscribed interest without real understanding of the social and legal consequences. One young man removed shoes of a particular pattern but of any size from shoe shops to add to his collection. Another set fire to his school as a result of his fascination with chemical interactions. They had a quality of innocence, in marked contrast to the knowingness of the delinquent sociable retarded adolescents.

Changes with Age

Follow-up into adolescence or early adult life (Wing, 1988) showed that all those with the triad in childhood retained the cluster of features as they grew older, though around 20 percent changed in the sub-type of impairment of social interaction, usually from aloof to passive or passive to odd. One or two retained only a subtle form of the impairment, but enough to give them problems in their social and working lives. A very few grew into a pattern of behavior more like Kanner's autism, whereas some who were autistic when young became less typical when older, though still with the triad. This underlines the difficulties of differentiating Kanner's autism from the rest.

We attempted to identify other named syndromes. At follow-up, a few fitted Asperger's description of his syndrome, but half of these had had

Kanner's syndrome when younger. It was possible to find individuals with patterns like those described by Earl (1934) and other authors mentioned earlier in this chapter, but the descriptions were too general for precision. Some children fitted more than one group and some fitted none.

Other Findings

There was an overall excess of boys with the triad, especially among those with the highest levels of ability. The lower the IQ, the smaller the boy to girl ratio (Wing, 1981). Like Lotter, we found reported age of onset in most cases to be before three years of age, but a very few were reported to have become abnormal between three and five years of age. The high prevalence of mental retardation, especially at the severe and profound level, noted by other authors was confirmed, as was the association with some condition in the history or present state likely to cause brain dysfunction (Wing and Gould, 1979; Wing, 1988a,b). It was of interest that Down's syndrome and cerebral palsy were rather unlikely to be associated with the triad, in contrast to a range of other conditions, mentioned earlier, that were likely to be associated with social impairment. The only point on which we disagreed with Lotter (1967) was that we found no evidence of higher social class among the parents of autistic children or of others with the triad (Wing 1980). Other recent papers on social class have also failed to confirm Kanner's view of a social class bias (Brask, 1972; Gillberg and Schaumann, 1982; Schopler, Andrews, and Strupp, 1979). It is not clear why Lotter's findings differed on this point from other epidemiological surveys.

Patterns of Impairments and Behavior

The study was also designed to assess levels of performance in a wide range of developmental skills. The reported tendency for an uneven profile of abilities in autistic children was confirmed, and the same was found in others with the triad. It was evident, from inspection of the profiles, that all kinds of combinations of skills and impairments could occur in association with the triad. Thus, it was possible for a child to be aloof, mute, unable to dress himself without help, but to be adept at jigsaw puzzles, making the most unlikely objects spin and climbing and balancing in the most unlikely places. Another child would be aloof sometimes and passive at others, with poor expressive speech, but slightly better comprehension, unable to read, but good at working with numbers, unable to cross the road safely on his own, but capable of cleaning and tidying the house without supervision. Yet another would be active but odd in social interaction, with good grammar and a large vocabulary, but repetitive in speech and poor in comprehension, able to read fluently with little understanding, hopeless at arithmetic, ill coordinated in most gross motor skills, but able to dismantle and put together again any spring-wound clock he could lay his hands on. The overall IQ level depended upon the range and severity of each child's impairment, though the presence of the triad was usually associated with poor use in practice of the skills that were available, probably because of lack of appreciation of the meaning of any activities.

Certain regularities could be discerned, such as aloofness associated with good visuo-spatial skills and ability in climbing and balancing, or active but odd interaction with a large vocabulary but poor motor skills. Nevertheless, it appeared that any combination could occur, even if some were much less frequent than others.

Formulation

The first step in the formulation to be put forward here is to discuss the nature of social interaction, communication and imagination. The use of the word "social," necessary though it is to convey the essence of the behavior concerned, can be misleading. It may suggest to some readers that the activities making up the triad must be learnt entirely from contact with other human beings, the first and most important of these being the mother. This assumption is wrong. Work carried out over the last two decades has demonstrated that the capacity to engage in social interaction, the desire to communicate feelings and ideas through non-verbal means in infancy (facial expressions, gestures, vocal intonation, bodily posture) and later through language, and the ability to develop imaginative understanding of other people are inbuilt in the human brain and unfold in sequence over time (Bretherton, McNew, and Beeghley-Smith, 1981; Bullova, 1979; Newson and Newson, 1975; Pawlby, 1977; Schaffer, 1979; Shantz, 1983; Trevarthen, 1974).

These inbuilt capacities are to be regarded as developmental skills, as are, for example, sucking, chewing, walking, understanding and using language, reading, writing, number work, and so on. Just like these more familiar skills, social interaction, communication, and imagination can be impaired for reasons that are genetic, or due to pre-, peri-, or post-natal events causing damage to the relevant parts or functions of the brain. It appears that these skills are markedly resistant to impairment by psychological factors alone, except perhaps in the most extreme cases of mental combined with physical deprivation (Clarke and Clarke, 1976).

As with all development disorders, impairment of the triad of social skills can occur in widely differing degrees of severity. The aloof, passive,

active but odd, and the most minor and subtle manifestations of impairment are steps along the continuum of severity from the most to the least
severe. At the top end of the scale, the continuum shades into eccentric
normality and then into the less sociable end of the normal range. The
question of where abnormality begins is, for practical, clinical purposes,
determined by whether or not the person is incapacitated by his impairments and needs help in managing his life. For purposes of research, more
rigid, precise operational criteria to define the borderlines may be needed,
but the different requirements of research and clinical work should never
be confused.

An Evolutionary Perspective

Waterhouse (1988) has speculated as to the evolutionary history of
human social behavior. She suggested that "co-regulation" of activities
between pairs and within groups arose in three stages. The first was the
pair bonding of mother-infant and of male-female, which involve close
physical contact and multiple co-regulation of physiological, motor, and
affective activities. The second was the stage of small group living in which
co-regulation is mediated by individual idenfication through face and body
recognition and mimicry of each other by the group members. This enabled
the group to engage successfully in joint activities such as hunting. The
third and most remarkable stage was the development of the capacity to
produce and understand abstract symbols, thus enabling humans to co-
regulate with the behavior of others in different places and at different
times. The most flexible use of this skill developed together with the
realization within each human that other people could understand and be
affected by these symbols.

It is tempting to link these stages of the evolution of co-regulation (social
behavior) to the different manifestations of social impairment. The most
aloof children could be seen as lacking the skills for all but the simplest
forms of pair-bonding (they usually enjoy being tickled and bounced up
and down and will manipulate their parents' hands to obtain such stimulation). The passive group have pair-bonded but have developed only to the
point of recognizing others and imitating them without understanding
(many of them have echopraxia as well as echolalia). The active but odd
group can imitate and have some idea of symbolic representation, but do
not know how to use this to influence other people. As suggested by
Baron-Cohen, Leslie, and Frith (1985), they lack the capacity to appreciate
that other people have ideas, thoughts and feelings, which these authors
sum up in the statement that they lack a "theory of mind." The group
with the most subtle form of the triad of impairments seem to have

developed through all three stages, but by a kind of rote learning, without an innate understanding of how to act in social situations.

Developmental Disorders Associated with the Triad

The triad of impairments can occur on its own as the only aspect of development that has gone wrong, but this is rare. Much more often it is associated with developmental disorders in other areas of function. Delay and deviance in language development is found in the great majority of cases (Ricks and Wing, 1975; Wing, 1981b). Peculiarities of motor coordination are equally common (DeMyer, 1976). However, all kinds of developmental disorders in any combination can occur in individual cases. Perhaps, eventually, one or more specific patterns of impairments will be proven to be associated with specific areas of brain dysfunction or even with specific causes, but no clear associations between cause and behavior pattern has yet been established. Even those cases with what appears to be a genetic trait differ in the details of the clinical picture, perhaps due to a combination of genetic tendency and peri-natal problems (see for example the triplets described by Burgoine and Wing, 1983).

At the moment, the most reasonable hypothesis appears to be that the different possible causes can affect the brain in various ways and in varying degrees of severity. The pattern of impairments in each case depends upon various factors as yet unspecified. The named syndromes happen to be particular combinations which impressed the authors who named them. Kanner's syndrome is a combination of the triad in a severe form, a severe or moderate impairment of language development, but reasonable visuo-spatial skills and rote memory. Asperger's syndrome is the triad in its least severe form, with poor motor coordination, excellent rote memory, some intact scholastic skills, such as mechanical reading, but problems in others, such as arithmetic. A case can be made that these combinations occur by chance, or because of proximity of certain brain areas or functions. Both Kanner's and Asperger's syndromes form only a small minority of all those with the triad. Wing and Wing made this formulation as long ago as 1971. The details of the suggested impairments would now be formulated somewhat differently, but the principle remains the same.

From the practical point of view of helping socially impaired people, there is little to be gained from a detailed concern with identifying syndromes within the whole range of these conditions, however necessary this is for research. It is nevertheless important to identify social impairment in any of its forms when this is causing problems to individuals.

All developmental disorders are a disadvantage to the child or adult concerned, but the triad of social impairments has more handicapping and far reaching effects than any of the others. The person affected needs sympathetic understanding, a structured, organized program for daily life, and education or occupation geared to his special problems. Sometimes, underlying social impairment is overlooked because the child has some other more obvious problem, such as a developmental receptive or expressive language disorder, some form of reading disability, motor clumsiness or visual or hearing impairments. In this situation, remedial treatment for any of these problems is unlikely to be helpful unless the social impairment is recognized and dealt with appropriately.

Recent discussions among linguists of the so called disorders of the pragmatic aspects of language (Conti-Ramsden and Gunn, 1986; McTear, 1985; Rapin and Allen, 1983) have raised a new aspect of the diagnostic problem. The descriptions of children with pragmatic disorders include the features of social impairment as found among people with the triad in its more subtle form. In particular they resemble Asperger's description of his group (Asperger, 1944; Wing, 1981a). It seems likely that some, if not all, of the pragmatic disorders as diagnosed by the linguists are part of the autistic continuum under another name.

The Nature of the Triad

The presence of the triad of impairments is manifested through overt behavior. It still remains to be seen whether the capacity to develop social interaction, communication and imagination can be analyzed into a set of simpler psychological functions, and, if so, do different patterns of impairments of these underlying functions relate to the different ways in which the triad can be manifested. Earlier views that the social impairments of autism are secondary to the language problems (Churchill, 1972; DeMyer, 1975; Ricks and Wing, 1975; Rutter, Bartak and Newman, 1971; Wing, 1969) have had to be modified in the light of the fact that severe developmental language disorders can exist without the autistic type of social impairment, and social impairment can occur without disorder of the formal aspects of language (Asperger, 1944; Gould, 1982; Wing, 1981a; 1988a). It is obviously of significance that language delay and disorder is so common in the autistic continuum, but the reasons for this remain to be discovered (Boucher, 1976).

Shah's (1988) finding that autistic people attend to the details rather than to the meaning of the visual displays used in her study suggests the possibility that a lack of concern with meaning is a general problem underlying the triad of impairments. Frith's (1970a,b; 1971) work showing that autistic children tend to impose simple, usually irrelevant, patterns on all kinds of sensory input raises the question of whether they impose the patterns because they fail to understand the meaning, or conversely, whether abnormal brain mechanism force them to impose simple patterns and therefore prevent them grasping the meaning of their experiences.

A new approach to the psychological dysfunction underlying social impairment in typical autism is to be found in the work of Baron-Cohen, Leslie, and Frith (1985; 1986), Leslie (1987), and Leslie and Frith (1988). The essence of this is that autistic people are impaired in development of the cognitive skills necessary for pretense and for recognition that other people have knowledge and ideas (the "theory of mind" mentioned earlier). The writers concerned consider that this impairment can explain all aspects of the triad.

Hobson (1986a; b) has suggested an underlying affective rather than cognitive explanation for the triad, reflecting Kanner's view of an "innate lack of affective contact." He hypothesized that autistic children have an innate inability to develop reciprocal relationships with other people that primarily involve feeling. Hermelin and O'Connor (1985) suggested that affect and cognition interact inseparably and that the disorder in autism is logico-affective in nature.

It seems to the present author that the argument whether the basic underlying dysfunctions are cognitive or affective in nature is purely semantic. The task for the future is to develop hypotheses that can be tested and that will eventually lead to identification of the underlying brain abnormality.

Terminology

Putting the findings of research together, it is now clear that it is inappropriate to apply the term "childhood psychosis," with its implication of illness occurring in a potentially normal child, to those with the triad of social impairments. The name for the whole group used in the American Psychiatric Association's Diagnostic and Statistical Manual, Edition III (APA, 1980) and the revised version of DSM III (APA, 1987) and in the tenth edition of the International Classification of Diseases (World Health Organization, 1987) is "pervasive developmental disorders." This is useful in emphasizing the developmental nature of the disorder, but unfortunate in that it suggests impairments in all areas, whereas it is uneven profiles that characterize people with the triad. For want of a better name, the present author prefers the term "autistic continuum," since it stresses the relationship with autism, but suggests a wider range of conditions than "childhood autism" alone.

Future Work

For the future, work should continue on the three themes that have characterized the studies carried out in the Unit. Further analysis is needed of the specific impairments to be found in developmental disorders and their relationship to overt behavior. The work should be concentrated upon elucidating the clinical phenomena of the autistic continuum and not upon current diagnostic sub-groups which may eventually be shown to have no validity. It would therefore be of interest to examine whether the experimental findings made in those said to have Kanner's autism also apply to children and adults with other patterns within the autistic continuum. Attempts to identify specific defects of psychological function that possibly underlie the social impairments should continue, as should the search for sub-groups based on specific aetiology or brain localization. Studies of social impairment in conditions other than the autistic continuum, such as the one currently under way in the Unit comparing people with schizophrenia and those with Asperger's syndrome, will help to elucidate further the nature of the components of the triad. The eventual aim must be to discover the links between underlying biological abnormalities and all the overt behavioral manifestations in the autistic continuum. Only then will it be possible to define diagnostic sub-groups with confidence.

The prevalence of the triad among adults is still unknown, and an epidemiological study is needed. Ongoing work in the Unit is examining the prevalence of social and communication disorders in a large group of children, most of whom are attending mainstream schools. New epidemiological work should cover the forms of social impairment seen in children of normal or high ability, including "Asperger's syndrome," since these have not always been included in previous studies.

Innovation and evaluation of services are required in the light of the basic impairments and needs of individuals with different handicaps and skills. The day is past when mental retardation can be regarded as a unitary condition and all mentally retarded people expected to fit into one pattern of services.

References

Akinsola, H.A. and Fryers, T. (1986) A comparison of patterns of disability in severely mentally handicapped children of different ethnic origins. *Psychological Medicine, 16,* 127–133.

American Psychiatric Association (1980) *Diagnostic and Statistical Manual of Mental Disorders.* 3rd Edition, Washington: APA.

Anthony, E.J. (1958a) An etiological approach to the diagnosis of psychosis in childhood. *Revue de Psychiatrie Infantile, 25,* 89–96.

Anthony, E.J. (1958b) An experimental approach to the psychopathology of childhood autism. *British Journal of Medical Psychology, 21,* 211–225.

Anthony, E.J. (1962) Low grade psychosis in childhood. *Proceedings of the London Conference Scientific Study of Mental Deficiency, Vol. 2,* London: May and Baker.

American Psychiatric Association (1987) *Diagnostic and Statistical Manual of Mental Disorders 3rd Edition Revised,* Washington: APA.

Asperger, H. (1944) Die autistischen psychopathen im kindesalter. *Archiv für Psychiatrie und Nervenkrankheiten, 117,* 76–136.

Baron-Cohen, S., Leslie, A.M. and Frith, U. (1985) Does the autistic child have a "theory of mind"? *Cognition, 21,* 37–46.

Baron-Cohen, S., Leslie, A.M. and Frith, U. (1986) Mechanical, behavioural and intentional understanding of picture stories in autistic children. *British Journal of Developmental Psychology, 4,* 113–125.

Bender, L. (1947) Childhood Schizophrenia: a clinical study of 100 schizophrenic children. *American Journal of Ortho-psychiatry, 17,* 40–56.

Boucher, J. (1976) Is autism primarily a language disorder? *British Journal of Disorders of Communication, 11,* 135–143.

Bradley, C. (1941) *Schizophrenia in Childhood,* New York: MacMillan.

Brask, B.H. (1972) A prevalence investigation of childhood psychoses. *In Nordic Symposium on the Comprehensive Care of the Psychotic Children,* Oslo: Barnepsykiatrist Forening.

Bretherton, T., McNew, S., and Beeghley-Smith, M. (1981) Early person knowledge as expressed in gestural and verbal communication: When do infants acquire a 'theory of mind'? *In* M.E. Lamb and L.R. Sherrod (eds.) *Infant Social Cognition,* Hillsdale, NJ: Erlbaum.

Bullowa, M. (ed.) (1979) *Before Speech: The Beginning of Interpersonal Communication,* London: Cambridge University Press.

Burgoine, E. and Wing, L. (1983) Identical triplets with Asperger's Syndrome. *British Journal of Psychiatry, 143,* 261–265.

Cantor, S. (1988) *Childhood Schizophrenia,* New York: Guilford Press.

Chess, S. (1971) Autism in children with congenital rubella. *Journal of Autism and Childhood Schizophrenia, 1,* 33–47.

Chess, S. (1977) Follow-up report on autism in congenital rubella. *Journal of Autism and Childhood Schizophrenia, 7,* 69–81.

Churchill, D.W. (1972) The relationship of infantile autism and early childhood schizophrenia to developmental language disorders of childhood. *Journal of Autism and Childhood Schizophrenia, 2,* 182–197.

Connolly, J. (1861–2) Juvenile insanity. *American Journal of Insanity, 18,* 395–403.

Coleman, M. and Gillberg, C. (1985) *The Biology of the Autistic Syndromes,* New York: Praeger.

Conti-Ramsden, G. and Gunn, M. (1986) The development of conversational disability: a case study. *British Journal of Disorders of Communication, 21,* 339–351.

Cox, A., Rutter, M., Newman, S. and Bartak, L. (1975) A comparative study of infantile autism and specific developmental language disorder: II Parental characteristics. *British Journal of Psychiatry, 126,* 146–159.

Creak, E.M. (1961) (Chairman) Schizophrenic syndrome in childhood: progress report of a working party (April 1961). *Cerebral Palsy Bulletin, 3,* 501–504.

Creak, E.M. (1964) Schizophrenic syndrome in childhood: further progress report of a working party (April 1961). *Developmental Medicine and Child Neurology,* *6*, 530–535.

Critchley, M. and Earl, C.J.C. (1932) Tuberose sclerosis and allied conditions. *Brain, 55,* 311–346.

DeMyer, M., Hingtgen, J., and Jackson, R. (1981) Infantile autism reviewed: a decade of research. *Schizophrenia Bulletin, 7,* 388–451.

DeMyer, M.K. (1975) Research in infantile autism: a strategy and its results. *Biological Psychiatry, 10,* 43–452.

DeMyer, M. (1976) Motor, perceptual-motor and intellectual disabilities of autistic children. *In* L. Wing (ed. *Early Childhood Autism (2nd ed.),* Oxford: Pergamon Press.

DeMyer, M.K. (1979) *Parents and Children in Autism,* Washington: Winston.

DeMyer, M., Barton, S. and Norton, J. (1972) A comparison of adaptive, verbal and motor profiles of psychotic and non-psychotic subnormal children. *Journal of Autism and Childhood Schizophrenia, 2,* 359–377.

DeMyer, M.K., Barton, S., DeMyer, W.E., Norton, J.A., Allen, J. and Steele, R. (1973) Prognosis in autism: a follow-up study. *Journal of Autism and Childhood Schizophrenia, 3,* 199–246.

De Sanctis, S. (1906) Sopra alcune varieta della demenza precoce. *Rivista Sperimentale di Freniatria e di Medicina Legale, 32,* 141–165.

De Sanctis, S. (1908) Dementia praecocissima catatonica oder Katatonie des fruheren kindesalters? *Folia Neurobiologica, 2,* 9–12.

Despert, J.C. (1938) Schizophrenia in children. *Psychiatric Quarterly, 12,* 366–371.

Earl, C.J.C. (1934) The primitive catatonic of idocy. *British Journal of Medical Psychology, 14,* 230–253.

Fish, B. (1977) Neurobiologic antecedents of schizophrenia in children. *Archives of General Psychiatry, 34,* 1297–1313.

Folstein, S.E. and Rutter, M.L. (1988) Autism: familial aggregation and genetic implications. *Journal of Autism and Developmental Disorders, 18,* 3–30.

Frith, U. (1970a) Studies in pattern detection in normal and autistic children: reproduction and production of colour sequences. *Journal of Experimental Child Psychology, 10,* 120–135.

Frith, U. (1970b) Studies in pattern perception in normal and autistic children: immediate recall of auditory sequences. *Journal of Abnormal Psychology, 76,* 413–420.

Frith, U. (1971) Spontaneous speech patterns produced by autistic, normal and subnormal children. *In* Rutter, M. (ed.) *Early Infantile Autism: Concepts, Characteristics and Treatment,* London: Churchill.

Gellner, L. (1959) *A Neurophysiological Concept of Mental Retardation and its Educational Implications,* Chicago: J.D. Levinson Research Foundation.

Gillberg, C. and Schaumann, H. (1982) Social class and infantile autism. *Journal of Autism and Developmental Disorders, 12,* 223–228.

Gillberg, I.C. and Gillberg, C. (1989) Asperger syndrome—some epidemiological considerations: a research note. *Journal of Child Psychology and Psychiatry, 30,* 631–638.

Gillberg, C., Steffenburg, S., Borjesson, B. and Anderson, L. (1987) Infantile autism in children of immigrant parents: a population-based study from Goteborg, Sweden. *British Journal of Psychiatry, 150,* 856–857.

Goldfarb, W. (1961) *Childhood Schizophrenia,* Cambridge, MA: Harvard University Press.

Gould, J. (1977) The use of the Vineland social maturity scale, the Merrill Palmer scale of mental tests (non-verbal items) and the Reynell development language scales with children in contact with the services for the severe mental retardation. *Journal of Mental Deficiency Research, 21,* 213–226.

Gould, J. (1982) *Social Communication and Imagination in Children with Cognitive and Language Impairments,* London: Ph.D. Thesis (Unpublished).

Hagberg, B., Aicardi, J., Dias, K. and Ramos, D. (1983) A progressive syndrome of autism, dementia, ataxia and loss of purposeful hand use in girls: Rett's syndrome: report of 35 cases. *Annals of Neurology, 11,* 471–479.

Hagerman, R. J. (1987) Fragile x syndrome. *Current Problems in Paediatrics, 17,* 623–674.

Haslam, J. (1809) *Observations on Madness and Melancholy,* 185–206, London: Haydon.

Hermelin, B. and O'Connor, N. (1985) Logico-affective states and non-verbal language. *In* E. Schopler and G. Mesibov (eds.) *Communication Problems in Autism,* New York: Plenum.

Hermelin, B. and O'Connor, N. (1970) *Psychological Experiments with Autistic Children,* Oxford: Pergamon Press.

Hobson, R.P. (1986a) The autistic child's appraisal of expressions of emotion. *Journal of Child Psychology and Psychiatry, 27,* 321–342.

Hobson, R.P. (1986b) The autistic child's appraisal of emotions: a further study. *Journal of Child Psychology and Psychiatry, 27,* 671–680.

Hulse, W.C. (1954) Dementia infantilis. *Journal of Nervous and Mental Diseases, 119,* 471–477.

Hunt, A. and Dennis, J. (1987) Psychiatric disorder among children with tuberous sclerosis. *Developmental Medicine and Child Neurology, 29,* 190–198.

Itard, J.M.G. (1801) Of the first developments of the young savage of Aveyron. *Reprinted in* Malson, L. and Itard, J.M.G. (1972) *Wolf Children and The Wild Boy of Aveyron,* London: NLB.

Itard, J.M.G. (1807) Report on the progress of Victor of Aveyron. *Reprinted in* L. Malson and J.M.G. Itard. *Wolf Children and the Wild Boy of Aveyron* (1972) London: NLB.

Jervis, G.A. (1963) The clinical picture. *In* F.L. Lyman (ed.) *Phenylketonuria,* Springfield: Charles C. Thomas.

Kanner, L. (1943) Autistic disturbances of affective contact. *Nervous Child, 2,* 217–250.

Kanner, L. (1949) Problems of nosology and psychodynamics in early childhood autism. *American Journal of Orthopsychiatry, 19,* 416–426.

Kanner, L. (1973) *Childhood Psychosis: Initial Studies and New Insights,* New York: Winston/Wiley.

Kanner, L. and Eisenberg, L. (1956) Early infantile autism 1943–1955. *American Journal of Orthopsychiatry, 26,* 55–65.

Kolvin, I. (1971) Studies in the childhood psychoses: I. Diagnostic criteria and classification. *British Journal of Psychiatry, 118,* 381–384.

Kushlick, A., Blunden, R. and Cox, G. (1973) A method of rating behaviour characteristics for use in large scale surveys of mental handicap. *Psychological Medicine, 3,* 466–478.

Leslie, A.M. (1987) Pretence and representation: The original of "theory of mind." *Psychological Review, 94,* 412–426.

Leslie, A.M. and Frith, U. (1988) Autistic children's understanding of seeing, knowing and believing. *British Journal of Developmental Psychology, 6*, 315–324.

Lockyer, L. and Rutter, M. (1969) A five to fifteen year follow-up study of infantile psychosis: III Psychological aspects. *British Journal of Psychiatry, 115*, 865–882.

Lotter, V. (1966) Epidemiology of autistic conditions in young children: I. Prevalence. *Social Psychiatry, 1*, 124–137.

Lotter, V. (1967) Epidemiology of autistic conditions in young children: II. Some characteristics of the parents and young children. *Social Psychiatry, 1*, 163–173.

Mahler, M.S. (1952) On child psychoses and schizophrenia: autistic and symbiotic infantile psychoses. *Psychoanalytic Study of the Child, 7*, 286–305.

Maudsley, H. (1867) Insanity of early life. *In The Physiology and Pathology of the Mind* First edition, New York: Appleton.

McTear, M. (1985) Pragmatic disorders: a case study of conversational disability. *British Journal of Disorders of Communication, 20*, 129–142.

Newson, J. and Newson, E. (1975) Intersubjectivity and the transmission of culture: on the social origins of symbolic functioning. *Bulletin of the British Psychological Society, 20*, 129–142.

O'Connor, N. (1989) The performance of the 'idiot savant': implicit and explicit. *British Journal of Disorders of Communication, 24*, 1–20.

O'Connor, N. and Hermelin, B. (1962) *Speech and Thought in Severe Subnormality*, London: Pergamon Press.

O'Connor, N. and Hermelin, B. (1984) Idiot-savant calendrical calculators: maths or memory? *Psychological Medicine, 14*, 801–806.

O'Connor, N. and Hermelin, B. (1988) Low intelligence and special abilities. *Journal of Child Psychology and Psychiatry, 29*, 391–396.

O'Connor, N. and Tizard, J. (1956) *The Social Problem of Mental Deficiency*, London: Pergamon Press.

O'Connor, N. and Hermelin, B. (1978) *Seeing and Hearing and Space and Time*, London: Academic Press.

Pawlby, S. (1977) Imitative interaction. *In* H.R. Schaffer (ed.) *Studies in Mother and Infant Interaction*, New York: Academic Press.

Pitfield, M. and Oppenheim, A.N. (1964) Child rearing attitudes of mothers of psychotic children. *Journal of Child Psychology and Psychiatry, 5*, 51–57.

Potter, H. W. (1933) Schizophrenia in children. *American Journal of Psychiatry, 12*, 1253–1270.

Rapin, J. and Allen, D. (1983) Developmental language disorders. *In* A. Kirk (ed.) *Neuropsychology of Language, Reading and Spelling*, New York: Academic Press.

Reynell, J. (1969) *Reynell Developmental Language Scales*, Slough, Bucks: N.F.E.R.

Ricks, D.M. and Wing, L. (1975) Language, communication and the use of symbols in normal and autistic children. *Journal of Autism and Childhood Schizophrenia, 3*, 191–221.

Rutter, M. (1968) Concepts of autism: a review of research. *Journal of Child Psychology and Psychiatry, 9*, 1–25.

Rutter, M. (1970) Autistic children: infancy to adulthood. *Seminars in Psychiatry, 2*, 435–450.

Rutter, M., Bartak, L. and Newman, S. (1971) Autism—a central disorder of cognition and language? *In* Rutter, M. (ed.) *Infantile Autism: Concepts, Characteristics and Treatment*, London: Churchill.

Schaffer, H.R. (1974) Early social behaviour and the study of reciprocity. *Bulletin of the British Psychological Society, 27,* 209–216.

Schopler, E., Andrews, C.E. and Strupp, K. (1979) Do autistic children come from upper middle class parents? *Journal of Autism and Developmental Disorders, 9,* 139–152.

Schopler, E. and Mesibov, G.B. (1987) *Neurobiological Issues in Autism,* New York: Plenum.

Shah, A. (1988) *Visuo-Spatial Islets of Abilities and Intellectual Functioning in Autism,* London: Ph.D. Thesis (Unpublished).

Shantz, C. U. (1983) Social cognition. *In* J.H. Flavell and E.M. Markmen (eds.) *Cognitive Development: A Handbook of Child Psychology,* Vol. 3, New York: Wiley.

Stutsman, R. (1931) *Merrill-Palmer Scale of Mental Tests,* New York: Harcourt, Brace & World.

Taft, L.T. and Cohen, H.J. (1971) Hypsarrhythmia and childhood autism: a clinical report. *Journal of Autism and Childhood Schizophrenia, 1,* 327–336.

Tantam, D. (1988a) Lifelong eccentricity and social isolation: I Psychiatric, social and forensic aspects. *British Journal of Psychiatry, 153,* 777–782.

Tantam, D. (1988b) Lifelong eccentricity and social isolation: II Asperger's syndrome or personality disorder? *British Journal of Psychiatry, 153,* 783–791.

Tizard, J. (1964) *Community Services for the Mentally Handicapped,* Oxford: University Press.

Tizard, J. (1966) The experimental approach to the treatment and upbringing of handicapped children. *Developmental Medicine and Child Neurology, 8,* 310–321.

Trevarthen, C. (1974) Conversations with a two-month old. *New Scientist, 62,* 230–235.

Van Krevelen, D.A. (1971) Early infantile autism and autistic psychopathy. *Journal of Autism and Childhood Schizophrenia, 1,* 82–86.

Waterhouse, L. (1988) Aspects of the evolutionary history of human social behaviour. *In* L. Wing (ed.) *Aspects of Autism: Biological Research,* London: Gaskell.

Wechsler, D. (1949) *Wechsler Intelligence Scale for Children: Manual,* New York: Psychological Corporation.

Wechsler, D. (1974) *Manual for the Wechsler Adult Intelligence Scale,* New York: The Psychological Corporation.

Wing, J.K. (1976) Kanner's syndrome: a historical introduction *In* L. Wing (ed.) *Early Childhood Autism,* Oxford: Pergamon.

Wing, J.K., Cooper, J.E. and Sartorius, N. (1974) *The Measurement and Classification of Psychiatric Symptoms,* Cambridge: Cambridge University Press.

Wing, L. (1969) The handicaps of autistic children—A comparative study. *Journal of Child Psychology and Psychiatry, 10,* 1–40.

Wing, L. (1971) Severely retarded children in a London area: prevalence and provision of services. *Psychological Medicine, 1,* 405–415.

Wing, L. (1979) Mentally retarded children in Camberwell (London) *In* H. Häfner (ed.) *Estimating Needs for Mental Health Care,* Berlin: Springer-Verlag.

Wing, L. (1980) Childhood autism and social class: a question of selection. *British Journal of Psychiatry, 137,* 410–417.

Wing, L. (1981a) Asperger's syndrome: a clinical account. *Psychological Medicine, 11,* 115–130.

Wing, L. (1981b) Language, social, and cognitive impairments in autism and severe mental retardation. *Journal of Autism & Developmental Disorders, 11,* 31–44.

Wing, L. (1988a) The continuum of autistic characteristics. *In* E. Schopler and G. Mesibiv (eds.) *Diagnosis and Assessment in Autism*, New York: Plenum.

Wing, L. (1988b) Autism: possible clues to underlying pathology. Clinical facts. *In* L. Wing (ed.) *Aspects of Autism: Biological Research*, London: Gaskell.

Wing, L. (ed.) (1988c) *Aspects of Autism: Biological Research*, London: Gaskell.

Wing, L. (1989) *Hospital Closure and the Resettlement of Residents: The Case of Darenth Park Hospital*, Aldershot: Gower.

Wing, L. and Wing, J.K. (1971) Multiple impairment in early childhood autism. *Journal of Autism and Childhood Schizophrenia, 1*, 256–266.

Wing, L. and Gould, J. (1979) Severe impairments of social interaction and associated abnormalities in children: epidemiology and classification. *Journal of Autism and Childhood Schizophrenia, 9*, 11–29.

World Health Organization (1977) *International Classification of Diseases: Ninth Revision*, Geneva: World Health Organization.

World Health Organization (1987) *International Classification of Diseases: Tenth Revision. Draft Research Diagnostic Criteria*, Geneva: WHO (Unpublished document).

II

Instrumentation in Social Psychiatry

7

Measuring and Classifying Clinical Disorders: Learning from the PSE

J. K. Wing

Introduction

It was suggested in Chapter 1 that a full grasp of the technicalities of diagnosis, in order to recognize or to exclude disease, is a central component of a doctor's expertise and one on which the more general social functions of doctors depend. Diseases are clinical constructs composed of elements (symptoms and signs, or phenomena) that represent deviations from some cycle or system of biological functioning. The more that is known of the forces that keep the system within normal limits, the more complete can be the theories of how and why deviations occur, the more precise the theories of prevention, treatment and prognosis, and also the more reliable and valid the recognition of the manifestations of biological deviation as symptoms and signs. To make a diagnosis, therefore, is not to specify the presence of a disease entity but to postulate, on the basis of an observable pattern or syndrome of symptoms and signs, that a disturbance in such a system will be found once the means of demonstrating it are available.

Successful disease theories of the disorders brought by patients and their families to psychiatrists have been hard to come by. This does not mean that the descriptive phenomenology of the past 150 years has been wasted. In the history of medicine, the recognition, definition, and labelling of a clinical syndrome has time and again proved to be of incalculable value and not only because it has provided a stimulus to the discovery of primary, secondary, and precipitating causes, or to the development of methods of treatment or rehabilitation. Once recognized, the afflicted person and the family can be given information about course or prognosis or means of coping. At the very least, the fact that the condition is known, that it has a name, that other people suffer from it and can give advice, and that its frequency, characteristics, and causes can be studied, is a consolation. The many charitable organizations set up to help those who have a named condition, such as the syndromes attributed to Alzheimer, Down, Kanner, and Rett, demonstrate the value placed on recognition even when there is no hard and fast knowledge about causes and no firm cure is available.

The syndromes are often described in the first place by an intuitive clinician. If the observations can be repeated accurately and independently, they appear to take on a "validity" of their own. The fact that their elements occur in an observable pattern, together or over time, suggests that there is a non-random structure, the nature of which can be investigated. However, it is less confusing to use terms such as "reliability" and "internal consistency" to describe these characteristics, because "validity" is usually assumed to mean that links to a biological pathology or substrate have already been demonstrated. Medical terminology ("symptoms" and "syndromes") is also used, however, when a biological basis has been postulated but not fully demonstrated.

The problems brought to psychiatrists are far from exclusively biological. Biological abnormalities can have social causes. Many biological systems depend for their proper functioning on interaction with the psychosocial environment. Social influences can amplify biological impairment. The extent to which an individual is socially disabled depends, in addition, on purely social factors such as disadvantage and public, family, and self attitudes. Finally, social definitions of "normality" must be distinguished from concepts of biological deviation.

Scientists must nevertheless try to keep the various factors contributing to social disablement theoretically separate, since they are likely to have different causes and practical effects and to require different types of intervention. Any research unit concerned with psychiatric problems must be interested in achieving the most accurate and comparable clinical assessments possible.

This conclusion can be applied to most psychiatric syndromes, from phobias to dementia. The more clearly "symptoms" are described, and the more precisely the rules for grouping them into syndromes are specified, the more comparable will be tests of hypotheses of all kinds. Validity, in terms of a demonstrable and replicable relationship to some independent criterion, can sometimes be demonstrated even when the manifestations are diverse and variable and can then be used to refine the syndrome, but it would not be sensible to rely only on that chance. This is why attempts have been made to reach a degree of consensus at least on the classifying rules.

It is essential to get clear at the outset the relationship between the top-down approach to diagnosis (using a set of rules to select one class from a complete nosological system) and the bottom-up approach (determining the set of clinical phenomena on which the rules operate). The provision of diagnostic guidelines, for example in the new tenth edition of the International Classification of Diseases (ICD10: World Health Organization, 1990), has focused attention on the top-down part of the problem by getting a common denominator of agreement between international member states on rules they find acceptable. But for any given condition the rules must be a compromise. They are different from those of DSM-IIIR, and different again from those of any individual expert. Their great advantage is that their use increases the comparability of research results and of administrative statistics. But only one component of variability, and perhaps the simplest, is reduced in this way.

A careful concern with systems of classification is appropriate for clinical psychiatry at its present stage of development. But the rules of systems such as ICD10 and DSM-IIIR need to be applied to a range of carefully defined symptoms that cover as many of the manifestations familiar to psychiatrists as is feasible. It will then be possible to apply other sets of rules as well and to compare the results of hypothesis testing. Public competition between diagnostic concepts is as essential in psychiatry as in other branches of medicine.

In retrospect, it is clear that members of the Social Psychiatry Unit in the early days almost invariably approached the problems of clinical measurement from the bottom up. This strategy developed from the exigencies of hypothesis testing, which most frequently demanded the measurement of symptoms or disabilities rather than disorders. Diagnoses were used, but only to obtain a sample for more detailed testing. Then they were obtained clinically or from case records. It was only later that the fallibility of such an approach was recognized and techniques for top-down standardization were introduced. This chapter is concerned with some of the lessons for diagnostics that can be derived from the continuity of hypothesis, experiment and reformulation of hypothesis during 25 years experience in a research unit.

The Development of the PSE

The Beginnings

The development of a set of instruments intended to serve these purposes was made necessary by the kind of work undertaken in the Unit during the first twenty years of its existence (O'Connor, 1968). Several useful scales were devised, for example, to measure the ward behavior of mentally handicapped and mentally ill people as seen through the eyes of ward nurses. An operational distinction could be made between paranoid and non-paranoid forms of schizophrenia, although the diagnosis itself was based on the unstandardized judgments of various clinicians (Venables, 1957; Venables and O'Connor, 1959). Developments of these were used in hypothesis-led studies of in-patient care during the late fifties and early sixties. At the same time, a simple descriptive categorization of chronic schizophrenia was constructed, based on four symptoms rated at interview that were commonly seen in patients in those days—flatness of affect, poverty of speech, incoherence of speech, and coherently expressed delusions and hallucinations (Venables and Wing, 1962; Wing, 1959, 1961, 1962). The latter was then extended in order to cover psychotic symptoms in detail, in effect producing the second edition of what became the "Present State Examination" (PSE).

J. R. Wittenborn (1955), and M. Lorr (1966) developed instruments with a broader spectrum. Check lists of items were rated on the basis of behavior observed in unstandardized situations and the results analyzed statistically in order to produce empirical groupings, such as "perceptual distortion." The results were relatively reliable and precise compared with clinical procedures (Foulds, 1965; Kreitman, 1961) but the categories did not look very different from the syndromes already in use.

It seemed unwise to assume that unreliability was inherent in the phenomena being observed, since similar problems had been noted and overcome in other fields of medicine, for example in the interpretation of chest X-rays and electro-cardiograms, and psychologists had produced encouraging results by operationalizing clinical concepts. Sections dealing with neurotic symptoms were added to the "second edition" to produce a third schedule which was actually given the designation "Present State Examination" (PSE).

PSE3 to PSE6

This was rapidly expanded and reorganized during intensive studies between 1963 and 1966, and the results of a wide range of tests of the third, fourth, and fifth editions of the PSE, based on interviews with 172 out-, day- and in-patients, were published (Wing et al., 1967).

The interview was based on "clinical cross-examination," a procedure that was well-accepted by patients, who recognized that their problems were being taken seriously by clinicians who had to rule out some possibilities as well as focus on others. The aim of the examiner was to discover whether each of a list of symptoms was present and, if so, with what degree of severity. For most symptoms a line of questioning was suggested but the examiner was free to depart from this, and from the order of questioning, if necessary, to obtain clarity. The symptom definitions were carried in the head of the interviewer. The examination, therefore, was based on a process of matching the respondent's behavior and descriptions of subjective experiences with the clinical concepts of the interviewer. The time period covered was limited to one month, chosen after experience with hospital patients at that time suggested that recall over a longer period could be unsatisfactory.

The conclusions derived from these studies still bear quotation, because they have remained true since and include the formulation of some principles that are still central to the PSE system:

> The flexibility of this approach, the incorporation of detailed cross-examination which allows changes in the order and wording of questions according to the way the interview is going, the freedom of the clinician to pursue some lines of enquiry while cutting off others, the fact that the examiner and not the patient makes the judgment as to whether a symptom is present, do not seriously impair the reliability of the procedure. When two raters assess the same interview there is a very high degree of agreement on provisional categorization and very high correlation coefficients between scores representing areas of symptomatology. When there are two interviews at an interval of several days, the provisional categorizations made by the two clinicians are still very similar, but the correlations on section scores fall somewhat.

The only score on which there was unsatisfactory reliability was anxiety, a problem that has continued to be evident since. A key point to note is that the "categorizations" referred to in the extract were clinical diagnoses, made independently of each other by the five psychiatrists taking part. The agreement was high, although no standardized definitions of the symptoms or specification of the classifying rules was attempted. The agreement was likely to have been due in part to the fact that all five had been trained in the same school of psychiatry and phenomenology, thus reducing inter-rater variability.

Another important factor was standardization of the set of symptoms on which the diagnosis was based, which also limited variation. This second factor was shown to be particularly important when reliability exercises conducted by the World Health Organization (WHO) included clinicians from many countries and diagnostic schools (Shepherd et al., 1968). The participants were able to rate symptoms from videotapes of standard interviews (a version of PSE6) with remarkably little disagreement, but their diagnostic formulations of the same cases were much more diverse.

The results did something to counter the skepticism of those who argued, from the poor showing made by clinical diagnosticians in tests of reliability based on unstandardized data, that only a fully standardized questionnaire approach, accepting the respondent's Yes or No and allowing as little as possible to clinical judgment, could produce agreement.

PSE7 and PSE8

The sixth edition of the PSE was modified for use in two large multinational studies then being devised. The first was the U.S.-U.K. Diagnostic Project (Cooper et al., 1972), which began wih the seventh edition (PSE7) and later changed to PSE8, in common with the WHO-sponsored International Pilot Study of Schizophrenia (IPSS, WHO, 1973). Reliability was satisfactory in both studies and in others conducted elsewhere (Cooper et al., 1972; Kendell et al., 1968; Luria and Berry, 1979; Luria and McHugh, 1974; Wing, Cooper, and Sartorius, 1974; WHO, 1973). Both studies were concentrated on the differential diagnosis of schizophrenia, particularly from affective disorder.

The central result of the New York-London study was that the team of research psychiatrists, examining patients on both sides of the Atlantic, diagnosed far fewer schizophrenic disorders than their hospital counterparts in the USA, while agreeing more closely with the latter in the U.K. The PSE profiles confirmed that New York hospital diagnoses of schizophrenia were substantially broader (including part of what, in London, would be called mania or depression or personality disorder). This has no implications for validity in the strict sense but does indicate that the boundaries of the disorder were, at that time, drawn so differently that the results of studies into causes, treatments, and outcomes might well not be comparable if based on hospital diagnoses in the two cities.

The IPSS investigators were a larger and much more diverse group than those of the U.S.-U.K. study. They came from Centers in Aarhus, Agra, Cali, Ibadan, London, Moscow, Prague, Taipei, and Washington. However, there was a very similar result. The Centers in Washington and Moscow used a much broader definition than the other seven when PSE profiles were studied. (The reason for the similarity between Moscow and Washington, so unlikely on casual inspection, is part of a different story.) It was clear that it would be possible to develop reliable research instruments for practical use in international psychiatric research.

From the point of view of improving the PSE, three major lessons were learned from the IPSS. The first was that a glossary of differential definitions of symptoms should be provided as a basis for training courses; the second, that additional schedules would be needed to allow the rating of previous episodes of disorder and possible causes and pathologies; the third, that rules of classification should be written, which could be applied to PSE data through a computer program in order to provide a standard of reference in addition to (not as a substitute for) clinical diagnosis.

PSE9

The ninth edition of the PSE was shorter than its predecessor: only 140 items, which could be derived by a simple formula from the much larger PSE7 and PSE8. Each item was given a differential definition in the Glossary. Together with a Syndrome Checklist, Aetiology Schedule, and CATEGO computer program, the new system filled in most of the gaps in the old (Wing, Cooper, and Sartorius, 1974). A fourth change was a major innovation, made subsequent to publication: the construction of a computer program, the Index of Definition (ID), providing a means of differentiating eight levels of confidence that sufficient symptoms were present to allow a diagnosis of one of the "functional" categories of the International Classification of Diseases, 8th revision, Chapter 5 (ICD8). These four changes involve principles that (together with the key problem of translation into languages other than English) receive separate discussion below.

Three other modifications were found useful for particular purposes: a "change rating scale," using PSE9 items, for monitoring clinical progress over time (Tress et al., 1987); a technique for ascertaining lifetime prevalence (McGuffin, Katz and Aldrich, 1986); and a brief form, using only ten questions to identify "cases" with remarkable success (Cooper and MacKenzie, 1981).

The Aims of the PSE-SCL-ID-CATEGO System

Publishing the PSE for the first time, after 10 years of development, provided an opportunity to state the aims of the system, summarize its limitations and advantages, and specify the relationships between the PSE9 text and glossary, representing the original bottom-up clinical orientation of the procedure and the top-down imitation of the ICD8 rules.

The first and most important aim was to describe clinical phenomena as clearly, precisely, and reliably as possible. If this could be achieved, the symptom and syndrome profiles and scores could be used to facilitate a wide range of research—epidemiological, biological, therapeutic, prognostic, and psychosocial.

A second aim was to apply computerized classifying rules (based on the glossary to ICD8 and therefore highly approximate) to the descriptive

PSE9 data provided by the clinical examination of an individual patient, in order to produce a category or profile of potential subcategories, that would always be identical and, to that extent comparable, no matter where they were produced, so long as the patient showed the same pattern of phenomena. The computer output could then be compared across studies in a way that clinical diagnoses could not. Comparisons between computer and clinical classification could also prove fruitful when modifying existing nosologies.

A third aim was dependent on the other two. Since the system was simply a standardization of a particular clinical approach, it could have educational as well as research and clinical uses. Many of those who used the PSE found that their style of interviewing, coverage, and ability to recognize accurately psychopathology increased; indeed, with its Glossary, the PSE has been used in university clinics as an introduction to phenomenology and clinical interviewing.

This use in professional training carried a potential disadvantage, in that there has been a tendency to regard the CATEGO output as a diagnosis, instead of a technical aid. That is far from the authors' intention. A central principle is that the system itself cannot "make a diagnosis." The people who use it are responsible for interpreting the results: (a) according to their judgment of the quality of the interview and the data recorded; (b) their choice of outputs from the computer analysis, most of which are profiles of scores or categories, with only the final one a single class tentatively representing an ICD8 rubric; (c) if they use this single class, their personal evaluation of the rules used to produce it.

PSE10 and SCAN

More than 15 years of experience with the PSE9 system provided a mass of suggestions for improvement. Preparations for a tenth edition of the PSE were started in 1980, in anticipation of the tenth edition of the ICD. The major emphasis of correspondents was on broadening the content, both by returning to the larger item-pool of PSE7 and PSE8, and by adding new sections to cover somatoform, dissociative and eating disorders, alcohol and drug misuse, and cognitive impairments. A second suggestion was that an extra rating point was needed to extend the 0-1-2 scales of severity used for most PSE9 items, allowing a mild or "sub-clinical" level to be used, particularly in population surveys. A third, very obvious, requirement was for a better system for rating episodes of disorder, adding other information relevant to the history and to the causes of disorder, and processing all the information by means of one set of computer programs. The publication and widespread use of DSM-III and later its revised version, DSM-IIIR, meant that one of these or, perhaps more usefully, an eventual DSM-IV, would require clinical supplements. Finally, users of PSE9 made it clear that they would wish any tenth edition to remain compatible, in the sense that PSE9 items could be derived from PSE10 ratings so that the CATEGO4 program could be applied to produce output comparable with data from earlier studies.

This work has been taken forward by a Task Force on Psychiatric Assessment Instruments, established within the framework of a World Health Organization (ADAMHA) project aimed at improving the accuracy and reliability of measurement and classification of psychiatric disorders (Jablensky et al., 1983).

An early version of SCAN (Schedules for Clinical Assessment in Neuropsychiatry) was used in a study of the service needs of long term attenders at day hospitals and day centers in Camberwell, southeast London (Brugha et al., 1988). This provided a severe test of the historical capacities of SCAN, since the attenders had been in contact with services for an average of fifteen years and nearly half did not have conditions that could be diagnosed from a present state interview alone.

This experience, together with suggestions from international reviewers whose opinions were canvassed by the Task Force, led to further modifications and additions. The February 1988 version of SCAN was then used in international field trials to test reliability between interviewer and observer and between two interviewers over time and general practicality in use across a wide range of disorders. Twenty centers were involved and new sections of PSE10, such as those for substance misuse and cognitive impairment, were thoroughly tested. Preliminary analyses suggest that PSE10 has much the same biometric characteristics as the predecessor system and that the extra components have not diminished feasibility or reliability. The CATEGO5 computer algorithms produce results for ICD10 and DSM-IIIR categories that can be predicted from a reading of these top-down systems of rules. Perhaps more important in the long run, they provide profiles of scores, item-groups, and sub-categories that can be used, in conjunction with ICD10 and clinical diagnoses, to test hypotheses concerning the relationship to normally functioning systems, the causes, the treatments, and the influences on the course of psychiatric disorders.

Ten years work on SCAN nevertheless leaves many questions unanswered. It was not undertaken only to produce a technically advanced version of clinical psychiatric expertise to serve the purposes of research and education, but to specify, and make available for public criticism, at least one version of the set of assumptions that underlie that knowledge. The top-down rules in ICD10 and DSM-IIIR and expressed in the CATEGO5 computer programs represent one kind of "knowledge base."

The bottom-up components of SCAN provide another. Both are necessary to test clinical theories.

The Lessons of the PSE:

Increasing Advantages and Decreasing Limitations

The foregoing summary of how the PSE developed into SCAN may help to illustrate both the advantages and the limitations of such a system and also indicate where further development could be useful. Within the limits which restrict interpretation the advantages are substantial, since SCAN provides a version of clinical description and classification whose assumptions are open to publlic inspection, criticism, and constructive modification. Some of the more obvious problems are considered in a broader context below.

Choosing, Defining and Interpreting PSE Items

What do PSE Items Measure? Most PSE items are regarded as "symptoms" of a putative deviation from a cycle or system of normal biological functioning. The greater the knowledge of the forces that keep the system within normal limits, the more complete can be the theory that links the cause of any deviation to the clinical manifestations. Theories of prevention, treatment, and rehabilitation then also have a better chance of succeeding.

In so far as it is possible, therefore, symptoms should be defined in terms that contain no social component. Shoplifting, for example, cannot be defined in this way. Nor can "evil" (Bentall, Jackson, and Pilgrim, 1988). Nor can a subcultural possession state. This does not mean that social criteria play no part in determining what phenomena are chosen as a focus of interest by clinical scientists. Criteria for potential musical genius, for example, could theoretically be laid down in purely psychological and biological terms, without recourse to any social judgment. Social attitudes (shared by clinicians) would not regard such indicators of prodigious talent as medically abnormal. But these social influences on the choice of what phenomena are regarded as "symptoms" should, ideally, play no part in the symptom definition itself. (The dangers of including criteria of social deviance in the definition of symptoms were illustrated in Chapter 1.) Moreover, there are instances where social value is attached to manifestations that can unequivocally be demonstrated to be manifestations of a harmful disease. Rene Dubos, for example, described a tribe of American Indians in which dyschromic spirochaetosis, a serious disease characterized by multicolored spots on the skin, was so common that those who did not have it were regarded as abnormal and excluded from marriage (Dubos, 1965).

These are good reasons why symptoms should be technically defined and differentiated both from other symptoms and from nonsymptoms. The PSE10 glossary can be examined to see how well this can be done. It should be read in conjunction with the PSE10 schedule, which contains brief definitions, suggests forms of questioning and provides numerous prompts as to how to conduct the interview.

The Glossary of Differential Definitions. The subjective experiences described to psychiatrists by patients, and the behavioral characteristics associated with them, particularly when personally distressing or socially disabling, provide the immediate but also the final target for preventive action. No matter how far "downstream" from possible genetic, neuroanatomical, and biochemical abnormalities, and no matter how diagnostic conventions change over the years, the chief aim is to prevent the phenomena occurring or to mitigate their severity, using whatever methods have been shown to be safe and effective. The phenomena may also provide clues to the nature of the underlying impairments. It is therefore necessary to continue efforts to make definitions as unambiguous and precise as possible, in order to promote comparability between tests of hypotheses about impairments, and thus also about causes, treatments, coping mechanisms and prognosis.

No selection of symptoms, and no set of definitions, will satisfy everybody. Nor should it, since few symptoms, at present, can be checked against external criteria. As Karl Koehler (1979) has observed, the only interesting question in such circumstances is whether divergent views about particular symptoms can be specified or not. Otherwise, one is led into interminable discussions about how many angels can dance on the point of a pin, a scholastic indulgence that Karl Jaspers and Kurt Schneider were careful to avoid. There is undoubtedly a risk in relying on criteria that are relatively straightforward and communicable (Berner, Gabriel, and Schanda, 1980, Berner and Kufferle, 1982). Concepts that cannot be explained may turn out to be valuable. Nevertheless, they must first reach the stage at which they can be understood and tested by others. Meanwhile, the more obscure the formulation, the less easy it is to test its significance.

Items that can only be defined vaguely or inconsistently tend to be excluded from schedules such as the PSE. *Praecox Gefühl*, for example, is regarded by some expert clinicians as an imprtant indicator for schizophrenia, and may indeed be so for them. It is indescribable, not because it is subjective but because it is idiosyncratic. Perhaps it can be handed down, ostensively, from professor to student, in which case it could be videotaped, analyzed, and standardized. The symptom may, in part, be based on flatness of affect, which can be defined behaviorally, but there are probably other elements, such as particular kinds of thought disorder, each of which can better be defined separately.

There must be good reasons for omitting symptoms, because the bottom-up approach requires the system to be over-inclusive, not simply aimed at the set of items specified by a particular nosology. The criteria suggested by C. M. Fisher (1983), for example, when he introduced neurologists to a syndrome he called *abulia minor* (a milder version of akinetic mutism), are all well known to psychiatrists because they were described by Kleist and Kretschmer before the war. They have to be included in order to allow tests of co-morbidity between so-called organic and so-called functional disorders.

A few examples may serve to illustrate these points.

DELUSIONS OF REFERENCE

The nature of a differential definition is illustrated by certain delusions of reference that can be mistaken for auditory hallucinations if the interviewer does not cross-examine when a respondent answers Yes to a question such as "Do you hear voices?" The proper continuation is to obtain a description in the respondent's own words before continuing to question in order to clarify the nature of the experience. The glossary definition of Delusions of Reference includes the following guidance: "If respondents think people are talking about them when in their presence, or making remarks intended for them to overhear, it is probable that they are misinterpreting, not hallucinating. Careful examination should enable the interviewer to judge whether one or the other symptom or both are present."

FEELING OF LOSS OF FEELING

The fact that subjective descriptions of a deficit in emotions do not have to be vague is illustrated by the symptom "feeling of loss of feeling," defined originally (as so often in phenomenology) by German writers, who regard it of major significance in the diagnosis of melancholia: *"Die Gefühllosigkeit wird gefühlt, die Erstarrung empfunden, die Leblosigkeit erlebt."* (Bleuler, E., 1983). This symptom was not included in PSE9 but it is added in PSE10. A draft of the glossary definition prepared by Paul Bebbington is as follows:

> Subjects complain that they have lost the ability to feel, to experience emotion. They can remember a time when they did have this capacity, though it might have been months or years ago, and are quite clear about losing it. A typical

example might be an elderly depressed woman who can no longer *feel* love for her grandchildren. She knows she does love them but the inability to feel the love causes distress. The symptom is commonly associated with a history of severely depressed mood and with other symptoms of depression but should be assessed on its own merits, irrespective of context. Differentiate from flatness of affect (q.v.).

The PSE schedule includes suggestions for questions to be used when the examiner reaches this item. They can be modified as necessary in accordance with the flow of answers to several previous items about mood: "Sometimes people don't describe sadness or depression as such but say they have lost the ability to feel any emotion at all. They can't feel sad or can't cry. Have you experienced such a lack?" Further probes follow if the answer is Yes. "What is it like?" "How severe has it been during . . . [period under review]?" "Have you been free of it at all?" "When did you last have ordinary feelings of happiness or sadness or other emotions?" A brief version of the definition is included in the text of the item: "This should be a definite loss compared with the normal state, but the loss need not have begun during the period under review." This is followed by a translation of Bleuler's words: "The loss of feeling is felt, the numbness perceived, the lifelessness experienced." The interviewer is free to ask as many more or as few questions as the context requires. It may occasionally happen that the respondent's spontaneous description, in answer to an earlier question, may provide all that is necessary for the decision.

In this way, the glossary definition, the suggested form and context of questioning, and the brief definition in the text, provide guidance to the examiner as to how to decide, from the respondent's description, whether the symptom is or is not present. The final decision rests with the examiner.

LOUD THOUGHTS

One of the symptoms that most obviously illustrates the importance of recognizing symptoms correctly is the subjective experience of hearing one's thoughts aloud, so loud, it would seem that someone standing nearby should be able to hear them. This experience may well provide a basis, when elaborated, for auditory hallucinations, and possibly for experiences such as thought insertion and thought broadcast. To test theories concerning its relationship to neurobiological functioning (e.g., Frith, 1987) requires reliable recognition.

WORRYING

"Loud thoughts" is a symptom taken from Part II of PSE10, which deals with psychotic, language, cognitive, and behavioral symptoms and signs. At the opposite end of the spectrum, an item such as "worrying" may play a significant part in a loose grouping of symptoms that can be associated with substantial social disablement and use of health services—an appropriate term for which might be "mental ill-health." Everybody worries if there is something to worry about. The definition excludes "normal" worrying by specifying three criteria: (a.) that there is a round of painful thought, which (b.) cannot be stopped simply by turning the attention elsewhere, and (c.) is out of proportion to the subject worried about. Use of the PSE by lay interviewers as a first screen in population surveys depends on training them to use such definitions (Wing, 1976).

The PSE9 glossary has now been incorporated into an implementation for lap computer, so that the definitions and instructions can be displayed on the screen whenever the interviewer is in doubt. A similar implementation is being developed for PSE10 and SCAN.

Reliability, and What it Means. The literature on how reliably items in successive versions of the PSE are rated is large and on the whole reassuring. The latest SCAN trials support this conclusion but the term "reliability" carries several possible connotations that should be distinguished. The reliability between interviewer and observer on a simple Yes or No answer to a clinical question is likely to be high but it is acquired at the price of uncertainty about the meaning of the answer. In the case of relatively common and easy to define items this should not be a serious problem. A question about autonomic symptoms of panic experienced when walking across a large empty space should be easy to understand and answer correctly. Interviews like the CIDI (Composite International Diagnostic Interview) (Robins et al., 1988) which restrict the interviewer to a series of designated questions and do not allow cross-examination about meaning, will nevertheless often obtain clinically appropriate as well as reliable information from ratings of these items. Similarly a short version of PSE9, consisting mainly of non-psychotic items, has been used with good reliability by lay interviewers in population surveys, and good agreement with subsequent clinical interview, though it was found that considerable attention had to be paid during training to prevent the threshold for rating being too low.

Obsessional symptoms, however, which are not within the experience of most people without special training, are difficult for lay interviewers to rate reliably. Many of the psychotic, cognitive, and behavioral items in Part II are well outside ordinary experience. Specialists need a good deal of training to recognize them.

A PSE symptom represents a concept that can be differentially defined with more or less clarity and accuracy. The definition is based on clinical descriptions that have been widely and frequently reported and, to that extent, verified. The technique of cross-examination matches what the respondent describes against the glossary definition. Reliability, in this sense, suggests more than agreement about whether the respondent answers Yes or No to a standard question. An important element in the variability of what different respondents understand by the question is also removed.

Classification

The Threshold for a "Case": Category and Dimension. Many surveys of general populations and of general practice settings have suggested a high prevalence of disorders, variously referred to as mental illness (Srole et al., 1962), preclinical neurosis (Taylor and Chave, 1964), minor neuroses (Shepherd et al., 1966), or depressive conditions (Brown et al., 1975), that are not referred for specialist advice (Goldberg and Huxley, 1980). During the course of a given year rather less than 1 percent of the population of countries with well-developed health services are referred for specialist advice or treatment (Wing and Hailey, 1972) whereas surveys of general practice in the U.K. suggest that 10–15 percent of those who visit their general practitioner during the course of a year complain about symptoms that can be regarded as psychiatric (Shepherd et al., 1966). Population surveys have suggested even higher proportions of undiagnosed "cases" (Srole et al., 1962).

The problems of diagnosis in this large group have been discussed by many authors, and methodological advance has been achieved by improving the reproducibility and reliability of the procedures used. The use of PSE9 to measure the presence of symptoms, syndromes, and disorders in samples of the general population provides further insight into its advantages and limitations and also gives rise to suggestions as to how the former can be increased and the latter reduced.

The Index of Definition (ID) incorporates a set of rules based on number, type, and severity of PSE9 symptoms that define eight levels of probability that sufficient information is available to allow a classification in terms of ICD8 (Wing, 1976; Wing et al., 1977, 1978). At the lowest level, there are no PSE9 symptoms at all. At level 4, there may be, for example, a single rating of moderately depressed mood without any further symptoms of a depressive disorder as defined by ICD8, with no other specific symptoms, and a total score, made up chiefly of non-specific symptoms, not higher than 10. At level 5, the minimum criteria for an ICD8 classification are met. Levels 6, 7, and 8 indicate increasing degrees of certainty and severity of disorder. The ID uses both categorical rules (loading of specific symptoms) and a dimensional criterion (total PSE9 score).

The results of studies using the ID (e.g., Bebbington et al., 1981; Brown and Harris, 1978; Henderson et al., 1979; Orley and Wing, 1979; Sturt et al., 1981; Urwin and Gibbons, 1979; Wing et al., 1981) must be interpreted within the usual limits—the purpose of the study, the quality of the interview, the presence of factors not covered by the PSE, the relevance of the previous clinical history, etc. Assuming that the project has been carried out with a full awareness of these factors, the ID provides a set of operational criteria for comparing samples drawn from a variety of populations, including all the levels of referral described by David Goldberg (Goldberg and Huxley, 1980). The comparisons can be made at below-threshold, as well as above-threshold, levels of probability, if that is required for the purposes of the project.

Comparison of the ID with global clinical judgment suggests that setting the threshold for a case at level 5 is in fairly good accordance with some clinical practice. The concordance can be improved by setting a PSE score of 15 rather than 10 as the dimensional part of the criteria for probability level 5, but at the expense of excluding a group with marginal conditions. Neither clinical judgment nor the application of operational criteria can answer the question "What is a case?," if the answer is understood to be a definition from left to right (see Chapter 1). The ID is useful only in so far as it helps to test theories, and that will usually require the use of the dimensional, the profile, and the categorical options of the PSE (Wing, Bebbington, and Robins, 1981).

The ID can be derived by a simple conversion program from PSE10 but only, at the moment, using the sections covered by PSE9.

Is Clinical Judgment a Disadvantage? Glyn Lewis and Paul Williams (1989) have argued that the use of clinical judgment in standardized interviews is a disadvantage because it reduces reliability and introduces observer bias. So far as unreliability is concerned the evidence provided is scanty; in fact the authors seem to agree that standardization reduces it. Their main concern is the distinction between depression and anxiety, which they think is made more sharply by doctors than would be the case in self-reports. The results of a complex statistical analysis of scores derived from the Clinical Interview Schedule (CIS: Goldberg et al., 1970) suggests that the clinical judgments made during the second part of the interview add little to the self-reported items in the first, so far as overall severity is concerned. Moreover, the clinicians' judgments on the presence of depression and anxiety show the two symptoms to be less correlated than is the case when the respondents' Yes or No is recorded.

The authors come to two conclusions about studies of "minor psychiatric disorders"—a categorical concept that they do not define but which must involve a differentiation from major disorders and possibly, the plural is ambiguous, between the minor disorders themselves. The first is that self-report scales should be used which provide sufficient information for the respondent to know "what is meant in psychiatric terms." Second, that self-report questionnaires or equivalent schedules administered by law interviewers are more useful for population surveys than instruments that incorporate clinical judgment.

So far as minor psychiatric disorder is concerned, a simple score is a useful measurement for many purposes. It correlates highly with a total PSE9 score. Using the latter when the former would do would be a clear case of the sledgehammer and the nut. But if the focus of enquiry were co-morbidity, for example the relationship of anxiety and depression in a population survey, the two concepts would have to be differentially defined. There is no evidence from the use of PSE9 in population surveys that psychiatrists are biased in their ratings one way or the other, compared with lay interviewers. Neither the CIS nor the GHQ would be more appropriate, since no definitions are supplied for the relevant items. Testing theories of depression like those of George Brown and Tirril Harris (1978) that are dimensional rather than categorical would require instruments that crossed these boundaries. Accepting the respondent's Yes or No to questionnaire items would not help much.

The authors assume that all "standardized interviews" are the same and end their paper with an unexceptional plea for a more exact specification of psychiatric phenomena. A comparison of the CIS and the CIDI shows how much progress has already been made. It could be postulated that the results of a survey using the CIDI would be similar to those obtained by lay or professional interviewers using the short version of PSE9, though the latter would probably take less time. The results of a survey of more severely ill people might turn out very differently. These are matters for empirical investigation. Meanwhile it is sensible to consider the psychometric characteristics and the practical track record of different instruments before choosing one that is particularly suited to the purpose of the project.

Validity: Cleaning the Syndromes, Measuring the Course, Finding Clues to Causes. Many of the issues discussed above are thought by the various protagonists to have a bearing on the validity of the diagnostic concepts used by psychiatrists. Lee Robins (1989) has pointed to ways in which standardized measuring techniques can remove ambiguities that must reduce validity simply by introducing noise into the diagnostic system. She is concerned chiefly with the clarification of inconsistent or vague diagnostic criteria and with the design of questions that, when asked by lay interviewers of lay respondents, will elicit Yes/No answers that indicate whether a target symptom is truly present or absent.

Whether such a procedure can be as successful with rare symptoms such as "loud thoughts," with which lay interviewers and respondents are unlikely to be familiar, as with common ones that everyone experiences, has been considered above. It is certainly true that cleaning the interview procedure will improve the accuracy with which a given symptom concept is recognized and that cleaning the diagnostic rules will improve the accuracy with which they operate on the symptoms to reach a classification. In fact, PSE10 has benefited from the experience of modifying some PSE9 items to a format suitable for insertion into the CIDI (Robins et al., 1988). Lee Robins' statement is also fair:

> At present we have no better standard for assessing psychiatric illness that the standardized interview. It may well be most accurate in the hands of a clinician, but it is not economically feasible to have all epidemiological studies carried out by psychiatrists, so long as lay interviewers do reasonably well.

Robert Kendell (1989) has addressed the problem of validity more directly, suggesting several strategies (leaving aside the appeal to the creative insight of great clinicians) for establishing validity. They boil down to three: using statistics to refine syndromes, predicting outcome, and finding biological correlates.

The statistical approach, both looking for internal consistency and seeking points of discontinuity between syndromes, has been quite energetically pursued without managing to prove or disprove very much. This may be due partly to the fact that symptoms appear and disappear over time, so that full syndromes are not displayed when measured in cross-section, although evident to the clinician who sees the course of the disorder. It must also be due in part to the hierarchy that seems to run through psychiatric classification, ensuring that disorders high in the hierarchy tend, in addition to their specific manifestations, to show the symptoms of disorders lower down (Foulds, 1965; Surt, 1981; Wing, 1978, chapter 3; Wing et al., 1974).

Outcome is a doubtful criterion for the same reasons and also, particularly in the case of disorders that may be reactive to adverse environmental influences (for example, if anxiety and depression are precipitated by different types of life events), because the respondent's circumstances change. Schizophrenia is problematic because of the difficulty of differentiating negative symptoms from other causes of lowered motivation (Wing, 1988). The fact that autism and schizophrenia appear to be distinct in almost every aspect of clinical course does not mean that there can be no element of shared aetiology, improbable though that appears (Frith and Frith, chapter 4).

The measurement of clinical course is a problem for standardized instruments. The CIDI solves it by producing a diagnosis for a range of time periods. SCAN concentrates on the clinical concept of "episodes," together with a Clinical Information Schedule that provides options for coding the presence of a broad range of contextual factors for a narrative summary in addition to symptom and syndrome scores and profiles, profiles of possible sub-categories, and diagnostic groupings according to the rules of ICD10 and DSM-IIIR.

Kendell suggests a number of indirect ways of studying aetiology and pathology, using clues from differential drug trials and kinship studies. These seem to present the most useful ways to refine and thus begin to validate syndromes.

Conclusion

The bottom-up tradition of the PSE has lasted continuously for over thirty years and the principles involved are more firmly embodied in its structure than ever. The database is comprehensively clinical.

A top-down perspective that was incorporated about twenty years ago has been given new solidity by the sponsorship of WHO and the link to the development of operational rules for ICD10. This, and the upcoming DSM-IV, are not, of course the only algorithms that will be applied.

The chief advantage of the SCAN system is the flexibility with which descriptive, dimensional, and categorical methods of analysis can be combined and interactions between them exploited for clinical scientific purposes. Diagnostic systems like ICD10 are by their nature ephemeral compromises and the next edition might reflect advances in understanding the nature of psychiatric disorders that require a radical modification of present diagnostic concepts. It is much less likely that the experiences and behaviors of people referred for specialist advice will change very much, though laboratory and other investigations will no doubt play a more specific part in diagnosis.

Systems such as SCAN seem likely to be found useful by at least one more generation.

References

American Psychiatric Association (1987) *Diagnostic and Statistical Manual of Mental Disorders,* third edition-revised. Washington, DC: APA.

Bebbington, P.E., Hurry, J., Tennant, C., Sturt, E. and Wing, J.K. (1981) Epidemiology of mental disorders in Camberwell. *Psychological Medicine* 11: 561–580.

Bentall, R.P., Jackson, H.F. and Pilgrim, D. (1988) Abandoning the concept of schizophrenia. *British Journal of Psychology* 27: 303–324.

Berner, P., Gabriel, E. and Schanda, H. (1980) Non-schizophrenic paranoid syndromes. *Schizophrenia Bulletin* 6: 627–632.

Berner, P and Kufferle, B. (1982) British phenomenological and psychopathological concepts: A comparative review. *British Journal of Psychiatry* 140: 558–565.

Bleuler, E. (1950) *Dementia Praecox or the Group of Schizophrenias*. Translated by Zinkin, J. from the 1911 edition. New York: International Universities Press.

Bleuler, E. (1983) *Lehrbuch der Psychiatrie*. Funfzehnte Auflage, neubearbeitet von Bleuler M,'s 233. Heidelberg: Springer-Verlag.

Brown, G.W. and Harris, T.O. (1978) *Social Origins of Depression: A Study of Psychiatric Disorder in Women*. London: Tavistock.

Brugha, T.S., Wing, J.K., Brewin, C.R., MacCarthy, B., Mangen, S., Lesage, A. and Mumford, J. (1988) The problems of people in long-term psychiatric daycare. An introduction to the Camberwell High Contact Survey. *Psychological Medicine* 18: 443–456.

Cooper, J.E., Kendell, R.E., Gurland, B.J., Sharpe, L., Copeland, J.R.M. and Simon, R. (1972) *Psychiatric Diagnosis in New York and London*. London: Oxford University Press.

Cooper, J.E. and McKenzie, S. (1981) The rapid prediction of low scores on a standardized psychiatric interview (PSE). In: *What is a Case?* (eds.) Wing, J. K., Bebbington, P. and Robins, L. N. London: Grant McIntyre.

Dubos, R. (1965) *Man Adapting*. New Haven: Yale University Press.

Fisher, C.M. (1983) Abulia minor versus agitated behavior. *Clinical Neurosurgery* 31: 9–31.

Foulds, G.A. (1965) *Personality and Personal Illness*. London: Tavistock.

Goldberg, D., Cooper, B., Eastwood, M.R., Kedward, H.B. and Shepherd, M. (1970) A standardized psychiatric interview for use in community surveys. *British Journal of Social and Preventive Medicine* 24: 18–23.

Goldberg, D. and Huxley, P. (1980) *Mental Illness in the Community: The Pathway to Psychiatric Care*. London: Tavistock.

Henderson, S., Duncan-Jones, P., Byrne, D.G., Scott, R. and Adcock, S. (1979) Psychiatric disorder in Canberra. A standardized study of prevalence. *Acta Psychiatrica Scandinavica* 60: 355–374.

Jablensky, A., Sartorius, N., Hirschfeld, R. and Pardes, H. (1983) Diagnosis and classification of mental disorders and alcohol- and drug-related problems. A research agenda for the 1980s. *Psychological Medicine* 13: 907–921.

Kendell, R.E. (1989) Clinical validity. *Psychological Medicine* 19: 45–55.

Kendell, R.E., Everitt, B., Cooper, J.E., Sartorius, N. and David, M.E. (1968) Reliability of the PSE. *Social Psychiatry* 3: 123–129.

Koehler, K. (1979) First rank symptoms of schizophrenia. Questions concerning clinical boundaries. *British Journal of Psychiatry* 134: 236–249.

Kraepelin, E. (1896) *Dementia Praecox*. Translated from fifth edition of Psychiatrie. In: Cutting, J. and Shepherd, M. (eds.) (1987) *The Clinical Roots of the Schizophrenia Syndrome*. Cambridge: University Press.

Kreitman, N. (1961) The reliability of psychiatric diagnosis. *Journal of Mental Science* 107: 876–886.

Lewis, G. and Williams, P. (1989) Clinical judgement and the standardized interview in psychiatry. *Psychological Medicine* 19: 971–979.

Lorr, M. (1966) *Explorations in Typing Psychotics*. London: Pergamon.

Luria, R.E. and Berry, R. (1979) Reliability and descriptive validity of the PSE syndromes. *Archives of General Psychiatry* 36: 1187–1195.

Luria, R.E. and McHugh, P.R. (1974) Reliability and clinical utility of the Wing PSE. *Archives of General Psychiatry* 30: 866–871.

McGuffin, P., Katz, R. and Aldrich, J. (1986) Past and present state examination. The assessment of 'lifetime ever' psychopathology. *Psychological Medicine* 16: 461–466.

O'Connor, N. (1968) The origins of the Medical Research Council Social Psychiatry Unit. In: Shepherd, M. and Davies, D.L. (eds.) *Studies in Psychiatry*. London: Oxford University Press.

Orley, J. and Wing, J.K. (1979) Psychiatric disorders in two African villages. *Archives of General Psychiatry* 36: 513–520.

Robins, L.N. (1989) Diagnostic grammar and assessment. Translating criteria into questions. *Psychological Medicine* 19: 57–68.

Robins, L.N., Wing, J.K., Wittchen, H-U., Helzer, J., Babor, T.F., Burke, J., Farmer, A., Jablensky, A., Pickens, R., Regier, D.A., Sartorius, N. and Towle, L.H. (1988) The Composite International Diagnostic Interview. *Archives of General Psychiatry* 45: 1069–1077.

Schneider, K. (1971) *Klinische Psychopathologie*. Stuttgart: Thieme.

Shepherd, M., Brooke, E., Cooper, J.E. and Lin, T.Y. (1968) An experimental approach to psychiatric diagnosis. *Acta Psychiatrica Scandinavica* Sup 201.

Shepherd, M., Cooper, B., Brown, A.C. and Kalton, G.W. (1966) *Psychiatric Illness in General Practice*. London: Oxford University Press.

Spitzer, R. and Endicott, J. (1968) Diagno: A computer program for psychiatric diagnosis utilizing the differential diagnostic procedure. *Archives of General Psychiatry* 18: 746–756.

Srole, L., Langner, T.S., Michael, S.T., Opler, M.K. and Rennie, T.A.C. (1962) *Mental Health in the Metropolis: The Midtown Manhattan Study*. New York: McGraw Hill.

Sturt, E. (1981) Hierarchical patterns in the distribution of psychiatric symptoms. *Psychological Medicine* 11: 783–794.

Taylor, S. and Chave, S. (1964) *Mental Health and Environment*. London: Longmans.

Tress, K.H., Bellenis, C., Brownlow, J.H., Livingston, G. and Leff, J.P. (1987) The PSE change rating scale. *British Journal of Psychiatry* 150: 201–207.

Urwin, P. and Gibbons, J.L. (1979) Psychiatric diagnosis in self poisoning patients. *Psychological Medicine* 9: 501–507.

Venables, P.H. (1957) A short scale for 'activity-withdrawal' in schizophrenics. *Journal of Mental Science* 103: 197–199.

Venables, P.H. and O'Connor, N. (1959) A short scale for rating paranoid schizophrenia. *Journal of Mental Science* 105: 815–818.

Venables, P.H. and Wing, J.K. (1962) Level of arousal and the subclassification of schizophrenia. *Archives of General Psychiatry* 7: 114–119.

Williams, P. (1986) The problem of diagnosis in psychiatric research. *Journal of the Royal Society of Medicine* 79: 1–2.

Wing, J.K. (1959) The measurement of behaviour in chronic schizophrenia. *Acta Psychiatrica et Neurologica* 35: 245–254.

Wing, J.K. (1961) A simple and reliable subclassification of chronic schizophrenia. *Journal of Mental Science* 107: 862–875.

Wing, J.K. (1962) Institutionalism in mental hospitals. *Journal of Social and Clinical Psychology* 1: 38–51.

Wing, J.K. (1976) A technique for studying psychiatric morbidity in in-patient and out-patient series and in general population samples. *Psychological Medicine* 6: 665–671.

Wing, J.K. (1976) Kanner's syndrome. A historical introduction. In: Wing, L. (ed.) *Early Childhood Autism*, chapter 1. Oxford: Pergamon.

Wing, J.K. (1978) *Reasoning about Madness*. London: Oxford University Press.

Wing, J.K. (1983) Use and misuse of the PSE. *British Journal of Psychiatry* 143: 111–117.

Wing, J.K. (1988) Comments on the long term outcome of schizophrenia. *Schizophrenia Bulletin* 14: 669–672.

Wing, J.K., Bebbington, P.E. and Robins, L.N. (1981) Theory testing in psychiatric epidemiology. In: *What is a Case? The Problem of Definition in Psychiatric Community Surveys*. (eds.) Wing, J.K., Bebbington, P.E. and Robins, L.N. London: Grant McIntyre.

Wing, J.K., Birley, J.L.T., Cooper, J.E., Graham, P. and Isaacs, A.D. (1967) Reliability of a procedure for measuring and classifying 'present psychiatric state.' *British Journal of Psychiatry* 113: 499–515.

Wing, J.K., Cooper, J.E. and Sartorius, N. (1974) *The Description and Classification of Psychiatric Symptoms: An Instruction Manual for the PSE and CATEGO System*. London: Cambridge University Press.

Wing, J.K. and Hailey, A.H. (eds.) (1972) *Evaluating a Community Psychiatric Service. The Camberwell Register 1964–1971*. London: Oxford University Press.

Wing, J.K., Nixon, J.M., Mann, S.A. and Leff, J.P. (1977) Reliability of the PSE (ninth edition) used in a population survey. *Psychological Medicine* 7: 505–516.

Wing, J.K., Mann, S.A., Leff, J.P. and Nixon, J.M. (1978) The concept of a 'case' in psychiatric population surveys. *Psychological Medicine* 8: 203–217.

Wing, L. (1981) Asperger's syndrome. *Psychological Medicine* 11: 115–129.

Wing, L. (1991) This volume, Chapter 6.

Wing, L. (in press) The relationship between Asperger's syndrome and Kanner's autism. In: Frith, U. (ed.) Asperger's syndrome.

Wittenborn, J.R. (1955) *Wittenborn Psychiatric Rating Scales*. New York: Psychological Corporation.

World Health Organization (1973) *The International Pilot Study of Schizophrenia*. Geneva: WHO.

World Health Organization (1990) *International Classification of Diseases*, tenth edition. Geneva: WHO.

8

The Measurement of Need

Steen Mangen and Chris R. Brewin

> *For the practitioner, the problem of managing clients becomes the problem of successfully managing the concept of social need. For the social scientist, the problem of understanding social need becomes, in part, the problem of understanding the management techniques that the practitioner employs*
>
> —Smith, 1980

Introduction

The relationship between need and resource allocation lies at the heart of social planning. But there are major difficulties in conceptualizing needs, and in the absence of reliable measurement there can be no proof of the allocative efficiency of public services. These shortcomings are also manifest in legislation on health and social services in which the concept of need tends to be treated as unproblematic. It is not surprising, then, to hear the view expressed that a complex bureaucratic organization such as the British National Health Service "cannot display a ready assessment of the effectiveness with which it is meeting . . . needs" (Griffith Report, 1988). Weaknesses of this kind have been exacerbated by the increasingly precarious nature of the funding of the mental health care system in the contemporary welfare state, the current planning basis of which has been characterized by Webb and Wistow (1986) as a "flight from need."

One consequence of the lack of reliable measurement of need is that much of the funding of psychiatric care may be mis-allocated. Moreover, the conflicting goals and the organizational constraints imposed by the complex of mental health services and allied provisions such as social security routinely lead to a mismatch of patients' needs with service provision. The lack of dynamism in the delivery of the total care package and the failure to coordinate monitoring to respond swiftly to an individual's changing needs reinforces the doubts that we are obtaining the best value for our money (Abel-Smith, 1976; Wing and Hailey, 1972). Similar views are expressed in the 1986 Audit Commission Report whose authors, in reviewing the transfer from hospital to community care, express wonder that any schemes were successful, given the bureaucratic complexity within which they had to work. Without remedial action, current government policies can be expected to make matters worse: the "mixed economy" of welfare, a care system encompassing public, voluntary and private services, as well as formal and informal care, significantly extends the number of agencies whose actions must be incorporated if planning for need is to have any feasibility. Funding policies in the eighties which prescribe a fuller exploitation of existing resource allocations, rather than a reliance on new ones, serve to add to the urgency of the problem (see, for example, DHSS, 1983).

Conceptualizing Need

Although the problem of psychiatric need has preoccupied researchers, planners and providers of mental health care, it is only comparatively recently that serious attempts have been made to elaborate the concept. Given the routine pressures of clinical practice, there has been an irresistible tendency to regard need as a given, and in much of empirical psychiatric research analysis there have typically been no more than desultory references to generalized "hierarchies" or "taxonomies" of need such as those developed by Maslow (1954) or Bradshaw (1972). Contemporary research interest is in part an attempt to redress the deficiencies of a precipitate rush to empiricism and also to meet the demands of planners for reliable planning instruments. Models of need which have been proposed more recently, some of which are reviewed here, have been concerned to advance conceptual clarity by addressing the problems of relativity and subjectivity of need and its conflation with "wants" and "demand."

Miller (1976) underpins his theory of social justice by utilizing what he terms a "plan of life," which, in part, forms the basis of an individual's sense of identity. According to Miller's scheme, essential needs which contribute to the fulfillment of this life plan and are left unmet cause that person "harm" and justify compensatory action. Miller has formulated three categories of need: "instrumental need" (x needs y in order to achieve z); "functional need" (needs which must be fulfilled in order that a function can be performed); and "intrinsic need" (principles of social and territorial justice). Miller's harm principle is a valuable means of distinguishing "want" from "need" (e.g., the alcoholic wants drink but needs drying out—an instrumental need) and, equally important, his model is sensitive to the individual subject and his or her sub-cultural norms.

Another valuable contribution, albeit again in a pre-operational state, is the theory of need formulated by Doyal and Gough (1984). These authors argue the futility of individualistic conceptions of need which fail to locate subjects within their social and historical contexts. The subjectivity and confusion between wants and need can be overcome, they claim, by defining "basic individual needs" for, on the one hand, survival and physical and mental health and, on the other, for autonomy and learning. These needs are essential to the person's creative consciousness and are basic in the sense that they have to be satisfied before other needs can be met. This initial component of their theory most closely approaches our own work. However, the authors go on to propose four societal needs which, if unfulfilled, will frustrate the individual's attempts to satisfy basic needs. These societal needs refer to production, reproduction, culture and communication, and political authority. Doyal and Gough interpret the interactive effect of successfully meeting these two levels of needs as promoting human liberation by maximizing individual and collective choice.

Analyses of the relationship between need and resource allocation have also been significant. At a general level, the efficiency of any social service must be judged in terms of the matching of need to resources. Effectiveness of psychiatric treatments then becomes subsumed under definitions of efficiency, since an ineffective service must automatically be considered a waste of scarce resources that could be utilized elsewhere. When evaluating options, the most efficient mental health provision must be the one that meets needs at the lowest level of resource consumption or, alternatively, the one that meets most needs at a fixed resource input. This discussion is taken up in more detail by Mangen (1988) and the conceptualization of efficiency is expanded by Davies and Challis (1986).

Rationing theory provides the conceptual link between need and resource allocation. Rationing criteria attempt to match need with resources in a way that promotes the highest level of allocative efficiency. Put another way, rationing is concerned with distributive justice, that is, with the reconciliation of competing claims for scarce resources. Thus, rationing is not narrowly confined to economic principles in administering the supply of goods and services, but incorporates social and ethical considerations such as equality of access to treatment. All these considerations are critically influenced by the personal predilections and professional ideologies of those determining the specific system of rationing process (Smith, 1980). Moreover, in practical application, the ability to plan and implement effective rationing strategies supposes a certain stability of resource inputs over time (Glennerster, 1985). In view of the current vagaries of funding health and social services, this is not an entirely unproblematic assumption.

The MRC Needs Assessment Procedure

Our current approach to measuring need in long-term psychiatric patients has been developed from the work of John Wing on the planning and evaluation of psychiatric services (Wing, 1972, 1978, 1986). The present model involves a four stage process. At the first stage, we identify the presence of *social disablement,* defined as lowered physical, psychological, and social functioning, compared with what would ordinarily be expected, in a particular society, of a typical individual. The second level is concerned with methods of *care* that are thought to be effective and acceptable means of reducing or containing the components of social disablement. The term 'care' is used in a broad sense to encompass all interventions from the most active treatment to the most passive form of shelter. At the third stage the therapeutic *agents* (e.g., psychiatrists, general practitioners, nurses etc.) capable of undertaking these interventions are identified. Finally, the appropriate organization of agents into *agencies* (e.g., self-help groups, day hospitals, hostels) for the coordinated delivery of care is considered. These agencies collectively form the total "need for service" of the individual patient.

Social disablement may be considered as a series of "wants" or "problems" presented by the individual patient. In some cases these are accompanied by the "wants" and "problems" of relatives who live with or take care of the patient. These wants and problems are then legitimized as "needs" for care and services by others—in this case by professionals who are afforded allocative discretionary powers through the exercise of their expertise. In many circumstances—particularly in non-technical areas—the individual's articulation of wants corresponds totally with the judgments of professionals concerning needs. Nonetheless, in our model, the individual cannot be the final arbiter of needs, for their resolution depends on (a) expert knowledge, (b) the integration of information from patients, families, and involved professionals, and (c) the reconciliation of competing wants. Our procedure, then, relies on professional judgment— "normative" need to use Bradshaw's (1972) terminology—and makes the assumption that a substantial clinical consensus among "experts" is achievable. It is an attempt to formalize and structure what is good clinical practice. This process is shown diagramatically in Figure 8.1

A previous study of the long-term mentally ill carried out in the Social Psychiatry Unit (Wykes et al., 1982) assessed needs for services and for broad categories of intervention under ten headings. Judgments of met and unmet need were made by a research team using information from patients, staff, relatives, and case records. Subsequent work has led to the development of separate instruments to measure needs for care and needs for services. The MRC Needs for Care Assessment (Brewin et al., 1987) was an attempt to standardize Wykes and colleagues' judgments, to increase the number of areas of functioning covered, and to extend the level of analysis down to more specific types of care. Another procedure was then devised for translating needs for care into needs for services. The following sections describe in detail the rationale behind and the methods used in the most recent versions of these assessments.

Measuring Needs for Care

Our definition of need is based on the principle that, for need to exist, some item of care must be identified that might reduce or ameliorate social disablement. In other words, actions by care staff are not legitimized simply by the existence of social disablement, but by a further set of rules indicating whether action is appropriate or inappropriate. This leads to the following definitions of need for care:

1. Need is present when (a) a patient's functioning (social disablement) falls below or threatens to fall below some minimum specified level, and (b) this is due to a remediable, or potentially remediable, cause.

2. A need (as defined above) is met when it has attracted some at least partly effective item of care and when no other items of care of greater potential effectiveness exist.

3. A need (as defined above) is unmet when it has attracted only partly effective or no item of care and when other items of care of greater potential effectiveness exist.

These definitions are represented in Figure 8.2, which specifies how assessments of social disablement and assessments of items of care are combined to yield judgments concerning need. Figure 8.2 implies the necessity for assumptions about which areas of social disablement are important, which interventions are appropriate for different types of social disablement, and what constitutes effectiveness. In effect, a set of such wide-ranging assumptions add up to a simplified model of ideal practice in the care of the long-term mentally ill, and we have deliberately attempted to mimic the process of decision-making as it might be carried out by a

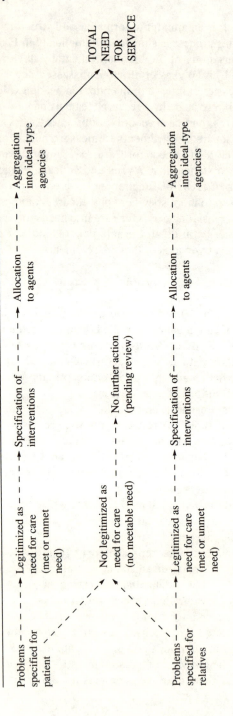

FIGURE 8.1
The MRC Needs Assessment Procedure

FIGURE 8.2
Assessment of functioning, assessment of interventions, and need status

Assessment of functioning	Assessment of interventions	Need status
No problem or mild problem	None employed	No need
Significant current or recent problem	None even partly effective	No meetable need
	Some potentially fully effective	Met need
	None fully effective: no alternatives	Met need
	None fully effective: alternatives available	Unmet need for treatment
Level of functioning not known		Unmet need for assessment

clinical team. We now briefly discuss these assumptions, which are presented in more detail in Brewin et al. (1987).

Assessing Social Disablement

Behind the definition of this concept lie notions of physical and psychological health, and of a *core of competence*. For our purposes, these notions were conceived as minimal acceptable levels of health and competence. Thus, health was defined in terms of the absence of various kinds of symptoms rather than in terms of the achievement of positive health goals. Similarly, the core of competence was defined in terms of the minimum skills required to function independently in the community, rather than in terms of higher level skills that might maximize the individual's autonomy and quality of life.

The symptoms and competencies covered in the second version of the MRC Needs for Care Assessment are shown in Figure 8.3. Ratings reflect whether symptoms are current (i.e., were present in the past month), absent in the past month but recently present, or completely absent. The distinction between "current" and "recent" symptoms is necessary in order that items of care offered for purely preventive purposes can be rated appropriately. In exceptional cases, for example, a slow-cycling manic-depressive disorder, patients can be rated as having a "recent" problem even though they have been symptom-free for two years or more.

FIGURE 8.3
Areas of functioning covered in Version 2 of the Needs for Care Assessment

Symptoms and behavior problems
Positive psychotic symptoms
Retardation (slowness and underactivity)
Side effects of medication
Neurotic symptoms
Organic brain disorder
Physical disease and disorders
Violence or threats to self/others
Socially embarrassing behavior
Distress about social circumstances

Personal and social skills
Personal cleanliness
Household shopping
Cooking or buying meals
Household chores
Use of public transport
Use of public amenities
Basic literacy and arithmetic skills
Occupational skills
Social interaction skills
Management of money
Management of household affairs

Our approach to the measurement of social functioning in this often severely impaired group has been to itemize the presence or absence of basic skills, such as cooking, shopping, and budgeting. Our original decisions about which skills were essential have been validated against the judgments of an independent group of rehabilitation care staff (Brewin et al., 1987). We also distinguish between *lack of competence* and *lack of performance*. Lack of competence means that a skill has never been acquired or has been lost, whereas lack of performance means that, in spite of knowing what to do, a person nevertheless fails to demonstrate skilled performance. This may occur through lack of interest, lack of opportunity, or some other reason. In determining the minimum acceptable levels of social functioning, it may be important not to insist that all patients should regularly perform all the skills listed. To do this would leave no room for freedom of choice on the part of patients and their relatives, and might create apparent need where none in fact existed. In our view, the minimum acceptable level of functioning is that the patient should possess competence in all basic social and personal skills, so that he or she can exercise choice about whether or not to perform them. Lack of competence is always, therefore, unacceptable. In certain rare cases, for example when acute symptoms disrupt functioning in an otherwise competent individual, lack of performance may also require intervention and this can be rated separately.

Choice of respondents is often crucial in assessing social disablement. Analysis of data from the Camberwell High Contact survey (Brewin et al., 1990) indicates that underactivity and impaired social interaction are more likely to be identified by day care staff than from a clinical interview with the patient, whereas neurotic symptoms are more likely to be identified by the clinical interview. Symptoms and behavior problems are more likely to be identified by interviewing relatives or hostel staff than by either of the two former methods. These data indicate that interviewing relatives or hostel staff is of critical importance for an accurate assessment of social disablement. A reasonable approximation of social competencies may, however, be obtained by interviewing patients themselves (MacCarthy et al., 1986).

Assessing Items of Care

In each area of social disablement, the Needs for Care assessment specifies a list of 2 to 8 appropriate items of care, covering such diverse types of care as medication, counselling, behavior programs, remedial education, and the provision of a sheltered environment. Our aim was to be over- rather than under-inclusive, and this meant including items of care not necessarily in widespread use, although we judged them to be generally acceptable to professionals. The original list of items of care was also validated against the judgments of rehabilitation care staff (Brewin et al., 1987), and has been slightly amended in the light of subsequent empirical work. In each area of social disablement there is the facility to add a specific item of care that seems appropriate but does not figure on the standard list.

Each item of care receives a single rating by the investigator that indicates whether or not it has been tried, how effective it was, whether or not it was acceptable to the patient, and whether or not it is currently appropriate. This rating is based on an interview with a key worker or with other appropriate staff. The investigator must determine whether items of care have received an adequate trial from a properly qualified or supervised person and must solicit evidence for the effectiveness or otherwise of the intervention. Rules exist to help decide how long to persevere with one form of care before trying another and to decide when ineffective or unacceptable items of care should be tried or offered again. Staff members are similarly questioned about the appropriateness of the various alternative items of care, but the final judgment on the rating is the investigator's.

Assessing Need Status

Need status in each area of social disablement is derived algorithmically from consideration of the level of disablement and the ratings given to items of care. The level of disablement is effectively matched with the level of care provided, permitting an estimate of under-, over-, or appropriate provision. Primary need status falls into four categories, "met need," "unmet need," "no need," and "no meetable need" (the last two categories have in previous reports been collapsed together as "no need"). "Met need" indicates that there is current or recent disablement but that the patient is receiving an effective or potentially effective item of care. When the items of care being employed are clearly insufficient, although worth continuing, a rating of "met need" indicates that no other potentially effective items of care exist. "Unmet need" indicates that there is current disablement, that no current items of care are fully effective, and that potentially more effective alternatives do exist. An "unmet need" for assessment is also rated when the presence or absence of current disablement is not known. Finally, "no need" indicates that there is no disablement, and "no meetable need" that there is disablement but there are no items of care currently feasible and appropriate.

The fact that wants or problems can only be legitimized as needs if there are currently feasible or appropriate interventions deserves further comment. This principle follows logically from our definition of need as a requirement for some specifiable form of care. Hence, if all forms of care are inappropriate, have proven to be ineffective, or have been refused by the patient, need cannot be said to exist. Instead, the individual will be rated by our methods as having a problem but no meetable need. An example from another area of medicine will illustrate this situation. Patients with terminal cancers may *want* a cure, but from the perspective of the service providers they do not have a meetable *need* for a cure so long as the cancer is untreatable by currently available methods. The same patients may, on the other hand, be in pain and distressed, two problems for which interventions do exist. It therefore makes sense to say that they have a need for pain relief and for counselling. To say that terminal cancer patients *need* a cure may be a useful statement for clinical researchers who can set about inventing or developing one. The statement has little meaning for clinicians or planners, however, since there are no immediate service implications.

Problems with no associated meetable needs do occur from time to time with the long-term mentally ill, and were found to account for approximately 6 percent of identified problems in the Camberwell High Contact Survey (Brewin et al., 1988). It seems to us essential to be able to distinguish in this way those problems for which no effective care can realistically be offered at present. While recognizing the limitations of current forms of care, this in no way vitiates the obligation of agents to develop new and more effective interventions or to persevere in the future with interventions that may have been unacceptable or ineffective in the past. Indeed, future repetitions of the Needs for Care Assessment would make this duty explicit. The concept of a problem with no meetable need highlights the very important fact that professional knowledge and practice are inadequate to meet all our patients' problems.

In addition to the primary need status, the assessment permits three secondary judgments to be made in each area of disablement. *Overprovision* is rated whenever one or more items of care are rated as being superfluous. In some cases this will be because an item of care continues to be given even though it is not aimed at a specific problem or appears to be completely ineffective. In other cases the rating reflects that the patient is in receipt of an item of care even though there has been no disablement for a considerable period of time, and there is no apparent danger of relapse. *Future need* can be rated when a patient is currently socially disabled but cannot receive the appropriate item of care because of incapacitating symptoms or other priorities for intervention. *Lack of performance* is rated when a patient is known to be socially competent in some area of functioning and is not receiving any care, but is not currently exercising that skill. The intention here is to draw attention to a possible area in which action might be required. In the Camberwell High Contact Survey (Brewin et al., 1988) instances of overprovision were found to be as common as were unmet needs for treatment, but future needs and "lack of performance" were relatively rare.

Reliability and Validity

Initial data on the reliability and validity of the assessment are presented in Brewin et al. (1987, 1988). Clearly, estimates of validity can only be limited ones given that, by definition, need involves the making of value judgments and that no other comparable definitions and measures of need exist. Validity is also likely to be limited by cultural factors, such as the appropriateness of acquiring such skills as cooking and housework in some Mediterranean societies (see Lesage et al., 1990). Perhaps the most practical approach to validity would be to have a group of patients independently assessed before and after an intervention phase in which the Needs for Care Assessment was used to structure the care provided. Ideally, patients would be randomly assigned to structured needs assessment versus a traditional review of their treatment.

Some recent data do, however, shed light on the reliability of the procedure. Lesage et al. (1990) employed an Italian version of the assessment in a study of psychiatric services in South Verona. The primary need status of sixty-one identified problems found in twenty patients was independently rated by one Camberwell-trained judge and by two Italian judges. The three judges showed a high level of agreement (kappa = .92, p < .0001), correctly identifying a relatively high level of unmet need among this subset of problems.

The needs of patients from two different geographical areas attending the same day hospital have recently been assessed in two independent studies. One group (N = 11) were assessed as part of the Camberwell High Contact Survey (Brewin et al., 1988; Brugha et al.,*1988) and the other (N = 66) as part of a survey of day care in an inner city (Wainwright et al., 1988). Both studies used the MRC Needs for Care Assessment, although whereas Brewin et al. had a team of independent investigators interviewing patient, day staff, and relatives, Wainwright et al. adapted the assessment for use by a single investigator interviewing patient and day staff only. Despite these procedural differences the results of the two studies were very similar. Brewin et al. identified a mean of 5.27 clinical and social problems per patient, of which 28 percent were rated as unmet needs. Wainwright et al. identified on average 6.4 problems per patient, of which 30 percent were rated as unmet needs. These two studies suggest that the measure has good reliability in the hands of suitably trained investigators, and is robust enough to tolerate minor procedural deviations.

The Needs of Relatives

The needs identified in the Needs for Care Assessment are those of the patient rather than those of the relatives or supporters with whom the patient may live. It is important to recognize that relatives and supporters may have quite separate problems and needs arising from their situation that are either complementary to, or may at times conflict with, the needs of the person with a psychiatric illness. Recent studies have documented the sometimes very considerable burden that relatives carry (Creer et al., 1982; Creer and Wing, 1974; Fadden et al, 1987; Kuipers and Bebbington, 1985), and that may have to be considered as part of a total care package.

A procedure was therefore developed to assess the problems and needs for care of relatives in a way analogous to that used with the patients (MacCarthy et al, 1989). Seven problems specifically related to living with a psychiatric patient were specified that, if present, might be expected to prevent a supporter from maintaining an adequate quality of life for themselves. These were: (a) unwillingness to reside with the patient; (b) financial hardship, failure to receive available social payments, or inadequate housing; (c) unavailability of holiday relief; (d) inadequate contact with care staff; (e) inadequate information and coping advice; (f) excessive emotional burden; (g) childcare difficulties brought about by the presence of the patient. Once a problem was identified, evidence was sought that an appropriate intervention had been tried within the past year, and the effectiveness of any interventions tried was assessed. This enabled judgments of "met need," "unmet need," and "no need" to be made and appropriate items of care to be considered as part of an overall package for patient and supporter.

Measuring Needs for Service

The aim of the Needs for Service procedure is to translate needs for care into requirements for interventions, agents, and agencies that collectively form the "ideal-type" needs for service for an individual patient. The assessment procedure identifies five areas for intervention: symptomatology, behavioral problems, and social skills deficits; occupational and industrial therapy requirements; interventions to combat deficits in leisure (these two latter need areas are intended to enhance creative skills); housing requirements; and deficits in material welfare. The underlying assumption is that service delivery should be oriented towards equipping patients for as "normal" and independent a lifestyle as their disablement permits, and one which, wherever possible, utilizes separate environments for work, leisure, and home.

As with the Needs for Care Assessment, the evaluation of needs for services takes into account short- and medium-term interventions. To circumvent difficult ethical problems surrounding needs such as sexual satisfaction, the profile encompasses only those needs which could potentially be met by a formal therapeutic agent, even though in practice, when particular circumstances permitted, many needs were treated as being appropriate for intervention by the patients themselves or by their families or friends.

According to the lexicon of our assessments, elements of care are provided by therapeutic *agents* who possess a set of differentiated roles. To facilitate and structure the interaction of these roles, the agents may organize into *agencies* which maximize the efficient distribution of specialist knowledge and thus contribute to the effective allocation of therapeutic resources. Agencies may be professional (e.g., hospitals or clinics) or informal (e.g., self-help groups) or mixes; they may be multi-agent (for example, a pluridisciplinary day hospital) or predominantly a single agent type (for example, a group of occupational therapists in a workshop). Individual interventions are therefore undertaken by one agent or a variety of agents who may be grouped into one or several agencies. These agencies form the total service package for the patient. Such services form networks according to the degree of coordination that is feasible. Significantly, in determining needs for services, the assessment procedure is not constrained by considerations of present forms of collaboration between agents, either within an existing agency or between agencies. Moreover, because the aim is to construct ideal-type services matched to the needs of individual patients, assessments are deliberately naive to local problems of organization, management, or professional politics that could render implementation difficult.

For each problem where a met or unmet need for care is established, one or more voluntary or professional agents are identified who can provide what we conceived as the "minimum effective therapeutic intervention" to alleviate or contain the presenting problem—something akin to a minimum therapeutic dose. These agents are also allocated in cases where there is no present need but where an intervention is required as a preventive measure. The agents specified range from the individual himself, his family, and mutual aid groups through to nurses, social workers, psychologists, and psychiatrists. Agents are classified in an order crudely approximating a broad notion of "opportunity cost," that is, the value of their intervention if put to alternative uses in mental health. Thus, volunteers are rated as "lower opportunity cost" agents compared with nurses who, in turn, are "lower opportunity cost" agents in relation to psychiatrists.

Even when "lower opportunity cost" agents seem suitable for the specified task, we take into consideration whether this solution is appropriate in the context of a wider therapeutic program. There are frequently situations where, although in isolation the need might suggest an intervention by a "lower opportunity cost" agent, the task is allocated to a "higher opportunity cost" agent because, for example, it contributes to the consolidation of a therapeutic relationship. In addition, we identify "secondary agents" who are essential in sustaining the activities of the prime intervening agents (for example, a community psychiatric nurse as principal agent might require regular consultative support from a psychiatrist as a secondary agent). For each care area an estimate is made of the frequency and duration of the intervention as well as the potential for short-term changes in the intensity of interventions. After consideration of each need for care, a total intervention profile emerges of the agents required currently or in the immediate future. In addition, the patient's residential requirements and the service needs of relatives are specified.

It may be that a type of agency currently existing is the most appropriate base from which to organize the total service to the patient (for example, a need for frequent interventions by a psychiatrist, nurse, and occupational therapist may indicate a need for some form of day hospital rather than a day center). However, in such circumstances the needs assessments do not necessarily imply that current practices (e.g., the specific therapies or attendance patterns) within them are recommended to continue. Alternatively, a needs profile may emerge that indicates a potentially new type of agency, because it calls for agents who under existing arrangements are organizationally discrete (for example, a total care package that includes a befriender, a community psychiatric nurse, and a remedial teacher). Judgments that organizationally discrete agents are required do not automatically lead to recommendations for new institutional arrangements—in many situations there are individual agents who do not need to be located permanently in the main service setting.

In making overall placement decisions, various optional ways of combining the different elements of the service package may be considered and "single-best" solutions avoided, although disposal decisions for each subject can be prioritized. Profiles of total needs for services that are broadly equivalent among patients suggest the existence of group needs. The extent to which these broad categories of group need emerge may be an indication of the viability of planning a "network" of services.

The assessment procedures are an attempt to incorporate both micro- and macro-level planning concerns; that is, they address issues of direct concern to clinical decision-making and to the planning of services at the health district level. Again, we should emphasize that our approach does not naively impose a rigidity of professional roles, and we accept that, in practical application, the patient's predicaments, the feasibility of delivering new interventions in the short term, and changing therapeutic relationships will heavily influence immediate disposal decisions. Clearly, since on the whole long-term care management is non-technical, there are a wide range of possible alternative ways of delivering required interventions. The aim of the MRC procedures is to make explicit allocative criteria and establish baseline measurements for outcomes, rather than to impose any kind of therapeutic "blueprint." In this way they are intended to contribute to the development of effective evaluation and monitoring, a task to which the Griffiths Report attaches the utmost significance.

Discussion

Our research has had two principal goals: to contribute to conceptual formulation and to offer assessments that have immediate practical planning uses by generating reliable empirical data. We have attempted to introduce greater specificity to the concept of need by distinguishing and defining needs for care and needs for services. By linking need to resource consumption, our intention is to operationalize need as a useful tool in the planning process. Our central task has been to analyze the need-resource relationship in terms of the inputs (e.g., personnel, buildings etc.) and outputs (e.g., number of interventions offered) and the potential outcomes achievable by psychiatric services. Each assessment takes into account the legitimacy of the problem as a need, the effectiveness of the appropriate intervention and the differential feasibilities of the agents undertaking the intervention. To achieve our research goals we have also made explicit the desired ends in terms of the minimum acceptable behavioral, psychological, or welfare outcomes. The criteria, of course, can be contended, but at least there are clear benchmarks by which to determine the relevance of empirical results for the planning of services elsewhere.

Our procedures focus on a specific set of needs critical to the promotion of mental health and the limitation of mental disability, and utilize a "bottom up" as opposed to "top down" planning strategy. Importantly, assessments of needs for care and for services are not constrained by current institutional practices, and determining the appropriate agent for the required intervention precedes identification of the agency and total service requirement. This allows investigators to consider combinations of agents not currently working together who collectively might be the most effective deliverers of the total care package. The approach avoids the circular logic of defining needs in terms of current practices, current availability of services, or current organizational structures.

The monitoring of needs is a sensitive exercise: scanning too wide or too often can lead to an inappropriate action on ephemeral or "low priority" problems that might remit spontaneously. An effective monitoring system, in any case, is likely to generate additional demand by identifying new and unmet needs which, in the absence of additional resources, may lead to stricter rationing criteria in subsequent assessments. An overzealous system can also be experienced by patients and families as oppressive, especially in situations where they feel they are being selected out as belonging to marginalized "at risk" populations in need of close management (Castel, 1981). The complaints of ethnic minorities about their treatment by mental health services bear on this issue. Equally, failing to monitor needs sufficiently regularly can lead to misuse of scarce resources, and to the danger that patients' autonomy will be reduced rather than enhanced. The Royal College of Psychiatrists recently expressed concern about these issues in a report on deinstitutionalization policies now gaining pace in Britain when it drew attention to the "fine line between liberty and neglect." Further research is required to determine whether the MRC procedures strike the right balance between identifying too few and too many needs.

Among the limitations of our procedures is that, in order to be useful clinically, they must be repeated at regular intervals. Needs for care in particular are not static but are expected to change in response to improvement and deterioration in clinical condition, to the coming and going of staff, to the formation or loss of significant relationships, and to many other factors. This suggests that for clinical purposes needs for care assessments should be repeated at biannual or yearly intervals. This would almost certainly be true of other similar assessments, however.

A second limitation is that relatively little attention appears to be paid to patients' own definitions of their "needs"—indeed, these would be labelled as "wants" rather than as needs in our terminology. We have explained that one reason for our preference for "expert-defined" need is because service providers allocate scarce resources and have to decide what is clinically feasible. We also believe it essential that services should start out with a clear idea of potential areas of need rather than relying solely on patients to articulate them. While some patients would be more than able to articulate their wants, it is unrealistic to expect all to do so regardless of such factors as their education, clinical condition, and expectations. We have therefore opted for a procedure that in almost all cases can use information supplied by the patient to identify potential problem areas, and recognizes patients' rights to veto suggested interventions. There is also scope for patients' unique problems, whether raised by themselves or by members of staff, to be included as additional needs.

From an organizational and clinical perspective, the monitoring of needs is an iterative process by which alternative solutions to eradicate patients' problems and ways of coordinating and effectively implementing the appropriate interventions are assessed. This may require new working styles and new forms of collaboration among the many agencies now involved in mental health. This raises problems of funding, administrative responsibility, therapeutic competence, professional territoriality and training—issues which were beyond the scope of the present approach. Funding implications will vary according to local circumstances but, in areas where community-based provisions are significantly below those officially recommended, there may be considerable scope to transfer resources from the inpatient to the community sector, at least in the middle run. The issue of administrative responsibility is not directly addressed by our approach, that is, whether new "ideal" service types should be managed by the public, voluntary or private sector.

Despite these limitations, the MRC Needs for Care Assessment does set explicit minimum standards of care and enables services to be evaluated and compared in a meaningful way. The Needs for Services schedule permits innovatory patterns of services to be considered by requiring the investigator to assess the degree of surrogacy that is feasible both at the individual agent and agency levels. Confronted by the many resistances to change, it has frequently been easier to create a new service and a new professional specialism than to change existing practices. In the present climate of the welfare state that option now seems luxurious, and flexibility both between and within agencies is manifestly high on the agenda of policy priorities.

References

Abel-Smith, B. (1976) *Value for Money in Health Services*. London: Heinemann Educational Books.

Audit Commission (1986) *Making a Reality of Community Care*. London: HMSO.

Bradshaw, J. (1972) A taxonomy of social need. In: G. McLachlan (ed.), *Problems and Progress in Medical Care* (Vol. 7). London: Oxford University Press.

Brewin, C.R., Veltro, F., Wing, J.K., MacCarthy, B. and Brugha, T.S. (1990). The assessment of psychiatric disability in day and residential settings. *British Journal of Psychiatry, 157*, 671–674.

Brewin, C.R., Wing, J.K., Mangen, S.P., Brugha, T.S. and MacCarthy, B. (1987) Principles and practice of measuring needs in the long-term mentally ill: The MRC Needs for Care Assessment. *Psychological Medicine, 17*, 971–981.

Brewin, C.R., Wing, J.K., Mangen, S.P., Brugha, T.S., MacCarthy, B. and Lesage, A. (1988) Needs for care among the long-term mentally ill: A report from the Camberwell High Contact Survey. *Psychological Medicine, 18*, 457–468.

Brugha, T.S., Wing, J.K., Brewin, C.R., MacCarthy, B., Mangen, S.P., Lesage, A. and Mumford, J. (1988) The problems of people in long-term psychiatric day care: An introduction to the Camberwell High Contact Survey. *Psychological Medicine, 18*, 443–456.

Castel, R. (1981) *La Gestion des Risques*. Paris: Editions de Minuit.

Creer, C., Sturt, E. and Wykes, T. (1982) The role of relatives. In: J. K. Wing (ed.), Long Term Community Care: Experience in a London Borough *Psychological Medicine* Monograph Supplement 2.

Creer, C. and Wing, J.K. (1974) *Schizophrenia at Home*, Surbiton, National Schizophrenia Fellowship.

Davies, B., and Challis, D. (1986). *Matching Resources to Needs in Community Care*. London: Gower.

D.H.S.S. (1983). *Health Services Development: Care in the Community*. Departmental Circular.

Doyal, L. and Gough, I. (1984) A theory of human needs. *Critical Social Policy, 10*, 6–38.

Fadden, G., Bebbington, P. and Kuipers, L. (1987) The burden of care: the impact of functional psychiatric illness on the patient's family. *British Journal of Psychiatry, 150*, 285–292.

Glennerster, H. (1985) *Paying for Welfare*. Oxford: Basil Blackwell.

Griffiths, R. (1988) *Community Care: Agenda for Action*. London: HMSO.

Kuipers, L. and Bebbington, P.E. (1985) Relatives as a resource in the management of functional illness. *British Journal of Psychiatry, 147*, 465–470.

Lesage, A., Mignolli, G., Faccincani, C. and Tansella, M. (1990) Standardised assessment of the needs for care in a cohort of patients with schizophrenic psychoses. (In press) *Psychological Medicine*.

MacCarthy, B., Benson, J. and Brewin, C.R. (1986) Task motivation and problem appraisal in long-term psychiatric patients. *Psychological Medicine, 16*, 431–438.

MacCarthy, B., Lesage, A., Brewin, C.R., Brugha, T.S., Mangen, S. and Wing, J.K. (1989). Needs for care among the relatives of long-term users of day care. *Psychological Medicine, 19*, 725–736.

Mangen, S.P. (1988) Assessing cost effectiveness. In: F.N. Watts (ed.), *New Developments in Clinical Psychology* (Vol. 2). Chichester: Wiley.

Maslow, A. H. (1954) *Motivation and Personality*. New York: Harper & Row.

Miller, D. (1976) *Social Justice*. Oxford: Clarendon Press.

Smith, G. (1980) *Social Need: Policy, Practice and Research*. London: Routledge & Kegan Paul.

Wainwright, T., Holloway, F. and Brugha, T.S. (1988) Day care in an inner city. In: A. Lavender and F. Holloway (eds.), *Community Care in Practice: Services for the Continuing Care Client*. Chichester: Wiley.

Webb, A. and Wistow, G. (1986) *Planning, Need and Scarcity*. London: Allen & Unwin.

Wing, J.K. (1972) Principles of evaluation. In: J.K. Wing and A.M. Hailey (eds.), *Evaluating a Community Psychiatric Service*. Oxford: Oxford University Press.

Wing, J.K. (1978) Medical and social science and medical and social care. In: J. Barnes and N. Connelly (eds.), *Social Care Research*. London: Bedford Square Press.

Wing, J.K. (1986) The cycle of planning and evaluation. In: G. Wilkinson and H. Freeman (eds.), *The Provision of Mental Health Services in Britain: The Way Ahead*. London: Gaskell.

Wing, J.K. and Hailey, A.M. (eds.) (1972) *Evaluating a Community Psychiatric Service*. Oxford: Oxford University Press.

Wykes, T., Creer, C. and Sturt, E. (1982) Needs and deployment of services. In: J.K. Wing (ed.), *Long-term Community Care: Experience in a London Borough*. Psychological Medicine Monograph Supplement No. 2.

9

Social Behavior and Psychiatric Disorders

Til Wykes and Jane Hurry

Introduction

The phenomenon of social performance covers a wide range of issues, and so in this chapter we have chosen to concentrate on two aspects: the use of the concept of social performance in relation to psychiatric disorder, from its milder to its most severe forms, and the different levels of measuring social functioning. The concept has been used in many different types of study in the field of psychiatric disorder. Examples include its relationship with the use of and the need for psychiatric services, its employment as a measure of the effectiveness of treatment, and as a predictor of outcome.

This chapter will clarify how social performance schedules have been used. It will also provide a rational taxonomy for categorizing these performance measures in order to make the choice easier for the clinician or researcher. However, we do not analyze the existing scales in detail, as there are several reviews of the sorts of schedules that are available, together with data on their psychometric properties (Weissman, 1975; Weissman et al., 1981; Platt, 1986). This chapter will also concentrate on how the measurement of social performance has been developed, especially within the Social Psychiatry Unit where we have both been based. Furthermore, we examine how these schedules have been used to widen our knowledge of the effects of psychiatric disorder and the measures that may alleviate or mitigate its effects.

What is Social Performance?

The definition of psychiatric disorder is broadly based on the subject's description of his or her symptoms. However, symptoms may not be the only indication of dysfunction. In general terms, the ability to perform the common tasks normally required of an adult (to work, to relate to others, to look after one's personal appearance and one's dwelling place) may also be affected. These social functions are of relevance to the subject and to all those involved with him or her. However, much confusion surrounds the concept of social performance. It has developed a range of meanings: performance in roles, social behavior, and social interaction impairment; and its measurement has been underpinned by a number of different concepts such as social adjustment, fulfilling expected roles, meeting community expectations etc. The relevance of this concept spans the whole spectrum of mental illness, but the requirements for measurement may vary dramatically with the severity of illness being experienced.

How to Measure Social Behavior

The existing measures can be categorized into three major areas: *social attainments, social role performance,* and *instrumental behavior.*

Social Attainments

Social attainments consist of easily identified, relatively objective achievements in the major role areas, e.g., marital history and status, employment history. This type of measurement is comparatively easy to collect and has therefore attracted sociologists attempting large scale epidemiological work. Dohrenwend and her colleagues have developed such a measure, the Psychiatric Epidemiology Research Interview (PERI, Dohrenwend et al., 1981). This self-report schedule collects data on three attainment measures: job attainment, marital attainment, and parental attainment. It also includes six performance and satisfaction measures: job performance, job satisfaction, house work, marital performance and satisfaction, parental satisfaction, single heterosexual relations. Job attainment is measured by employment status over the preceding year and marital attainment by whether the subject of over thirty years is currently married or not. But this is a rather crude measure. Being unemployed or unmarried may signify a variety of things unrelated to social disability.

Dohrenwend and her colleagues were quite aware of this difficulty, noting that "a population's level of social functioning may be strongly influenced by social conditions, so that some people with no psychiatric symptoms are functioning poorly. For example, in his studies of the population of a section of Baltimore, Lemkau noted that during the economic depression of the 1930s lack of a steady job could not be assumed to be related to psychopathology (1948, p. 408). In such situations social functioning might not be significantly better in the general population than among mental patients'' (1981, p. 184).

In a review of sixty-eight outcome studies over an eighty year period, Warner (1985) concluded that there was a large negative correlation between the amount of unemployment in the general population and recovery rates in schizophrenia (recovery here denoting return to independent social and economic functioning). So, local environmental and social factors seem to play a role, in both mild and severe disorders, in affecting this type of measurement of social performance.

As well as the interaction between environmental and other pressures, there is a further problem which pervades much social functioning research, and is particularly relevant here. This is the use of factors, such as level of occupation and length of marriage, that are also frequently regarded as independent socio-demographic variables of possible aetiological significance. This confusion underlies the uncertain direction of causality in the association between psychiatric disorder and variables such as social class and marital status. It is a point raised in more detail elsewhere in this chapter.

These attainment measures are also coded as either present or absent, for example, married or not, employed or not etc., without any regard to actual functioning within the role. A man who, for instance, beats his wife cannot be considered as performing well in the role of husband.

This area of measurement is the least specific and contains no information on actual performance in any of the categories. Despite this, the fact that a person has been able to form an attachment that results in marriage or has been able to persuade an employer to offer him or her a job does, in general, indicate some social skills. However, social attainments will not provide the fine detail for much research and clinical work.

Social Role Performance

Social role performance is measured by asking either subjects or their associates how they cope in the major role areas of work, relationships, home, and self-management. There has been a considerable degree of consensus on the role areas to be studied (Katz and Lyerly, 1963; Weissman, 1975; Barrabee et al., 1955; Mandel, 1959; Hogarty and Katz, 1971; Paykel et al., 1971; Gurland et al., 1972; Platt et al., 1980; Platt, 1986).

In her review of social adjustment measures, Weissman (1975) outlines the most important aspects of content in instruments of this type:

1) the areas assessed should be extensive and have broad coverage;
2) these areas should be assessed individually rather than globally;
3) within each role area, functions can be further subdivided into instrumental and affective tasks, or behavior and attitudes in roles.

She writes, "a rating instrument that assesses many of these discrete components of social adjustment offers more precision and may have greater ability in classifying or differentiating treatment effects" (p. 358).

The performance in any particular role has to be measured in terms of the expectations of the cultural group. This is particularly true when one considers how good performance should be scored. Expectations of performance in a role, for example, within marriage, may differ from culture to culture. Even within one culture, expectations will differ with respect to age, sex, and social class in a complex fashion. For instance, the expectation of the contribution of a husband to housework or child care will be different if we know he is twenty-five or sixty years old.

The establishment of norms against which to measure deviation has, because of their cultural specificity, always proved a dilemma for researchers (Ruesch and Brodsky, 1968). The norms established in SSIAM (Gurland et al., 1972) are derived from the clinical assessments of social maladjustment made by four practicing psychotherapists. Other studies (Cochrane and Stopes-Roe, 1977; Williamson, 1976) create norms on the basis of the profile of responses obtained from the samples studied. Clare and Cairns (1978) used information derived from Government Statistics; for example, people's use of disposable income (after payment of rent) as laid down by the Department of Health and Social Security. In the MRC Social Role Performance Schedule (SRP), the threshold of disability is set in such a way that behavior classified as a problem would be considered abnormal across cultural and sub-cultural boundaries. This is reinforced by the fact that 87 percent of a general population sample were found to have no serious problem in any of the role areas measured (Hurry and Sturt, 1981).

The first edition of the SRP was constructed by Wing and Stevens at the MRC Social Psychiatry Unit and was used in studies of psychotic patients (Hirsch et al., 1973; Stevens, 1972, 1973; Leff and Vaughn, 1972; Wing et al., 1972). Using this experience, a second edition was prepared by Sheila Hewett and tested in a survey of the problems of relatives of schizophrenic patients (Creer and Wing, 1974). It incorporated a number of features, such as definitions, obligatory questions, probes, and cut-off points. With some modifications, a third version has also been used in a community survey and a sample of outpatients with predominantly mild affective disorders (Hurry and Sturt, 1981; Hurry et al., 1983; Hurry et al., 1987; Hurry, 1989). Later, it was also used in a study of severely disabled patients in hospital-based settings such as wards and day hospitals (Sturt and Wykes, 1987). Wing has recently traced these MRC schedules (and those described in the next section) in order to make their chronology and nomenclature clear (Wing, 1989). He has designated these three versions of the social role performance schedule as SRPS1–3, corresponding to the three versions cited above.

Many other different social performance scales have been used (Weissman, 1975; Weissman et al., 1981) and, even where they broadly conform to the structure outlined by Weissman, there are inevitable variations in item inclusion. The SRP differs from scales like the Social Adjustment Scale (SAS), used by Paykel and Weissman in a series of studies (Paykel et al., 1971; Paykel et al., 1973; Weissman et al., 1971; Weissman et al., 1974; Weissman and Paykel, 1974), and the Structured and Scaled Interview to Assess Maladjustment (SSIAM) (Gurland et al., 1972a, 1972b) in its avoidance of measurements of subjects' *feelings* about their performance. The SRP relies as much as possible on objective behaviors. This is intentional in order to reduce the overlap between the measure of social performance and the measure of psychiatric disorder. The SRP attempts to measure "performance" rather than "adjustment," although, as it relies on a person's accounts of their behavior rather than the behavior itself, there is inevitably an element of subjectivity.

The main problem affecting this category of measures appears to be the cultural bias built into some schedules and the possibility of obsolescence when used in cultures with changing norms. Weissman and colleagues (1981) pointed out one major failing, that the role of women had changed considerably since the late fifties and early sixties, but that this has not been reflected in the design or instructions for schedules. Although the adoption of normative approaches to measurement has its drawbacks, researchers are generally agreed on the role areas to be studied. However, use of measures based on a dysfunction or disability principle (e.g., the MRC Schedules) may help to overcome some difficulties. Social role performance measures do have one major strength over those of social attainment: they offer much greater precision, which is especially useful with less severely disabled subjects.

Instrumental Behavior

As well as the general roles described above, a more detailed description of social behavior is appropriate for two sorts of study. The first sort is the investigation of people for whom many of the roles will be inapplicable, for example, patients in long stay institutions, or members of a religious community where many of the roles would be unavailable. The second type of study is one with a requirement for a more detailed analysis of behavior, for instance, in a treatment trial or evaluation of outcome. For these purposes a measure is needed which is relatively culture-free and provides detailed data which are sensitive to differences both over time and between people. Within psychogeriatrics there has been a tradition of such measures, for example, CAPE (Pattie and Gilleard, 1976). They are described under the rubric "instrumental behavior" because they seem to encompass various activities prerequisite to an independent social life, such as being able to initiate conversation. As these schedules were developed for use with severely disabled subjects, they are rarely based on self report, most relying on third person ratings. We lack good data on the use of these scales in the general population.

Within the Social Psychiatry Unit, there has been a tradition of measuring behavior, based on the work of the Unit in the late fifties and early sixties (Venables, 1957; Wing, 1960a, 1960b). This work culminated in the development of Wing's Ward Behavior Rating Scale (Wing, 1961). This was used to measure the difficulties of patients in industrial rehabilitation programs, and formed a basis for comparison in Wing and Brown's (1970) seminal study of institutionalism and schizophrenia. The ward behavior rating scale was sociometrically sophisticated, in that it had clear instructions for use and a defined time period for measurement, and both inter-rater and test-retest reliability was assessed. When Hall (1980) published his review of twenty-nine rating scales, only four performed well on all of his criteria: two of these scales were published by Wing. The original questionnaire was published with two subscales supported by factor analyses. The subscales were the basis of an influential distinction between two sorts of behavior—social withdrawal and socially embarrassing behavior. The social withdrawal scale measured general behaviors that were quite frequent such as slowness, underactivity, and lack of conversation. The socially embarrassing behavior subscale was highly loaded on less frequent items such as threats of violence, odd mannerisms, and talking to one's self. The Wing scale used senior nurses as informants, thus enabling the less frequently observed but highly important behaviors to be rated.

In the twenty-seven years since publication, many studies have used this simple scale. Indeed, there have been more than one hundred references to the original scale over the past fifteen years in the Science Citation Index, and in 1988 four further studies have either used the scale or based an assessment on it. Within the Social Psychiatry Unit, it has been further developed to produce a second version that reflects the concerns of relatives (e.g., Creer and Wing, 1974), and a third version which reflects the concerns of hostel staff (e.g., Ryan, 1979). The standard version of the Social Behavior Schedule was published in 1986, together with current measures of its reliability and validity (Wykes and Turt, 1986). The schedule now covers twenty-one behaviors, including items on self care, initiating conversation, and violence. Items were included on the basis of frequent mention by staff as problems that contributed to a continuing dependency on psychiatric care. All but one item were rated as a problem by at least 5 percent of the populations studied. The schedule is still geared toward measuring the difficulties of patients with severe disabilities. The two subscales derived from the first version of this schedule, social withdrawal and socially embarrassing behavior, have not been distinguished on purely statistical grounds in later versions. This may be a result of the change in the population of patients investigated (from "old long stay" to the "new long stay" and community samples), and the slightly changed items and scoring procedure. It is, however, possible to formulate the contrast on a combination of clinical judgment and statistical procedures (Wykes, Sturt and Creer, 1982a).

Another scale which has been successful in assessing instrumental behavior is REHAB (Hall and Baker, 1983). This scale is also based on the Wing Ward Behavior Rating Scale, and is thus very similar in content to SBS. The only differences are in the time scale on which some items are measured and the inclusion of items on money management, care of possessions, and use of community facilities. The development of the scale is well described, as are its reliability and validity. Unlike the SBS, the development of the REHAB scale relies heavily on the distinction between socially embarrassing and socially withdrawn behavior. The factor analyses of this scale produced two main measures: a general behavior score and a deviant behavior score. The deviant behavior score is a measure of relatively infrequent behavior such as threats of violence and is thus measured over a longer time scale. This particular factor, as with the socially embarrassing subscale of the Wing form, is not as reliable as the other parts of the schedule. There is in fact little to choose between the two schedules, except that the SBS has been used more widely in community settings and, as Shepherd (1988) pointed out, is cheaper.

Both these scales measure disturbances in functioning rather than specifying "ideal" social functioning. One recent schedule that appears to be based on ideal functioning is the Self Care Measurement Schedule (Barnes and Benjamin, 1987). However, in common with other such measures, the norms are culture-specific. For example, problem behaviors include eating a meal in bed, not getting up before 10:00 A.M., and not going shopping.

Both authors of this chapter would certainly have scored on several of these "deviant behavior" items.

The main problems of using this category of measurement is the lack of self-report versions and the necessity for relying on third person accounts. In fact, MacCarthy and colleagues (1986) indicate that long term patients can be good informants. These measures were originally designed to study patients with severe disorders and in a great deal of contact with psychiatric services—inpatients, day hospital attenders, and so on. Since the move into the community, patients have been in much less contact with psychiatric personnel. Many do not have relatives and may only be supported by nurses whose infrequent contact may not allow reliable ratings to be made. There are several current projects aimed at producing or testing schedules for use with this new community. Hogg and colleagues (1988) have outlined the problems of one such project with homeless but severely disabled people, and have so far not arrived at an agreed solution. Anthony and Farkas (1982) in their review also found problems with schedules designed for the assessment of instrumental behavior. They pointed out that in thirty-one schedules reliability and validity were not well described, and that very few measures had been standardized on a severely psychiatrically disabled population. Many of these schedules were also developed out of particular institutional needs and are not designed for less unique environments (Cohen and Anthony, 1984).

Why Measure Social Behavior?

Psychological disturbance is multi-dimensional and is inadequately characterized by symptoms alone (Remington and Tyrer, 1979). Assessments of other dimensions, for example, relative burden, subjective satisfaction, can be a useful part of any clinical or research endeavor. Important among these dimensions is social functioning, as access to psychiatric services is gained only when psychiatric illness is accompanied by poor levels of functioning. Two factors may confound the measurement of social functioning. The first is environmental disadvantage, poverty, stigma, and so on. The second is the development of adverse attitudes, such as loss of confidence and lack of motivation. Both concepts have been described in more detail elsewhere by Wing (1972) in his model of impairments, disabilities, and handicaps. Below we briefly review the relationship of social functioning to three areas of research to illustrate how social functioning measures have been used. These areas really merit chapters in their own right, but, as a preliminary, it is important to establish the independence of social performance from psychiatric disorder, as this will clearly affect the interpretation of research results.

Independence of Social Functioning and Psychiatric Disorder

Psychiatric symptoms and social disablement are not logically synonymous. Poor social performance might reflect many things, such as low self esteem, poverty, or a persistent character disturbance, rather than a reaction to illness. However, in practice, the two variables are closely linked.

The definitions of symptoms in measures of psychiatric disorder such as the Present State Examination (PSE, Wing et al., 1974; Wing et al., 1978) are constructed so as to minimize the importance of any social component. So, for example, depressed mood and "free-floating" anxiety are rated solely on the intensity and frequency of the experiences described by the subject. Theoretically, it would be possible for someone to carry out expected social functions as well during periods of anxiety or depression as when mood is normal. However, other symptoms imply an almost necessary reduction in social functioning. Subjective anergia and psycho-motor retardation, for example, although not rated on social criteria, can hardly be severe without interfering with everyday activities. Prolonged sleeplessness is likely to have the same effect. Similarly, symptoms such as worrying and loss of interest or concentration are difficult to rate without taking social behavior into account, although the rating of the symptom is based essentially upon subjective experience.

A substantial correlation between symptoms and social disablement would therefore be expected. This was demonstrated quite clearly in a community survey and in a study of psychiatric outpatients carried out in South London by the Social Psychiatry Unit (Hurry and Sturt, 1981). Correlations between SRP and PSE of .68 and .57 respectively were reported. It was particularly amongst the depressive disorders, as defined by the CATEGO program (Wing and Sturt, 1978), that a strong relationship existed. In the general population, nine out of the fourteen subjects diagnosed as anxious were not socially disabled, and in the outpatient sample six out of fifteen patients suffering from an anxiety state had no social performance deficits. Mechanic and Greenley (1976) found a correlation of .43 between social disablement and psychiatric impairment. Weissman and colleagues (1978) in their follow-up study of a community sample from New Haven, Connecticut found correlations between their measure of social adjustment and psychiatric symptoms of .57 and .59 on two self-report symptom measures and of .44 with the Ruskin clinical symptom measure. However, in a study of female patients suffering from depression, the relationship between social adjustment and the overall severity of depressive symptoms during the depressive episode was so weak that the two sets of variables were virtually independent (Paykel et al., 1978). Finally, Dohrenwend and her colleagues report significant but small correlations between symptoms and social functioning in an Israeli community survey using the PERI (Dohrenwend et al., 1983).

Within psychiatric patient populations, both Paykel et al. (1973, 1978) and Hirsch et al. (1979) have found that psychiatric symptoms and deficit in social performance improve at differing rates, the latter being more intractable. Cohler (1975) also reported that an aftercare program had little effect on the social adjustment of hospitalized women.

There are also consistent differences in the demographic correlates of psychiatric symptoms and social disability, which suggests that although the two measures are closely correlated, they are not identical. In particular, the marked predominance of women amongst those suffering from mild affective disorders is not observed amongst the socially disabled (Weissman et al., 1978; Hurry et al., 1983; Richman, 1984). Most authors, including ourselves, would agree with Paykel that "much of the social impairment appears symptom related, subsiding with symptom reduction. A small, but definite, portion reflects underlying personality disturbance. It should be noted that even the symptom related portion cannot be regarded as merely an unimportant epiphenomenon. The severity and pervasiveness of the disturbances and their slow improvement render them important in their own rights both in assessment and in treatment" (Paykel and Weissman, 1973, p. 662).

With more severe, long lasting, disorders the argument for the independence of symptoms and social behavior is harder to sustain. Some symptoms, especially in the more chronic forms of illness are, by definition, virtually synonymous with absences of social functioning, e.g., social withdrawal. Some symptom measures use decrements in social functioning as an indicator of symptom severity (e.g., GAS, Spitzer and Endicott, 1978). However, when this hypothesis was tested recently (Sturt and Wykes, 1987) no relationship was found between levels of current symptoms (the total PSE score) and social performance measures, either as role functioning or instrumental behavior. Patients exhibiting florid symptoms, such as delusions or hallucinations, showed social performance right across the spectrum, as did those who reported experiencing neurotic symptoms: some were working in a community workshop and living at home, others residing in a long stay ward with no interest in any occupation.

A further problem is the use of social performance both as a dependent and as an independent variable in mental health research. When social functioning is taken as an independent variable, its contribution to the development of mental disorders, help-seeking, and recovery are measured, but in other instances the range of function of patients suffering from a particular illness is itself under examination. In other words, social performance may be associated with the development of mental disorders (independent variable) or it may be the result of mental disorder (dependent variable). The second use of social performance requires more detailed measurement than the first. Most researchers agree with Paykel (Paykel and Weissman, 1973, quoted above) that social performance measures are messy variables because of the contributions from stable, underlying characteristics which produce vulnerability and from the direct effects of current symptoms. Both aspects are modified by an environment that encourages learning and practicing the various skills needed to fulfill social attainments, social roles, and instrumental behaviors.

Confounding arises between the two uses of social performance measurements in so far as the prediction and assessment of outcome may employ similar or identical measures. The large correlations between these two sets of variables in many studies is therefore not surprising. In fact, nearly all prognostic scales, for example, Vaillant (1964), Phillips (1953), Stephens et al. (1966), Strauss and Carpenter (1974a) and Ullman and Giovannoni (1964), mix up information about social attainments, symptoms and chronicity of illness. These social attainments are frequently regarded as independent variables of possible aetiological significance. For instance, Phillips (1968) argued that a deficiency in social competence made the onset of pathology more likely. He interpreted the finding of Hollingshead and Redlich (1958) that those of higher social class were more heavily represented amongst neurotic as opposed to schizophrenic patients as a support for this thesis. Hollingshead and Redlich took their findings to mean something quite different, namely that those of higher social class were more readily accepted for treatment than those of low social class. In fact, there are few data on the changes in social functioning over time in the general population, making it extremely difficult to interpret post-illness functioning, especially in patients who have been ill for some time. Although in cases where dramatic decreases in functioning follow an episode of psychiatric illness it may be safe to infer a causal connection, qualification of the actual effect of mental illness must rely on much more sophisticated methods. Thus it is possible to control for the initial level of performance by entering it into analysis as a co-variate and trying to explain the remaining variance using other factors. An alternative is to look at the correlation between social performance time 1 − social performance time 2 and social performance time 1 + social performance time 2. The distinction between independent and dependent variables has been given little attention in reviews of social functioning.

Use of Psychiatric Services

Goldberg and Huxley (1980) have characterized the pathway to psychiatric care as a series of "filters" governing the passage to different levels of care. Examples of the filters include the decision to consult the general practitioner and referral from nonspecialist to specialist care. Each of these filters is determined by a variety of possible factors, including impairments in social performance.

The Decision to Consult. Symptoms are primarily a reflection of internal psychological or physical states, though they have a consequence in social relations. It has been argued that interference with our practical affairs caused by social disability is central to our personal definition of illness (Herzlich, 1973; Gordon, 1966; Foulds, 1976). Based on clinical experience, Schwab and his colleagues (1979) wrote that many persons seeking mental health care did so mainly for interpersonal problems. The argument is that only when we are so psychologically disturbed that we can't work or wash the dishes do we start to think of ourselves as ill. If this is true, social disability should be a significant factor in the decision to seek treatment, perhaps even more so than the level of symptoms. Mechanic and Greenely (1976) did indeed find, in a sample of American students, that the inability to continue with normal activities was at least as predictive of psychiatric health service use as the presence of psychiatric symptoms. It must be noted, however, that their social disability measure relied on the single question, "How often do your (psychological) problems prevent you from doing things you would like to do?", with six response categories ordered by frequency of occurrence. In a community survey in South London, it was found that those people who had seen their GP for "their nerves" in the year preceding interview were considerably more socially disabled than those who had not (Hurry et al., 1987; Hurry, 1989). Even amongst those who were psychiatric "cases" (ID level 5 or above of the Present State Examination; Wing and Sturt, 1978), the GP group were more disabled. However, social performance and total symptom score were highly correlated in this study (Hurry and Sturt, 1981) and, not surprisingly, symptom level was the major determinant of service use at all levels studied. Indeed, when symptom level was taken into account, the power of social performance as a discriminant of service use was non-existent.

Referral from GP to Psychiatric Clinic. The patient has considerable influence at this stage too (Mowbray et al., 1961; Fink et al., 1969). However, separate studies also found social disablement to be of importance to English GPs in the decision to refer to a specialist (Kaesar and Cooper, 1971; Mowbray et al., 1961). Both studies found that the presence of behavior disturbances, serious social difficulties, and abnormalities of conduct or social problems in the patient were given as the reason for psychiatric referral as frequently as diagnosis was. Casey and his colleagues (1985), in a more recent study of primary care using a measure of social performance broadly similar to the SRP, found that social functioning was a more important determinant of referral to psychiatric services than psychiatric symptomatology (as measured by total PSE score). In the MRC study, a random sample of outpatients was more socially disabled than the community cases, but most of this difference was explained by the higher symptom score in the treated cases. Social performance did, however, have a small independent effect (Hurry, 1989; Hurry et al., 1987).

Inpatient/Day Hospital Admission. Out of the seventy-four outpatients in the MRC study, twelve were admitted to a ward or day hospital during the year following interview. Those who were admitted had significantly higher levels of social disability at the initial interview. However, a stepwise discriminant analysis showed that the relationship between social performance score and admission to a ward or day hospital disappeared when symptom score (which accounted for 15 percent of the variance) was controlled.

If the social functioning of patients in short stay psychiatric wards is compared with that of patients in other residential care settings (e.g. hostels, group homes, etc.), the problems in social performance picked up by the SBS are much greater (Wykes et al., 1982a). However, the prevalence of problems varies widely (0–57 percent), so there is a great deal of overlap between the groups. Spitzer et al. (1970) also found that it was possible to distinguish inpatients from outpatients on the basis of role functioning. In addition, they found that poorer functioning characterized the more chronic, schizophrenic groups. Similarly, Baker and Hall (1988) report that REHAB scores were able to discriminate day hospital attenders from patients in long-stay wards.

Patients who are admitted to hospital or day hospital seem to have more problems in social functioning than those not admitted. They also appear to be less disabled than patients who have gravitated to longer stay highly supervised inpatient care, for example, hospital-hostels. But it is not clear whether all these differences can be accounted for merely by differing levels of symptoms between the groups.

Discharge from Inpatient Facilities. At the point of discharge, especially in the case of patients who have been inpatients for some time, social performance becomes a central factor. Clinicians have to face the practical issues of assessing the degree of independence that might be achieved. Birley (1974) has suggested that we should provide the minimal dose of psychiatric support, and other clinicians have suggested a balance between a patient's independence and the level of psychiatric input, maximizing the former whilst minimizing the latter (Bennett, 1978).

REHAB, the instrumental behavior schedule designed by Hall and Baker (1983), actually includes rules for distinguishing those patients who have a potential for discharge, although little work has yet been done on the validity of this cut-off.

Surveys of patients using the SBS have described the sorts of problem behaviors that different patient populations portray. These groups of patients include hostel residents, people in group homes, and those attending day hospitals and day centers, as well as those who are out of touch with formal services such as the destitute (Hewett et al., 1975; Ryan, 1979; Wykes et al., 1982a; Leach and Wing, 1980). The levels of problem behaviors in these groups are rather what one would expect. People in services which require high levels of supervision have the highest level of social performance difficulties, but there is considerable overlap between groups. It does, however, look as if there are broad criteria for acceptance into different sorts of care. If different groups of patients are compared on the same version of the Social Behaviour Scale, they show characteristic levels of problems (see Figure 9.1).

Patients who have graduated towards services providing high levels of support have higher levels of problem behaviors than those who are maintained in services with lower levels of support, such as group homes. This correlation holds for both day and residential care. The decision to

FIGURE 9.1
Social Behavior Problems

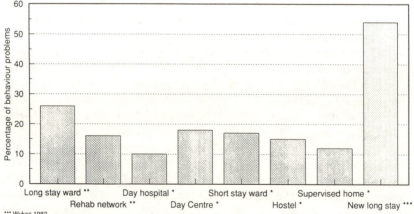

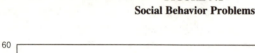

*** Wykes,1982
** Netherne series, Wykes and Sturt (1986)
* Camberwell series, Wykes et al. (1982)

discharge therefore seems to be based on social behavioral criteria. Further evidence to support this comes from Sturt and Wykes (1987). They compared symptoms, social role performance, and instrumental behaviors in community care and hospital samples. As expected, social role performance and instrumental behavior were highly correlated, but neither were related to the level of (largely florid) symptoms elicited by the PSE. Both SRP and SBS differentiated the long stay from the rehabilitation group, but the symptom measures did not distinguish these groups. When the measures were entered into a multiple regression analysis, social role performance (SRP) emerged as the only significant independent factor which differentiates those in traditional long stay wards from those in the rehabilitation network.

Differentiation would, however, be better if there were no ceiling or floor effects. Inspection of the SRP distributions within settings indicates considerable overlap of scores, and this has also been found with social behavior measures. Many of the patients in the wards were on or close to the maximum deficit score on SRP, and this clearly impedes the possibility of differentiating between the more severely disabled groups.

In summary, social functioning appears most important in the later stages of the chain of referral. In the early stages, for example the decision to consult the family doctor, impaired social performance appears to have no effect beyond what could be expected from its association with psychiatric symptoms. Controlling for the severity of symptoms virtually eliminates the predictive power of social performance. However, it does have an effect over and above symptom severity on placements within the specialist psychiatric resources.

Social Performance as a Predictor of Outcome

Phillips (1968) has quoted a large number of studies which report positive findings concerning "coping potential" (which would be categorized here under social attainment), both as a predictor of recovery rate and as an outcome of psychiatric disorder. However, many other studies relating social attainments to outcome have suggested that very little of the overall outcome variance (social, employment, service dependence etc.) is accounted for by any individual factor. Though there are large correlations between predictor and outcome measures of the same sorts (e.g., employment history predicting future employment: Strauss and Carpenter, 1974a; Watts and Bennett, 1977), there may be little relationship across different role areas. This is consistent with the finding that individual levels of social attainment are not highly correlated between different areas of life, for example, work and family, in either community or patient populations

(Dohrenwend et al., 1981). However, in the International Pilot Study of Schizophrenia (WHO, 1979; Hawk et al., 1975) social contacts prior to the first evaluation not only predicted social contacts at follow-up but also had predictive value for nearly all outcome measures. Social isolation was associated with a poor outcome, as was the marital category of widowed, divorced, or separated. Being married was associated with a good outcome. Sturt (1984) and Bland and colleagues (1978) also found that the presence of a viable marriage related favorably to outcome in more severely disabled groups. In one recent study, employment duration and quality of social contacts accounted for a significant amount of outcome variance (viz. 55 percent; Gaebel and Pietzcker, 1987).

In Strauss and Carpenter's study (1974a), as in many others that followed, chronicity is, not surprisingly, the one variable with general significance (for a review of these data see Kokes et al., 1977 and Klorman et al., 1977).

Wallace (1984), reviewing a number of studies that tested the significance of interpersonal functioning (an aspect of role functioning), concluded that, given poor functioning predates the onset of the disorder, it is predictive of future outcome and might be uniquely characteristic of patients with severe disorders, for example, schizophrenic patients. Fenton and McGlashan (1987) also used a measure of social functioning in their prognostic scale for a chronically disabled group. Their composite scale was reasonably predictive of several different outcome variables, including unemployment and poor social relations.

There are, of course, many other studies of outcome that are not reviewed here. The majority have picked out social functioning variables as important factors. However, as in the papers cited above, the variance in outcome accounted for is small.

Social Performance as a Measure of the Effectiveness of Treatment

Social performance has also been used in studies of the effectiveness of pharmacological, behavioral, and familial treatments.

The stimulus to develop social performance measures in the Social Psychiatry Unit was the need to study the effectiveness of new social and pharmacological treatments. The first version of the SBS schedule was used as a measure of outcome when patients in an industrial therapy unit were provided with extra stimulation: when patients were given encouragement, their output increased. Although workshop behavior improved each time a period of extra stimulation was provided, this was not mirrored in ward behavior. However, during the hours spent in the rehabilitation unit there was an overall reduction in social withdrawal, but not in socially embarrassing behavior, as rated by ward staff. This discrepancy between settings is one of the first examples of the difficulty of generalizing from a situation of extra stimulation to other settings (Wing and Freudenberg, 1961).

The relationship between social milieu and the level of handicap continued to be a focus for the Unit, and several studies subsequently investigated their interaction using social behavior as one outcome measure. In Wing and Brown's (1970) study, social measures of this type were used both to assess outcome and as a basis for comparison in investigating the effects of change in social care on schizophrenic patients within three psychiatric hospitals. The hospitals were found to have very different approaches to patient care, ranging from a wide variety of off-the-ward activities to virtually no alternative activity. In one hospital, Netherne, only 6 percent of patients remained on the ward during the day, whereas 87 percent at Severalls did so. Wing and Brown established that less restrictive forms of institutional care had an effect on the social withdrawal scores of patients. Those in the lest restrictive environments, where more activity was provided and less time was spent doing nothing, had the lowest scores. Patients also improved with changes in the social environment towards fewer restrictions and more activity, even though the use of drugs was not materially different over the study period. One interesting finding of this study was that some mildly handicapped patients actually got worse when social conditions improved. This was particularly apparent in increased socially embarrassing behavior. The explanation suggested by the authors was that the institutionalized behavior exhibited by this group of patients was a protective measure to decrease the amount of stimulation or stress that impinged on the patient. When placed in a situation of more social contact, the return of florid symptoms was precipitated.

The SBS has also been used in pharmaceutical research. Stevens (1973) used it to assess the effects of fluphenazine decanoate vs. placebo in a group of chronic patients. She reported an increase in problems of social functioning and burden on relatives in the placebo group compared with the medicated group.

In addition, the SBS has been employed in formal evaluations of the provision of improved social and domestic surroundings for severely disturbed patients. Two studies of new long stay provision ('a ward in a house') were carried out independently, using versions of SBS as part of a controlled evaluation (Wykes, 1982; Hyde et al., 1987). In both, patients were found to improve in a hospital-hostel which provided less restrictive, more domestic accommodation that that found on a traditional hospital ward. Improved social behavior was seen as one of the beneficial non-financial effects of moving the service outside the hospital framework.

REHAB has been used in several studies of behavior in the context of some external service change, for example, nurses giving up wearing a uniform, and in comparisons of services, for example, a community skills program vs. a standard psychiatric hospital regime (Baker, 1986; Baker and Hall, 1988). In this and other studies, the main changes were seen in the general behavior (GB) scores rather than in deviant behavior (DB), confirming the results cited above.

This review of studies has been necessarily brief, allowing only an introduction to the use of social functioning measures in assessing treatment effectiveness. We have therefore chosen to concentrate mainly on British studies. It is nevertheless clear that detailed social functioning measures, for example, instrumental behavior schedules, are able to differentiate between treated and non-treated groups.

Planning Services and Assessing Needs

Although it would not be difficult to use social attainments or social role functioning to assess needs for services as an aid to planning, very few studies have done so. With the move from hospital to community care came the need to devise some method of estimating the numbers of patients in the severely disabled group needing different forms of care. One of the first surveys employing the Wing Ward Behavior rating scale used it to assess service need. It was carried out at Netherne Hospital by Catterson, Bennett, and Freudenberg (1963). In this study, the scale provided a description of the behavioral difficulties of patients for the purpose of distinguishing a group who might easily be transferred to the community. Out of their sample of 150 patients, only 13 percent were possible candidates for immediate resettlement into the community, although some of the remaining group might have been eligible after a lengthy period in a transitional facility and the provision of support services outside the hospital.

The tradition of using social behavior measures to identify need was continued by Mann and Sproule (1972) and Mann and Cree (1976), who used a form of the SBS when they scanned the "new long stay" populations, initially in the Camberwell area, and later across England and Wales. The researchers used these behavioral data together with information from staff to divide the population into three main groups. These were: those requiring further hospital care; those needing a new service, the hospital-hostel; and the remainder, who needed other types of residence. The researchers found that this group of patients contained many with severe disabilities, and even the patients who were judged as requiring non-hospital accommodation were more disabled than a group of hostel residents investigated in a later study by Hewett, Ryan, and Wing (1975).

The evaluation of needs for services was converted into a slightly different concept, the "need for care," firstly in a study of long term patients in the Camberwell community services (Wykes et al., 1982b, 1985), and later expanded and refined by Brewin and colleagues (1987, 1988). In their studies, the SBS was used to supplement data from staff, patients, and relatives in order to distinguish a series of needs for care, such as that for medical and social assessment. This type of assessment allows an evaluation of current service provision and of its effectiveness in catering for the needs of patients, together with the formulation of novel services to fulfill unmet need.

The specification of service needs and needs for care should be extremely useful in a time when deinstitutionalization in the United States and community care in Britain have acquired a new impetus. Both measures have benefitted from the development of reliable social functioning measures.

Conclusions

We are now in a position to identify appropriate measures of social functioning for clinicians and researchers. Apart from factors such as the choice of informant and the time scale covered by items, which may be of relevance in individual studies, we make the following recommendations:

1. The use of social attainment measures, despite the crude nature of the information they provide, should be considered in large-scale studies where an overall view of functioning level is required.

2. Longitudinal, outcome, and effectiveness of treatment studies need the detail provided by social role and instrumental behavior measures. We recommend considering both types of scales as they provide complementary information. However, if this is not possible, a choice should be made on the basis of the level of severity of disability. Unlike symptom measures, neither role performance nor instrumental behavior span the spectrum of disorder. Social role performance measures suffer from a ceiling effect when used with patients with severe disabilities, as most will score at the maximum level of disability. This cannot be accounted for merely by role attrition. In contrast, instrumental behavior measures suffer from a "floor effect"—many people with less severe disorders do not rate as having any problems at all. Nevertheless, they probably cover a wider range of psychiatric disorders, and so will often be the first choice (e.g., REHAB, SBS) where a choice must be made. If the study is confined to

the less severe end of the spectrum, social role performance may be more appropriate.

3. Studies where behavior is likely to change slowly need a level of detail that is currently only found in schedules of instrumental behaviors.

Apart from the criticisms of the various measures made earlier, there are several general points we would like to make here. We made no attempt to review individual scales, as their number must run into hundreds, and information on their reliability and validity is very variable. Despite this profusion, many workers continue to adapt scales without carrying out further reliability studies, making it impossible to build up a general pattern of social functioning related to diagnosis and severity of psychiatric disorder. This expansion of instruments should be abandoned. If, as is sometimes the case, an available schedule does not quite fit the needs of the study, it should be augmented with a brief addendum rather than modified.

There is also a need for more basic information about social functioning instruments, for example, how do they measure changes in individuals over time? Longitudinal information is sparse, and the collection of such data would enable the developmental course of disorders to be charted. If such information were available for the general population, it would allow further inferences on the causal link between social functioning and disorder to be drawn.

Researchers have frequently failed to clarify whether social functioning is the independent or the dependent variable: they should make clear exactly how it is being used. If social functioning is treated as an independent variable, it is important to collect information on symptom levels so that their effects can be controlled.

We concur with Morrison and Bellack (1987), who state in their recent paper on social functioning and schizophrenia that, "Despite the convincing evidence on the poor overall social functioning of schizophrenic patients, there is surprisingly little data on the precise nature of the basis of their difficulties." This also applies to other groups of patients, and we conclude that one of the main reasons for this ignorance is the conceptual ambiguity of the scales and the lack of general agreement on the applicability of different schedules.

Twenty years ago, a similar problem inhibited research on symptomatic and diagnostic assessment. It was overcome by the development of standardized methods of establishing symptoms and of using them as the basis for classification. Although no one set of procedures has gained universal acceptance at the expense of the others, the credible choice is now restricted to two or three, and comparison between studies has been greatly facilitated. This is not the case for methods for measuring social functioning: further development depends crucially on the establishment of a consensus within and between research cultures, without which definitive measures will not be forthcoming. Such concensus is long overdue.

References

Anthony, W. and Farkas, M. (1982) A Client Outcome planning model for assessing psychiatric rehabilitation interventions, *Schizophrenia Bulletin, 8,* pp. 13–38.

Baker, R. (1986) The Development of a Behavioural Assessment System for Psychiatric Patients. Final report to the Grampian Health Board Department of Psychology, Royal Cornhill Hospital, Aberdeen.

Baker, R. and Hall, J. (1988) REHAB: A new assessment instrument for chronic psychiatric patients, *Schizophrenia Bulletin, 14,* pp. 97–111.

Barnes, D. and Benjamin, S. (1987) The Self Care Assessment Schedule SCAS—I. The purpose and construction of a new assessment of self care behaviours, *Journal of Psychometric Research, 31,* pp. 191–202.

Barrabee, P., Barrabee, E.L. and Finnesinger, J.E. (1955) A normative social adjustment scale, *American Journal of Psychiatry, 112,* pp. 252–259.

Bennett, D. (1978) Social forms of psychiatric treatment, in: Wing, J.K. (ed.) *Schizophrenia: Towards a New Synthesis,* pp. 211–231 (London, Academic Press).

Birley, J. (1974) A housing association for psychiatric patients, *Psychiatric Quarterly, 48,* pp. 568–571.

Bland, R., Parker, R. and Orn, H. (1978) Prognosis in schizophrenia: Prognostic predictors and outcome, *Archives of General Psychiatry, 35,* pp. 72–77.

Brewin, C., Wing, J., Mangen, S., Brugha, T. and MacCarthy, B. (1987) Principles and practice of measuring needs in the long term mentally ill, *Psychological Medicine, 17,* pp. 971–981.

Brewin, C., Wing, J., Mangen, S., Brugha, T., MacCarthy, B. and Lesage, A. (1988) Needs for Care among long-term mentally ill: a report from the Camberwell High Contact Survey, *Psychological Medicine, 18,* pp. 457–468.

Casey, P., Tyrer, P. and Platt, S. (1985) The relationship between social functioning and psychiatric symptomatology in primary care, *Social Psychiatry, 20,* pp. 5–9.

Catterson, A., Bennett, D. and Freudenberg, R. (1963) A survey of long-stay schizophrenic patients, *British Journal of Psychiatry, 109,* pp. 750–757.

Clare, A. and Cairns, V. (1978) Design, development and use of a standardized interview to assess social maladjustment and dysfunction in community studies, *Psychological Medicine, 8,* pp. 589–604.

Cochrane, R. and Stopes-Roe, M. (1977) Psychological and social adjustment of Asian immigrants to Britain: a community survey, *Social Psychiatry, 12,* pp. 195–206.

Cohen, B. and Anthony, W. (1984) Functional assessment in psychiatric rehabilitation, in: Halpern, A. and Fahrer, M. (eds.) *Function Assessment in Rehabilitation,* pp. 79–100 (Baltimore, Brookes).

Cohler, B.J. (1975) Social adjustment and psychopathology among formerly hospitalized and non-hospitalized mothers. I. Development of Social Role Adjustment Instrument, *Journal of Psychiatric Research, 12,* pp. 1–18.

Creer, C. and Wing, J.K. (1974) *Schizophrenia at Home* (London, National Schizophrenia Fellowship).

Dohrenwend, B.S., Cook, D. and Dohrenwend, B.P. (1981) Measurement of social functioning in community populations, in: Wing, J.K., Bebbington, P. and Robbins, L. (eds.) *What is a Case?*, pp. 183–201 (London, Grant McIntyre).

Dohrenwend, B.S., Dohrenwend, B.P., Link, B. and Levav, I. (1983) Social functioning of psychiatric patients in contrast with community cases in the general population, *Archives of General Psychiatry, 40,* pp. 1174–1182.

Fenton, W. and McGlashan, T. (1987) Prognostic scale for chronic schizophrenia, *Schizophrenia Bulletin, 13,* pp. 277–286.

Fink, R., Shapiro, S., Goldensohn, S. and Daily, E. (1968) The Filter-Down process to psychotherapy in a group practice medical care program, *American Journal of Public Health, 59,* pp. 256–260.

Foulds, G. (1976) *The Hierarchical Nature of Personal Illness* (London, Academic Press).

Gaebel, W. and Pietzcker, A. (1987) Prospective study of course of illness in schizophrenia: Part II. Prediction of outcome, *Schizophrenia Bulletin, 13,* pp. 299–306.

Goldberg, D. and Huxley, P. (1980) *Mental Illness in the Community; The Pathway to Psychiatric Care* (London, Tavistock Publications).

Gordon, G. (1966) *Role Theory and Illness, A Sociological Perspective* (New Haven, Connecticut, College and University Press).

Gurland, B.J., Yorkston, N.J., Stone, A.R. and Frank, J.D. (1972a) The Structured and Scaled Interview to Assess Maladjustment (SSIAM) 1. Description, Rationale and Development, *Archives of General Psychiatry, 27,* pp. 259–264.

Gurland, B., Yorkston, N.J., Goldberg, K., Fleiss, J.L., Sloane, R.B. and Cristol, A.H. (1972b) Structured and Scaled Interview to Assess Maladjustment (SSIAM) 2, *Archives of General Psychiatry, 27,* pp. 264–267.

Gurland, B., Stone, A. and Frank, J. (1974) *Structured and Scaled Interview to Assess Maladjustment (SSIAM)* (New York, Singer).

Hall, J. (1980) Ward rating scales for long-stay patients: a review, *Psychological Medicine, 10,* pp. 277–288.

Hall, J. and Baker, R. (1983) *REHAB, a Users Manual* (Aberdeen, Vine Publishing Company).

Hawk, A.B., Carpenter, W.J. and Strauss, J.S. (1985) Diagnostic criteria and five year outcome in schizophrenia: A report from the International Pilot Study of Schizophrenia, *Archives of General Psychiatry, 32,* pp. 343–347.

Herzlich, C. (1973) *Health and Illness* (London, Academic Press).

Hewett, S., Ryan, P. and Wing, J.K. (1975) Living without mental hospitals, *Journal of Social Policy, 4,* pp. 391–404.

Hirsch, S., Platt, S., Knights, A. and Weyman, A. (1979) Shortening hospital stay for psychiatric care: effect on patients and their families, *British Medical Journal, 1,* pp. 442–446.

Hirsch, S.R., Gaind, R., Rohde, P.D., Stevens, B.C. and Wing, J.K. (1973) Outpatient maintenance of chronic schizophrenic patients with long-acting fluphenazine, *British Medical Journal,* pp. 633–638.

Hogarty, G. and Katz, M. (1971) Norms of adjustment and social behavior, *Archives of General Psychiatry, 25,* pp. 470–480.

Hogg, L., Cullington, A., Marshall, M. and Hall, J. (1988) Assessing Pathways of Chronic Psychiatric Patients Through Different Care Facilities, Paper presented at World Congress of Behaviour Therapy, Edinburgh.

Hollingshead, A.B. and Redlich, F.C. (1958) *Social Class and Mental Illness* (New York, John Wiley & Sons).

Hurry, J. (1989) Social Factors and the Use of Psychiatric Services, Unpublished Ph.D. Thesis (University of London).

Hurry, J. and Sturt, E. (1981) Social performance in a population sample: relation to psychiatric symptoms in : Wing, J.K., Bebbington, P. and Robbins, L. (eds.) *What is a Case?*, pp. 202–213 (London, Grant McIntyre).

Hurry, J., Bebbington, P.E. and Tennant, C. (1987) Psychiatric symptoms, social disablement and illness behaviour, *Australian and New Zealand Journal of Psychiatry, 21*, pp. 68–73.

Hurry, J., Sturt, E., Bebbington, P. and Tennant, C. (1983) Socio-demographic associations with social disablement in a community sample, *Social Psychiatry, 18*, pp. 113–121.

Hyde, C., Bridges, K., Goldberg, D., Lawson, K., Starling, C. and Faracher, B. (1987) The evaluation of a hostel ward: A controlled study using modified Cost-Benefit Analysis, *British Journal of Psychiatry, 141*, pp. 805–812.

Kaesar, A.C. and Cooper, B. (1971) The psychiatric patient, the general practitioner, and the out-patient clinic: An operational study and a review, *Psychological Medicine, 1*, pp. 312–325.

Katz, M.M. and Lyerly, S.B. (1963) Methods for measuring adjustment and social behaviour in the community: I Rationale, description, discriminative validity and scale development, *Psychological Reports, 13*, pp. 503–535.

Klorman, R., Strauss, J. and Kokes, R. (1977) Premorbid adjustment in schizophrenia. Part IV some biological approaches to research on premorbid functioning in schizophrenia, *Schizophrenia Bulletin, 3*, pp. 226–239.

Kokes, R., Strauss, J. and Klorman, R. (1977) Premorbid adjustment in schizophrenia. I measuring premorbid adjustment: The instruments and their development, *Schizophrenia Bulletin, 3*, pp. 186–213.

Leach, J. and Wing, J.K. (1980) *Helping Destitute Men* (London, Tavistock).

Leff, J. and Vaughn, C. (1972) Psychiatric patients in contact and out of contact with services: A clinical and social assessment, in: Wing, J.K. and Hailey, A.M. (eds.) *Evaluating a Community Psychiatric Service*, pp. 259–274 (London, Oxford University Press).

MacCarthy, B., Benson, J. and Brewin, C. (1986) Task motivation and problem appraisal in long term psychiatric patients, *Psychological Medicine, 16*, pp. 431–438.

Mandel, N.G. (1959) *Mandel Social Adjustment Scale* (Minneapolis, University of Minnesota).

Mann, S. and Cree, W. (1976) 'New' long-stay psychiatric patients: a national sample survey of fifteen mental hospitals in England and Wales 1972/3, *Psychological Medicine, 6*, pp. 603–616.

Mann, S. and Sproule, J. (1972) Reasons for a six month stay, in: Wing, J.K. and Hailey, A.M. (eds.) *Evaluating a Community Psychiatric Service*, pp. 233–245 (London, Oxford University Press).

Mechanic, D. and Greenely, J. (1976) The prevalence of psychological distress and help seeking in a college student population, *Social Psychiatry, 11*, pp. 1–14.

Morrison, R. and Bellack, A. (1987) Social functioning of schizophrenic patients: Clinical and research issues, *Schizophrenia Bulletin, 13*, pp. 715–725.

Mowbray, R.M., Blair, W., Jobl, L. and Clarke, A. (1961) The general practitioner's attitude to psychiatry, *Scottish Medical Journal, 6,* pp. 314–321.

Pattie, A. and Gilleard, C. (1976) The Clifton Assessment Schedule—further validation of a psychogeriatric assessment schedule, *British Journal of Psychiatry, 129,* pp. 68–72.

Paykel, E.S. and Weissman, M. (1973) Social adjustment and depression: A longitudinal study, *Archives of General Psychiatry, 28,* pp. 659–663.

Paykel, E.S., Klerman, G.L. and Di Mascio, A. (1973) Maintenance antidepressants, psychotherapy, symptoms and social function, in: Cole, J. O., Friedhogg, A. and Freedman, A. (eds.) *Psychopathology and Psychopharmacology,* pp. 205–218 (Baltimore, Johns Hopkins University Press).

Paykel, E.S., Weissman, M.M. and Prusoff, B.A. (1978) Social maladjustment and severity of depression, *Comprehensive Psychiatry, 19,* pp. 121–128.

Paykel, E.S., Weissman, M., Prusoff, B.A. and Tonks, C.M. (1971) Dimensions of social adjustment in depressed women, *Journal of Nervous and Mental Disease, 152,* pp. 158–172.

Phillips, L. (1953) Case history data and prognosis in schizophrenia, *Journal of Nervous and Mental Disease, 117,* pp. 515–525.

Phillips, L. (1968) *Human Adaptation and Its Failures* (New York, Academic Press).

Platt, S. (1986) Evaluating social functioning: A critical review of scales and their underlying concepts, in: Bradley, P. and Hirsch, S. (eds.) *The Psychopharmacology and Treatment of Schizophrenia,* British Association for Psychopharmacology Monograph No. 8, pp. 263–285 (London, Oxford University Press).

Platt, S., Weyman, A., Hirsch, S. and Hewett, S. (1980) The Social Behaviour Assessment Schedule (SBAS): Rationale, contents, scoring and reliability of a new interview schedule, *Social Psychiatry, 15,* pp. 43–55.

Remington, M. and Tyrer, P. (1979) The social functioning schedule—a brief semi-structured interview, *Social Psychiatry, 14,* pp. 151–157.

Richman, J. (1984) Sex differences in social adjustment: Effects on sex role socialization and role stress, *Journal of Nervous and Mental Disease, 172,* pp. 539–545.

Ruesch, J. and Brodsky, C.M. (1968) The concept of social disability, *Archives of General Psychiatry, 13,* pp. 36–44.

Ryan, P. (1979) Residential care for the mentally disabled, in: Wing, J.K. and Olsen, R. (eds.) *Community Care for the Mentally Disabled,* pp. 60–89 (London, Oxford University Press).

Sartorius, M., Jablensky, A. and Shapiro, R. (1977) Two year follow-up of the patients in the WHO International Pilot Study of Schizophrenia, *Psychological Medicine, 7,* pp. 529–541.

Schwab, J.J., Bell, R.A., Warheit, G.J. and Schwab, R.B. (1979) *Social Order and Mental Health: The Florida Health Study* (New York, Brunner/Mazel).

Shepherd, G. (1988) Evaluation and service planning, in: Lavender, A. and Holloway, F. (eds.) *Community Care in Practice,* pp. 91–115 (Chichester, Wiley & Sons).

Spitzer, R.L. and Endicott, J. (1978) *Schedule for Affective Disorders and Schizophrenia—Life-Time Version* (3rd edition) (New York State Department of Mental Hygiene, New York State Psychiatric Institute, Biometrics Research).

Spitzer, R.L., Endicott, J., Fleiss, J. and Cohen, V. (1970) The Psychiatric Status Schedule: A technique for evaluating psychopathology and impairment in role functioning, *Archives of General Psychiatry, 23,* pp. 41–55.

Stephens, J.H., Astrup, C. and Mangrum, J.G. (1966) Prognostic factors in recovered and deteriorated schizophrenics, *American Journal of Psychiatry, 122*, pp. 1116–1121.

Stevens, B.C. (1972) Dependence of schizophrenic patients on elderly relatives, *Psychological Medicine, 2*, pp. 17–32.

Stevens, B. (1973) Role of fluphenazine decanoate in lessening the burden of chronic schizophrenics in the community, *Psychological Medicine, 3*, pp. 141–158.

Strauss, J.S. and Carpenter, W.T. (1972) The prediction of outcome in schizophrenia, *Archives of General Psychiatry, 27*, pp. 739–746.

Strauss, J.S. and Carpenter, W.T. (1974a) The prediction of outcome in schizophrenia II relationships between predictor and outcome variables: A report from WHO International Pilot Study of Schizophrenia, *Archives of General Psychiatry, 32*, pp. 37–42.

Strauss, J.S. and Carpenter, W.T. (1974b) Evaluation of the outcome in schizophrenia, in: Ricks, D.F., Thonmas, A. and Roff, M. (eds.) *Life History Research in Psychopathology, 3*, pp. 313–335 (Minneapolis, University of Minnesota Press).

Sturt, E. (1984) Community care in Camberwell: a two year follow-up of a cohort of long-term users, *British Journal of Psychiatry, 145*, pp. 178–186.

Sturt, E. and Wykes, T. (1987) Assessment schedules for chronic psychiatric patients, *Psychological Medicine, 17*, pp. 485–493.

Ullman, L. and Giovannoni, J. (1964) The development of a self report measure of the process-reactive continuum, *Journal of Nervous and Mental Disease, 138*, pp. 38–42.

Vaillant, G. E. (1964) Prospective predictions of schizophrenic remission, *Archives of General Psychiatry, 11*, pp. 509–578.

Venables, P.H. (1957) A short scale for 'activity withdrawal' in schizophrenics, *Journal of Mental Science, 103*, pp. 197–199.

Wallace, C. (1984) Community and interpersonal functioning in the course of schizophrenic disorders, *Schizophrenia Bulletin, 10*, pp. 233–259.

Warner, R. (1985) *Recovery from Schizophrenia. Psychiatric and Political Economy* (London, Routledge and Kegan Paul).

Watts, F. and Bennett, D. (1977) Previous occupational stability as a predictor of employment after psychiatric rehabilitation, *Psychological Medicine, 7*, pp. 709–712.

Weissman, M. (1975) The assessment of social adjustment by patient self report, *Archives of General Psychiatry, 32*, pp. 357–365.

Weissman, M. and Paykel, E. (1974) *The Depressed Woman: A Study of Social Relations* (Chicago, University of Chicago Press).

Weissman, M., Sholomkas, D. and John, R. (1981) The assessment of social adjustment: An update, *Archives of General Psychiatry, 38*, pp. 1250–1258.

Weissman, M., Paykel, E., Siegel, R. and Klerman, G. (1971) The social role of depressed women: Comparisons with a normal group, *American Journal of Orthopsychiatry, 41*, pp. 390–405.

Weissman, M.M., Klerman, G.L., Paykel, E.S., Prusoff, B. and Hanson, B. (1974) Treatment effects on the social adjustment of depressed out patients, *Archives of General Psychiatry, 30*, pp. 771–778.

Weissman, M., Prusoff, B., Thompson, W., Harding, P. and Myers, S. (1978) Social adjustment by self report in a community sample and in psychiatric out patients, *Journal of Nervous and Mental Disease, 164*, pp. 317–326.

Williamson, R.C. (1976) Socialization, mental health and social class. A Santiago sample. *Social Psychiatry, 11*, pp. 69–784.

Wing, J.K. (1960a) The measurement of behaviour in chronic schizophrenia, *Acta Psychiatrica Scandinavica, 35*, pp. 245–254.

Wing, J.K. (1960b) Pilot experiment in rehabilitation of long-hospitalised male schizophrenic patients, *British Journal of Preventative and Social Medicine, 14*, pp. 173–180.

Wing, J.K. (1961) A simple and reliable subclassification of chronic schizophrenia, *Journal of Mental Science, 107*, pp. 862–875.

Wing, J.K. (1972) Principles of evaluation, in: Wing, J.K. and Hailey, A. (eds.) *Evaluating a Community Psychiatric Service*, pp. 283–308 (London, Oxford University Press).

Wing, J.K. and Brown, G. (1970) *Institutionalism and Schizophrenia* (Cambridge, Cambridge University Press).

Wing, J. and Freudenberg, R. (1961) The response of severely ill chronic schizophrenic patients to social stimuli, *American Journal of Psychiatry, 118*, pp. 311–322.

Wing, J.K. and Sturt, E. (1978) The PSE-ID-CATEGO System: A Supplementary Manual (London, Institute of Psychiatry).

Wing, J.K., Cooper, J. and Sartorius, N. (1974) *The Measurement and Classification of Psychiatric Symptoms: An Instruction Manual for the PSE and CATEGO System* (Cambridge, Cambridge University Press).

Wing, J.K., Mann, S.A., Leff, J.P. and Nixon, J.M. (1978) The concept of a 'case' in psychiatric population surveys. *Psychological Medicine, 8*, pp. 203–217.

Wing, L., Wing, J.K., Griffith, D. and Stevens, B. (1972) An epidemiological and experimental evaluation of industrial rehabilitation for chronic psychotic patients in the community, in: Wing, J.K. and Hailey, A.M. (eds.) *Evaluating a Community Psychiatric Service*, pp. 283–308 (London, Oxford University Press).

World Health Organization (1979) *Schizophrenia. An International Follow-Up Study*. John Wiley.

Wykes, T. (1982) A hostel-ward for 'new' long stay patients: an evaluative study of a ward in a house, in: Wing, J.K. (ed.) *Long-term Community Care: Experience in a London Borough*, Psychological Medicine Monograph Supplement No. 2, pp. 57–97 (Cambridge, Cambridge University Press).

Wykes, T. and Sturt, E. (1986) The measurement of social behaviour in psychiatric patients: An assessment of the reliability and validity of the SBS Schedule, *British Journal of Psychiatry, 148*, pp. 1–11.

Wykes, T., Sturt, E. and Creer, C. (1982a) Practices of day and residential units in relation to the social behaviour of attenders, in: Wing, J.K. (ed.) *Long Term Community Care: Experience in a London Borough*, Psychological Medicine Monograph Supplement No. 2, pp. 15–27 (Cambridge, Cambridge University Press).

Wykes, T., Creer, C. and Sturt, E. (1982b) Needs and deployment of services, in: Wing, J.K. (ed.) *Long Term Community Care: Experience in a London Borough*, Psychological Medicine Monograph Supplement No. 2, pp. 41–55 (Cambridge, Cambridge University Press).

Wykes, T., Sturt, E. and Creer, C. (1985) The assessment of patients' needs for community care, *Social Psychiatry, 20*, 0p. 76–85.

10

Studies of Residential Environments: Lessons from the Past and Pointers to the Future

Ian Sinclair and Ronald V. Clarke

Introduction

In 1970, John Wing and George Brown summarized eight years of research in their book *Institutionalism and Schizophrenia.* In the book they made an important distinction between the primary impairments which were the direct consequences or manifestations of the patients' disease and the secondary handicaps which reflected the way they were treated. The study compared the symptoms of patients in three different hospitals, and also examined the relationship between changes in the patients' symptoms and changes in hospital regime. In these ways, it produced evidence that some of the characteristics of people with schizophrenia that might have been ascribed to an illness seemed rather to arise from the patients' environment.

Wing and Brown's book was concerned with theories of cause and effect, which were tested empirically. It showed that there were important variations between residential settings, that the consequences of these variations could be researched, and that the findings of this research could have implications beyond the study of institutions, in this case for the understanding of what is of the essence of schizophrenia and what is accidental to it. This chapter takes up similar themes in the fields of social welfare and criminology. It seeks to outline the main approaches to studying residential care in these fields and to illustrate their relevance to arguments about cause and effect. It also aims to show that these arguments can have important implications for understanding the impact of environment on human behavior.

The examples used in the chapter mostly come from research undertaken in the sixties and seventies. The research described was concerned with relating the way institutions were run to the outcomes they achieved. Thus by 1975 there was already considerable evidence in the children's field about the relationship between the overall aims of an institution, its organization, the behavior of the staff, and the response of the residents (Tizard et al., 1975). By contrast the 1980s have seen excellent descriptive studies of children's homes, old people's homes, and residential homes for the adult physically handicapped (Berridge, 1985; Canter, 1981; Godlove, 1982; Weaver et al., 1985; Willcocks et al., 1982) but in these fields only Booth (1986) and arguably Evans et al. (1981) have deliberately set out to test hypotheses about cause and effect. As a result, the hypotheses arising from the earlier work on residential care for children have neither been tested further nor extended to other areas of residential care. By drawing on examples from this earlier work, the chapter may point to its potential.

One final point by way of introduction concerns the practical importance of studying residential care as well as the more fashionable community care outside residential establishments. Residential care serves diverse interests including those of:

Relatives—Parents may prefer a residential home to fostering, because the homes are more welcoming than competitive foster parents and find it easier to accommodate more than one child from the same family (Aldgate, 1977; Rowe and Lambert, 1973). The mental health of relatives caring for very disabled or confused old people may improve if the old person is removed to residential care (Gibbins, 1986; Levin et al., 1989; Whittick, 1985).

"Society"—Asylums provide a "culturally legitimate alternative" for the "awkward and unwanted" (Scull, 1982); Community Homes with Education (CHEs) may be seen as protecting society and punishing the delinquent.

The welfare system—Old people's homes may relieve the pressure on hospital beds, and children's homes may act as a necessary buffer for the foster home system (Parker, 1988).

Perhaps for these reasons, attempts to reduce rather than reform residential care have sometimes led to the rise of other forms of residential units—for example to the increase in the number of youth custody orders which has accompanied the fall in the number of CHEs. Residential care is here for the foreseeable future. Typically, its clients have become so at someone else's behest, and it is important that they are not further disadvantaged by living in homes which are badly run but rather that their quality of life is enhanced.

Three Approaches to Studying Residential Settings

The ways of studying residential settings are as varied as those in any other field of social research. For the purpose of this chapter it is convenient to distinguish three groups of studies:

- Case studies of single establishments
- Descriptive studies of a number of establishments
- Evaluative studies of more than one establishment

As will be seen these different approaches shade into each other and most of those undertaking case or descriptive studies have wished to pass some sort of evaluative judgment on what they describe. Nevertheless the three groups can be distinguished and each has distinctive advantages and disadvantages.

Case Studies of Single Establishments

Many of the famous studies of residential settings have been single case studies. The obvious example is Goffman's (1961) book on asylums which drew on a wide range of experience but was fundamentally influenced by his experience of a single institution. It is quite possible to undertake quantitative research within a single institution (Clarke and Martin's 1971 study of absconding discussed below contains examples of this), but the typical case study has used "anthropological" methods. The researchers have set out to soak themselves in the life of an establishment and tried to describe and make sense of what they observe.

The advantages of this method are apparent from its success. The studies are vivid and interesting. They may arouse indignation and convey conviction in a way which generally eludes more statistical work. They identify the key issues of residential life and are fruitful sources of hypotheses. In this way, they act as a check on more arid statistical enquiry, and set the agenda for future research. Even researchers who differ from Goffman over his conclusions and adopt very different resarch designs have had to tackle the questions he raised and operationalize his concepts (e.g., King, Raines, and Tizard, 1971).

Despite these advantages, the case study, in common with all research, has its defects. One difficulty arises because the researchers typically concentrate on the behavior, views, and experiences of residents and front line staff. This may lead them to ignore or misinterpret other influences (e.g., those connected with organization) which they do not experience in so direct a way. A more serious danger is that researchers may be led to generalize too widely on the basis of a single institution. Polsky (1963), for example, described a small unit in an American correctional school and saw it as a pecking order of roles whose essentially exploitative character would remain whatever the character of those who filled them. The staff had little choice; they could condone the system, or fight it and lose control. Polsky subtitled his book "The Social System of Delinquent Boys in Residential Treatment," thus implying that any unit which took in delinquent boys would exhibit a similar social system irrespective of its size, staff, organization, or theoretical orientation. More generally, Goffman's model of asylums concentrated on what he took to be the common features of residential institutions, and is largely incapable of accounting for differences or change.

Descriptive Studies of More than One Establishment

An obvious solution to the difficulty of generalizing from one example is to study more than one institution. The intention here may be *descriptive*—to find out, for example, what kind of residents a set of institutions receives—or *evaluative*—to compare the impact of one type of institution with that of another or of some community treatment. As already implied, the descriptive studies are also likely to be in a sense evaluative. The researcher is interested in appraising what he describes in light of current views of good practice (e.g., the principles of normalization) or stated policy. Nevertheless, the research design is essentially concerned with description rather than assessing what "causes" good results.

An early and outstanding example of this descriptive approach was provided by Peter Townsend in his study of residential establishments for old people (Townsend, 1962). Townsend combined detailed vignettes of individual institutions with the collection of statistical information on such things as the physical characteristics of old people's homes, and the disabilities and attitudes of their residents. He showed that many old people were housed in shocking accommodation, had entered residential care because somebody else thought they should, and were not so disabled that they could not with appropriate housing and services have maintained themselves in the community. Since the publication of this study, and partly, perhaps, because of it, the fabric of old people's homes has greatly improved. In other respects most subsequent research has simply served to reinforce the picture which Townsend presented. Most residents still enter these establishments when they are reluctant to do so, know little about where they are going, and are not so disabled that they require more or less constant care (Sinclair, 1988).

Although Townsend illustrates the great variety in old people's homes at the time of his study, the point he really wishes to make is about old people's homes as a whole, namely that they are unnecessary and undesirable. However, this disregard for the differences among residential units is not an inevitable consequence of the descriptive approach. Other researchers, while still essentially concerned with description, have paid more attention to differences and sought to classify establishments or identify ideal types to which they are more or less approximate. Well known examples include Miller and Gwynne's (1972) description of the "warehousing" and "horticultural" models of residential care for the physically handicapped, and Berridge's (1985) classification of children's homes as "family-group," "hostel," and "multi-purpose."

These classifications allowed the authors to compare establishments in terms of such things as physical facilities and the time spent by staff on different tasks. Such comparisons can be illuminating but can only be called evaluative if there is already agreement on "good ways" of running institutions. Often there is, but not always. There are real differences of opinion over, for example, the best way to run residential units for autistic, delinquent, or disturbed children, and these differences cannot be resolved simply by recording how these children are treated.

Evaluative Studies

From a research point of view the identification of better ways of running residential establishments depends on comparing them in terms of desirable outcomes or criteria. Different ways of achieving the necessary comparisons include:

Experimental designs—ideally involving the random allocation of suitable residents to one or more different kinds of establishment, as for example in Cornish and Clarke's (1972) evaluation of a "therapeutic" unit in an approved school. "Before and after" studies which look at changes in residents who move from one setting to a new experimental one (e.g., Gibbons, 1986) might be included here.

Quasi-experimental designs—comparisons of outcomes between different kinds of residential unit allowing for differences in their intake by means of matching or other appropriate statistical techniques (as for example in Mannheim and Wilkins' (1955) study of the effects of open and closed borstals).

Cross-institutional designs—comparing a number of different residential units and seeking to explain differences in outcomes by means of variations between the units along a small number of dimensions (as, for example, in the studies collated by Tizard et al. (1975), or in Booth's (1985) more recent study of old people's homes). As in quasi-experimental designs, allowances have to be made for differences in intake.

In general, experimental designs would be ideal if the main aim was to determine the likelihood that two or more units were producing different outcomes. Unfortunately, the price of achieving this aim is often uncertainty over what leads to better outcomes and how they can be reproduced. Practical considerations usually make it very difficult to carry out a random allocation experiment which involves more than two units, and these will necessarily differ in a wide variety of ways (e.g., in their staff, residents, regimes, and buildings) any one of which could result in one being more effective than another. Moreover, the mere existence of an experiment could result in a superior performance on the part of an experimental unit which would not be reproduced if the unit's regime was more widely adopted.

Quasi-experimental designs can more easily encompass a large number of units, and rely on natural variation which should make it easier to generalize their results. Unfortunately, they pay for these advantages over true experiments by allowing greater uncertainty over whether differences in outcomes arise from differences in intake. For example, Mannheim and Wilkins (1955) showed that, after allowing for differences in intake, open borstals (reformatories) had lower reconviction rates than closed ones. Unfortunately, however, they could not prove that they had taken into account all the characteristics which may have been considered by those allocating youths to the two kinds of borstal and which may have been related to outcome. Moreover, they could not show that it was openness per se, rather than some characteristic associated with it, which led to the apparently superior performance of the open borstals.

Cross-institutional designs overcome some of these problems, being specifically intended to link particular outcomes to particular aspects of residential regimes. Like quasi-experimental designs, they may be criticized on the grounds that they have failed to allow fully for differences in intake. Moreover, there is always the possibility that particular aspects of regimes which are found to correlate with "good outcomes" are not those which cause the apparent success. For this reason, the design is inappropriate when differences between regimes "cluster" so that it is difficult to disentangle the effect of one aspect of a regime from those of another. Nevertheless, the accumulation of evidence in a cross-institutional study can often make a causal inference plausible. Dunlop (1974), for example, in a study of eight approved schools, showed that the residents in all schools valued trade training, and that those schools which laid particular emphasis on it had, after allowing for differences in intake, significantly lower reconviction rates. The combination of these two findings strengthened her suggestion that the emphasis on trade training caused a reduction in reconviction.

The possibility of linking aspects of regime and aspects of outcome is not confined to cross-institutional designs. Studies of "hospital hostels," for example, have typically compared the behavior of residents on long-stay wards in psychiatric hospitals with the behavior of similar or the same people living in special hostels. The differences in the behavior of the residents in the two environments seem to be more plausibly related to differences in the environments themselves than, for example, to the passage of time or a "Hawthorne Effect" (Garety and Morris, 1984; Gibbons, 1986; Goldberg et al., 1985; Wykes, 1982).

More commonly perhaps, convincing causal inferences are made on the basis of a combination of designs. Tizard (1975), for example, examined the language development of young children placed in residential nurseries. Using a cross-institutional design, she showed that in nurseries where staff were given more autonomy, they were more likely to talk "informatively" to children who, in turn, were more likely to make gains in verbal IQ. Similar gains were not made in non-verbal IQ, reinforcing the view that the children were making the verbal gains because of the quality of their verbal exchanges with staff. The nurseries which gave more autonomy received children similar to the others, but did have higher staffing ratios and an older staff. In order to rule out the possibility that these differences rather than greater autonomy were leading to differences in the verbal behavior of the staff, Tizard used an argument not based on a cross-institutional comparison. She showed that in the nurseries as a whole the staff talked more informatively to children when they did not have a superior present, and were thus in a more "autonomous" position.

Generalizing from Studies of Residential Care: Two Examples

As should be clear, studies of residential care do not always aim at understanding or generalization. Some investigators seek only a careful description of a particular situation in order to show, for example, that a set of institutions are not serving the clientele for whom they were intended, or have inadequate buildings, or an undertrained staff. In most cases, however, the investigator wishes to generalize from his or her results. Barbara Tizard, for example, used her study of residential nurseries to suggest that previous hypotheses about the ill effects of institutions may have been ill founded. In her view, the poor social and emotional development of institutionalized children found in previous studies may have been due not to maternal deprivation consequent on removal to residential care, but to remediable defects in the residential units themselves. This argument is clearly important, both for the way residential units are run and for general theories of child development. This section of the paper gives two further examples of the wider relevance of studies of residential care, this time from the field of criminology.

The first study was carried out by one of the authors in the 1960s, and focused on hostels for youths on probation (Sinclair, 1971). At the time, these were small establishments catering to about twenty probationers who, depending on the hostel, were aged between fifteen and eighteen, sixteen and nineteen, or seventeen and twenty-one. Each hostel was run by a husband and wife team (the warden and matron), who were helped by one or two assistant wardens, and domestic staff. The youths were generally sent to the hostels for one year as a condition of their probation order, and while at the hostel they went out to work and were subject to a more or less strict regime (being required, for example, to hand over their wages to the staff).

The study was dominated by the remarkable variations between the hostels in their "failure rates" (the proportion of boys who left the hostel prematurely as the result of an absconding or offense), and with the remarkable influence on these rates of the married couples in charge of the hostels. The four main stages of the research involved:

1. *Analysis of records on 4,343 consecutive entrants to hostels over a ten year period.* Under different wardens failure rates varied from 15 percent to 78 percent. The variations were not explained by differences in the way abscondings or offenses were treated; and they were as great between successive wardens in the same hostel as between wardens in different hostels, thus suggesting that factors connected with the hostel (size, age range, environment, policy of local court or police force) were not important in explaining them.

2. *A survey of 429 probationers admitted to hostels in one year, using the information (probation reports) available to those selecting for hostels.* The survey sought among other things to determine whether high, medium, or low failure rate hostels were taking probationers with different risks of offending/absconding (they were not).

3. *Case studies of the five most and fourteen least successful regimes out of the forty-six on which data were available.* The successful regimes were run by wardens perceived as firm but kindly, and who agreed with their wives on the running of the hostel. In the unsuccessful regimes, the

wardens were seen as harsh or as weak disciplinarians or as in disagreement with their wives.

4. *A cross-institutional study of fourteen hostels designed to test the hypotheses arising from the case studies.* This showed that "successful" wardens tended to be strict (as measured by the number of rules in hostel), warm (as measured by an attitude questionnaire) and agreed with their wives on the running of the hostel (as measured by the number of agreements on their two attitude questionnaires).

These findings suggested that the delinquent behavior of probationers is strongly influenced by their current residential environment, and in particular by the adults in that environment. This suggestion was reinforced by a number of other findings. The staff seemed to influence not only how many probationers "failed," but also which ones were likely to do so (under some wardens, for example, older boys were more likely to fail and under others, younger ones). Moreover, the number of abscondings doubled in months when the warden and matron were away. Neither of these findings could be plausibly explained by selection.

Further evidence on the importance of the immediate environment came from the finding that probationers from particularly unsatisfactory families were less likely than others to be reconvicted while in the hostel but more likely to be so on return home. Moreover, with the exception of one regime there was no evidence that the massive variations in failure rates for the year the probationers were in the hostel were reflected in similar variations in reconviction rates after the probationers had left. Apparently, it was possible to have a major effect on the delinquent behavior of probationers by placing them in a residential setting with some similarities to a family: as a corollary, the families they had left exerted a similarly powerful influence on them on their return. Strikingly the features of the probation hostels which seemed to discourage delinquency (firm discipline, kindness, and consistency of approach) were precisely paralleled by the features of families associated with absence of reconviction among probationers (Davies, 1969), and, in the case of the hostel, the association could not be explained by invoking heredity, early childhood experiences, or family reputation.

More or less simultaneously with the probation hostel study, a different project, in which the second author of this chapter was involved, led to similar conclusions about the importance of the immediate residential environment. Clarke and Martin (1971) set out to study what distinguished children who absconded from approved schools from those who did not. Despite extensive investigations, they found no differences in the build, school attainments, intelligence, home backgrounds, psychiatric histories, or work records of the two groups. Nor could they find any differences in "personality" as judged by a wide range of different tests. There was, however, some evidence that absconders had appeared in court for the first time at an earlier age, and they were much more likely to have absconded from another setting. It seemed therefore that absconders and non-absconders differed in remarkably few respects except absconding itself.

Following these findings, Clarke and Martin turned their attention to factors in the school environment which might encourage absconding. They showed that some schools had absconding rates which were five or six times as high as others catering for boys of a similar age. They were also able to show that the likelihood of boys' absconding was greater if their house was particularly full, if unusually large numbers of boys had recently been admitted, if they were admitted close in time to a boy who had absconded from somewhere else, if they had not been recently visited by their parents, and if the most recent absconder had not been caned for doing so. There was also a seasonal variation, with two and a half times as much absconding in November as in June.

Clarke and Martin interpreted their results in the light of what they called "social learning theory." Boys would be motivated to abscond by unhappiness arising, for example, because their parents had not visited them. Absconding, however, was not the only possible response to unhappiness. Whether or not an unhappy boy absconded rather than, for example, talked to the staff, would depend on "cues" in the environment and in particular on the opportunities to abscond which would be greater when the evenings were darker and provided cover. Absconding predicted future absconding not because absconders differed from others in personality but because absconding became a learned behavior whose likelihood increased with its repetition. In the light of their theory they predicted that persistent absconders would show a "learning curve" and abscond at shorter and shorter intervals. Their predictions in this respect were born out.

Clarke and Martin's conclusions suggest that, if residential care is to have an effect on a resident's subsequent behavior, it will be through its effect on the resident's behavior while in residence. This hypothesis was explored in a cross-institutional study (Sinclair and Clarke, 1973), which showed that approved schools with high absconding rates had, after allowances had been made for differences in the previous convictions and IQs of their intake, unusually high reconviction rates. Differences in absconding rates, however, accounted for only a small proportion of the variation in reconviction rates. A more general conclusion of these studies was that it was likely to be very difficult to ensure that law-abiding behavior learned in one setting would transfer to another. Subsequent English research and research reviews have largely born out this view (e.g., Brody, 1974; Clarke and Cornish, 1972; Fowles, 1978).

Faced with this difficulty, one solution would be to see residential care as a bridge to a life in a new setting rather than time out from a previous one. There is some evidence for the potential of this approach. The one warden in the probation hostel study who was apparently able to influence the subsequent reconviction rates of his charges had established a sort of satellite colony of former residents around his hostel and stayed in close touch with them. A very different strategy was pursued by the former approved schools which trained youths for the merchant navy, and which had significantly lower reconviction rates than others (Clarke, 1965). The apparent success of both the warden and the merchant navy schools may have arisen from their encouragement of former residents not to return home. Such a strategy would depend for its success on close attention to the processes of discharge from an institution, and one study did find that long-term prisoners who were randomly selected for more intensive pre-discharge counselling were significantly less likely than their controls to be reconvicted (Shaw, 1974; Sinclair et al., 1974).

A different approach, but one still consistent with the findings discussed above, would be to see residential care as an additional support to a potential resident in his or her current environment. An obvious example of this approach would be the core and cluster homes developed for the mentally ill and the mentally handicapped, or family centers or elderly persons' support units which include a short-term residential component. The approach which does not seem to be viable is to regard people with behavioral problems as "damaged individuals" who can be taken from one setting, reformed, and returned as new beings to the setting from which they came.

Unfortunately, the approach just described as ineffective is precisely the one followed by the legal system. It is the person, not the setting, who is seen at fault, and treatment, in so far as this exists, is focused on offenders rather than their families. Reflections of this kind, combined with evidence on the limitations on the police in preventing or detecting crime (Clarke and Hough, 1980; Morris and Heal, 1981) led the Home Office Research Unit to consider other ways than policing or treating offenders for reducing the volume of crime. Clarke and his co-workers in the Unit drew on the concept of opportunity found useful in the absconding studies to develop what came to be known as the "situational" approach to prevention (Clarke and Mayhew, 1980). Essentially, this consists of identifying factors that make houses liable to burglary, cars to theft, public telephone boxes to vandalism, schools to break-ins, Underground passengers to mugging and so forth, with the purpose of modifying these factors to make crime less likely. Evidence now exists (much of it gathered in studies utilizing essentially "cross institutional" designs) that crime can be prevented through, for example, defensible space architecture, vandal-resistant materials and design, supervision of children's play on housing estates, flat-fare and "no change" systems on public transport, steering column locks on cars, screening of airline passengers and a variety of other situational measures.

The Home Office has now established a Crime Prevention Unit to promulgate the situational approach, and a stream of useful projects has resulted. This work has produced its own scientific problems, however, relating particularly to the concept of displacement—the idea that reduced opportunity to commit one crime leads to an increase in others. It turns out that this occurs only to the extent that some other easy opportunity exists for the offender to achieve his particular ends, whether for money, sexual release, or the acclaim of his peers. Research has shown that not only is displacement far from inevitable, but the benefits of situational measures may sometimes "spill-over" beyond their intended targets. Thus, steps taken to protect the more vulnerable dwellings on a council estate [public housing] were found to reduce the risk of burglary for all houses on the estate, possibly because the estate as a whole no longer offered such easy pickings for the less determined offenders (Forrester et al., 1988).

A final development traceable to the absconding research concerns work on preventing opportunities for suicide. While studying displacement, Clarke came across research suggesting that the 40 percent fall in the suicide rate of England and Wales in the 1960s and 1970s was due to the elimination of carbon monoxide from the gas supply. This made it all but impossible to use domestic gas for suicide, and the resultant decline in the suicide rate provided startling confirmation of the power of opportunity. Given that the motives for suicide are usually deep, it may have been surprising that so little displacement to other lethal agents occurred. However, domestic gas has distinct advantages as a method of death and many people seem to have been unwilling or unable to use some other method. This case study provided powerful support for the concept of situational crime prevention; if suicide could be greatly reduced by limiting opportunities, then surely so could crimes, most of which are much less deeply-motivated. It also stimulated further research into the potential for reducing suicide through controls on other lethal agents such as firearms, drugs, car exhaust gases, and jump sites (Clarke and Lester, 1989).

Conclusion

This article suggests that it is possible for research to identify the effects of different ways of running residential units on residents, and that research of this kind can be of considerable practical and theoretical interest. Our conclusion summarizes why we hold this view.

In the first place, for those seeking to establish causal links, it is a particular advantage of residential establishments that their residents are rarely born in them. For example, a large number of studies have shown that disagreements between parents are associated with delinquency in adolescents. This association could be explained through heredity, through the effects of quarrelling between parents on young children which becomes apparent in adolescence, or on the grounds that unruly adolescents incline the most united parents to strife. In the probation hostel study, however, the association of staff disagreements with delinquency among the residents could not be explained on the grounds of heredity or early upbringing. This suggested that delinquency is very much related to an adolescent's immediate home environment—an idea which received further support from the fact that delinquent behavior on discharge reflected the home to which the probationer returned more than the hostel he left.

A second advantage in the study of residential homes lies in their variety which makes them an ideal subject for "natural experiments." The homes differ in their aims, staffing, clientele, methods, and facilities. They organize themselves in different ways, keep their residents for longer or shorter periods, and allow them greater or lesser contact with the outside world. Variations in the behavior and experiences of residents in different establishments are also very great. Research instruments exist which are capable of capturing these diverse aspects of residential life, and there are research designs capable of linking the characteristics of a residential unit to its outcomes. Examples given in this chapter show how it is possible to link the different levels of residential life, for instance the degree of autonomy given to staff, their behavior and the linguistic development of children.

A third advantage in the study of residential care lies in the possibility of studying the same residents before, during, and after their time in an establishment and, in some cases, over a time of change in an establishment. The use that can be made of this opportunity has been illustrated in the probation hostel study and in the "before and after" studies of hospital hostels. To return to our earliest example, the persuasiveness of Wing and Brown's analysis of the influence of the environment on the behavior of people with schizophrenia depends only partly on the comparison of different hospitals. They were also able to show that changes in the behavior of patients over time in the same hospital could be explained by changes in the hospital environment, and that this explanation was consistent with the hypotheses arising from comparisons between hospitals.

From the point of view of residential care, such research is important. To take the examples just quoted, Wing and Brown's research provides important pointers for the environments that health and social services more generally should seek to provide for people afflicted by schizophrenia; Barbara Tizard provided evidence on the way residential nurseries should be organized; the probation hostel study emphasized the crucial importance of selecting, supporting, and, if ultimately necessary, removing staff. If similar conclusions about the role of staff hold good in old people's homes, the current emphasis on improving the homes through inspection will have little effect unless it is accompanied by appropriate policies on personnel.

More generally such research can provide the raw material for discussions of what residential care can and cannot achieve and how its achievements are possible. The examples given above make it less likely that residential care can have a major impact on delinquency, particularly if the method of doing so is to allow a certain level of "acting out" and if the delinquent is returned to the environment from which he came. Similar findings may hold in the field of mental health where some studies suggest that the patient's environment, both at home and in the hospital, can have an effect on the course of his illness (Goldstein and Caton, 1983; Brown et al., 1972; Vaughn and Leff, 1976; Wing and Brown, 1970). Such findings seem to support the view that residential units should be closely related to their residents' subsequent careers. In other words they would support attempts to use wards as back-ups for discharged patients (Mitchell and Birley, 1983), to tackle the family problems of patients discharged home (Leff et al., 1982), and to arrange that some patients do not return home but are given appropriate skills and accommodation to manage in the community (Mosher and Menn, 1978).

Finally, the studies on which we have been drawing have a relevance outside the field of residential care—Barbara Tizard's for the development of linguistic ability in children, our own, we hope for the sources of criminal behavior, and Brown and Wing's for the understanding of schizophrenia. Their practical implications can be wide; for example, the concept of opportunity which was highlighted for one of us by a study in the now defunct approved schools has proved useful in work on crime prevention and suicide.

For these reasons, we believe that the advantages of studies of residential care have been unwisely neglected. More of them are needed.

References

Aldgate, J. (1977) *The Identification of Factors Influencing Children's Length of Stay in Care*, Ph.D., University of Edinburgh. Also summarized in J. Triseliotis (ed.), (1980) *New Developments in Foster Care and Adoption*. London: Routledge and Kegan Paul, 22–40.

Berridge, D. (1985) *Children's Homes*. Oxford: Blackwell, 41.

Booth, T. (1985) *Home Truths*. Aldershot: Gower.

Brody, S.R. (1976) *The Effectiveness of Sentencing*. Home Office Research Study No. 35. London: H.M.S.O.

Brown, G.W., Birley, J.L.T. and Wing, J.K. (1972) Influence of Family Life on the Course of Schizophrenic Disorders: A Replication, *British Journal of Psychiatry, 121,* 241–258.

Canter, H., Barnitt, R. and Buckland, S. (1981) *This is Their Home: A Study of Residential Homes for Adults with Physical Disablement,* unpublished report, DHSS.

Challis, D., Chessum, R., Chesterman, J., Luckett, R. and Woods, B. (1987). Community care for the frail elderly: an urban experiment, *British Journal of Social Work, 18* supplement, 13–42.

Clarke, R.V.G. (1965) Success Rates of HMS Formidable in *Approved Schools Gazette* December, 369.

Clarke, R.V.G. and Martin, D.N. (1971) *Absconding from Approved Schools*. London: H.M.S.O.

Clarke, R.V.G. and Hough, J.M. (eds.) (1980) *The Effectiveness of Policing*. Farnborough, Hants: Gower.

Clarke, R.V.G. and Mayhew, P. (eds.) (1980) *Designing Out Crime*. London: H.M.S.O.

Clarke, R.V. and Lester, D. (1989) *Suicide: Closing the Exits*. New York: Springer Verlag.

Cornish, D.B. and Clarke, R.V.G. (1975) *Residential Treatment and Its Effects on Delinquency*. Home Office Research Study No. 32. London: H.M.S.O.

Cornish, D.B. and Clarke, R.V. (1988) *The Reasoning Criminal*. New York: Springer Verlag.

Davies, M. (1969) *Probationers in their Social Environment*. London: H.M.S.O.

Dunlop, A.B. (1974) *The Approved School Experience*. London: H.M.S.O.

Evans, B., Hughes, B. and Wilkin, D., with Jolley, P. (1981) *The Management of Mental and Physical Impairment in Non-Specialist Residential Homes for the Elderly*. Manchester: University of Manchester, Department of Psychiatry and Community Medicine.

Forrester, D., Chatterton, M., Pease, K. and Brown, R. (1988) *The Kirkhold Project, Rochdale*. Crime Prevention Unit Paper 13. London: Home Office.

Fowles, A.J. (1978) *Prison Welfare: An Account of an Experiment at Liverpool*. Home Office Ressearch Study No. 45. London: H.M.S.O.

Gibbins, R. (1986) *Oundle Community Care Unit: An Evaluation of an Initiative in the Care of the Elderly Mentally Infirm*. Northampton: Northamptonshire Social Services Department, Joint Research Steering Group.

Gibbons, J.S. (1986) Care of 'new' long-stay patients in a district general hospital psychiatric unit, *Acta Psychiatrica Scandinavica, 73,* 582–588.

Godlove, C., Richard, L. and Rodwell, G. (1982) *Time for Action: An Observation*

Study of Elderly People in Four Different Care Environments. Sheffield: University of Sheffield, Joint Unit for Social Services Research.

Goffman, E. (1961) *Asylums: Essays on the Social Situations of Mental Patients and Other Inmates.* Chicago: Doubleday.

Goldberg, D.B., Bridges, K., Cooper, W., Hyde, C., Sterling, C. and Wyatt, R. (1985) 'Douglas House: a new type of hostel ward for chronic psychotic patients,' *British Journal of Psychiatry, 147,* 383–388.

Goldstein, J.M. and Caton, L.M. (1983) The effects of the Community Environment on Chronic Psychiatric Patients, *Psychological Medicine, 13,* 193–199.

King, R.D., Raynes, N. and Tizard, J. (1971) *Patterns of Residential Care.* London: Routledge and Kegan Paul.

Leff, J., Kuipers, L., Berkowitz, R. and Sturgeon, D. (1982) A controlled trail of social intervention in the families of schizophrenics, *British Journal of Psychiatry, 141,* 121–134.

Levin, E., Sinclair, I.A.C. and Gorbach, P. (1989) *Families, Services and Confusion in Old Age.* Aldershot: Gower.

Mannheim, T. and Wilkins, L.T. (1955) *Prediction Methods in Relation to Borstal Training.* London: H.M.S.O.

Miller, E.J. and Gwynne, G.V. (1972) *A Life Apart.* London: Tavistock Publications.

Mitchell, S.F. and Birley, J.L.T. (1983) The Use of Ward Support by Psychiatric Patients in the Community, *British Journal of Psychiatry, 142,* 9–15.

Morris, P. and Heal, K.H. (1981) *Crime Control and the Police: A Review of Research.* Home Office Research Study No. 67. London: H.M.S.O.

Mosher, M.D. and Menn, A.Z. (1978) Community Residential Treatment for Schizophrenia: Two-Year Follow-up, *Hospital and Community Psychiatry, 29,* 715–723.

Parker, R.A. (1988) Residential Care for Children. In Sinclair, I.A.C. (ed.) *Residential Care: the Research Reviewed.* London: H.M.S.O.

Polsky, H.W. (1963) *Cottage Six, the Social System of Delinquent Boys in Residential Treatment.* New York: Russell Sage Foundation.

Rowe, J. and Lambert, L. (1973) *Children Who Wait,* Association of British Adoption Agencies.

Scull, A. (1982) *Museums of Madness: The Social Organisation of Insanity in Nineteenth-Century England.* Harmondsworth: Penguin.

Shaw, M. (1974) *Social Work in Prison: an Experiment in the Use of Extended Contact with Prisoners.* London: H.M.S.O.

Sinclair, I.A.C. (1971) *Hostels for Probationers.* London: H.M.S.O.

Sinclair, I.A.C. and Clarke, R.V.G. (1973) Acting out and its significance for the residential treatment of delinquents, *Journal of Child Psychology and Psychiatry, 14,* 283–91.

Sinclair, I.A.C. and Clarke, R.V.G. (1974) The Relationship between Introversion and Response to Casework in a Prison Setting, *British Journal of Social and Clinical Psychology, 13,* 51–60.

Sinclair, I.A.C., Shaw, M.J. and Troop, J. (1974) The relationship between introversion and response to Casework in a Prison Setting, *British Journal of Social and Clinical Psychology, 13,* 57–60.

Tizard, J., Sinclair, I.A.C. and Clarkes, R.V.G. (1975) *Varieties of Residential Experience.* London: Routledge and Kegan Paul.

Tizard, B. (1975) Varieties of Residential Nursery Experience. In Tizard, J.,

Sinclair, I.A.C. and Clarke, R.V.G. (eds.) *Varieties of Residential Experience.* London: Routledge and Kegan Paul.

Townsend, P. (1962) *The Last Refuge: A Survey of Residential Institutions and Homes for the Aged in England and Wales.* London: Routledge and Kegan Paul.

Vaughn, C. and Leff, J. (1976) The influences of family and social factors on the course of psychotic illness, *British Journal of Psychiatry, 141,* 121–134.

Weaver, T., Willcocks, D. and Kellaher, L. (1985) *The Business of Care: A Study of Private Residential Homes for Old People,* Report No. 1. London: The Polytechnic of North London, Centre for Environmental and Social Studies in Ageing.

Whittick, J. (1985) The impact of psychogeriatric day care on supporters of the elderly mentally infirm. In *Dementia Research Innovation and Management.* Edinburgh: Age Concern Scotland.

Wilcocks, D.M., Peace, S. and Kellaher, L. with Ring, A.J. (1982) *The Residential Life of Old People: A Study in 100 Local Authority Old People's Homes, Volume I,* Research Report No. 12. London: Polytechnic of North London, Survey Research Unit.

Wing, J.K. and Brown, G.W. (1970) *Institutionalism and Schizophrenia.* Cambridge: Cambridge University Press.

Wykes, T. (1982) A hostel-ward for 'new' long-stay patients. In Wing, J.K. (ed.) Long-term community care: experience in a London borough, *Psychological Medicine,* Monograph Supplement 2.

III

From Research to Practice

11

Transcultural Psychiatry: A Question of Interpretation

R. Geil

Introduction

In recent years transcultural psychiatry has seen important changes and developments. There has been a demystification of culture-bound syndromes, although interest in their occurrence has certainly not waned. Furthermore, coordinated by the World Health Organization, various cross-cultural epidemiological investigations demanded the application of standardized research instruments, which required careful translation and evaluation. These studies resulted in an awareness of the universality of the more important mental disorders such as schizophrenia and the affective psychoses and, indeed, also of minor mental disorders. This finally led to demands for the extension of professional mental health care to areas of the world which had hitherto been dependent only on popular and folk healing systems. Most recently, there has been a resurgence of doubt regarding the universal applicability of professional mental disease categories as originated in the technically advanced countries.

In this chapter these developments will be briefly discussed. I will then use somatization disorder as an illustration of transcultural issues.

The Culture-Bound Syndromes

As a considerable improvement on section V of ICD-9 and its glossary, published by WHO in 1978, DSM-IIIR appears to have conquered the world right from its publication in 1981. This has happened almost as if semantic and methodological problems were minor (Kroll, 1988) in comparison to what stood to be gained by its use in transcultural research. Kapur (1987) objected strongly to the arbitrariness and reductionism involved in fitting culture-bound syndromes into illness categories assumed to be universal primarily by investigators from the Western world. Nevertheless, Simons and Hughes (1985) have successfully reviewed the world literature on "unfamiliar ways of being crazy" or "instances of deviant deviance," while trying to fit them into the categories of DSM-IIIR. They wanted to find out whether standard diagnostic categories are inadequate because they themselves are conceptually culture-bound, whether the exotic syndromes are simply unusual rather than pathological, or if there is such semantic confusion that meaningful discussion is altogether impossible. If one accepts that culture shapes ideation and psychomotor behavior, they argue, then it follows that at the phenomenological level there can be culturally distinctive ways of being mentally disordered regardless of the extent even of specific organic involvement. In the same way, anatomical and neurological factors provide the substrate and mechanism for speech, which expresses itself in culturally programmed language. The question then concerns the cultural context of norms and conceptualizations of illness relevant to the experience and behavior of the patient. For example, there may be typical social situations or disadvantaged roles that, over time, foster or predispose toward temporary or chronic disorder, as does the role of the established beggar in many African countries (Giel et al., 1974; Baasher et al., 1983). In this sense, the syndromes are more culture-reactive than culture-bound (Hughes, 1985). Indeed, the majority of non-culture-bound syndromes are not really qualitatively different in this respect.

While trying to separate accounts of meaning from accounts of unusual experience or behavior, Simons (1985) found that meanings may vary markedly from site to site, but that the salient features of those experiences and behaviors are sometimes surprisingly similar in historically unrelated and culturally dissimilar times and places. This led him to sort the syndromes into seven sets, or taxa: the startle matching taxon, the sleep paralysis taxon, the genital retraction taxon, the sudden mass assault taxon, the running taxon, the fright illness taxon and the cannibal compulsion taxon. This kind of sorting based on seemingly more exotic behavior or experience sometimes brings out additional features which the members of a taxon appear to share, although they are logically unconnected with those on which the sorting was based. The point is to find a formulation to explain the taxon. Simons emphasized that a distinction should be made between features which account for a syndrome's descriptive features and those which account for its being endemic to one site and absent from another (shape versus distribution). Factors which determine why a syndrome occurs in one place and not another are not necessarily the same as those which account for its descriptive features.

The West Indian anthropologist Wooding (1984) described the case of a man from Surinam, aged forty-four years, who had "inherited" a jungle spirit. He shared certain phenomena with some of his sisters and brothers, the sensation of waking up in the middle of the night with someone sitting on his chest and trying to smother him. The victim felt powerless and paralyzed. Traditional healers had not been able to help this man who suffered this indignity once or twice a month. The same phenomena are quite common in Ethiopia and Egypt (Giel, 1968; Kahane, 1984), where they are assumed to be caused by "Zar-spirits," inhabitants of the supernatural world. There they are not always malevolent, because they sometimes offer women in particular an escape from daily hassle and hardship through the trance state they induce when possessing their victim. More unpleasant is their tendency to visit someone who is about to fall asleep or wake in the middle of the night and sit on his chest trying to smother him. The victim feels paralyzed and very fearful, and may have threatening visions.

Similar observations have been made at other distant sites. For example, in Alaska where the experience has been noted amongst Eskimos (Bloom and Gelardin, 1985). The spirit world continues to exist as a reality for many Eskimo people, for whom dreaming is conceived as the wandering of the soul, while the concept of separation of body and soul also relates to death. An Eskimo woman aged thirty years provided the following description of an attack, related by Bloom and Gelardin: "Just before going to sleep and waking up, I get paralyzed. Sometimes it starts with a buzzing. Sometimes I can almost see something and it scares me. My grandparents told me it was a soul trying to take possession of me, and to fight it. After the buzzing sound I can't move. Sometimes I really start feeling like I am not in my body anymore, like I am outside of my body and fighting to get back. If I don't get back I never will. I really get panicky."

The woman became very anxious, remained dissociated for some length of time and had to be admitted.

Ness (1985) described how the victims of "Old Hag" or "Ag Rog," descendants of immigrants from the English West Country to the northeast coast of Newfoundland, suddenly awake feeling unable to move or speak. The experience occurs most frequently shortly after falling asleep. Concurrent with paralysis, victims often feel as though a heavy weight is pressing on their chest. Some report seeing the figure of an animal or a human astride their chest. Witnesses of such an attack report that some victims groan and that their eyes may be open or closed. The person's body is motionless and breathing appears normal. After the attack the victim usually perspires heavily and appears exhausted.

In this Newfoundland community, common explanations of "being hagged" are that the blood stagnates, especially if a person sleeps on his back; or when a person has worked too hard, for example, pushing himself too far at a lumber camp; or precipitated by another person who harbors hostile feelings toward the victim. The latter explanation is expressed by older people in the community. Ness found that Old Hag is not considered an illness or a symptom of illness by people. It was hardly ever mentioned by patients of the regional health center. He also established that respondents with a history of Old Hag did not report significantly more emotional or physical complaints, as measured with the Cornell Medical Index, than respondents with no history of attacks. In other words, it did not seem to generate the same terrifying experience it caused in an Eskimo or Ethiopian.

The frightening representation of sleep paralysis in certain cultures appears to be a culture-reactive syndrome resulting from its specific meaning in those cultural settings, while on the other hand it trancends cultural boundaries as a common phenomenon because of its biomedical genesis. In this respect, the concept of a taxon helps to demystify the culture-bound syndromes. However, it could also provide an opportunity to demystify some of the generalizations of DSM-IIIR, for example, by considering the cultural specificity of agoraphobia, anorexia nervosa, or somatization disorder, which, contrary to Old Hag, do find a place in DSM-IIIR.

In the next section of this chapter somatization disorder will be discussed, not within the context of a taxon, but as a transcultural issue which has come to the foreground as a result of the professional reinterpretation of complaints commonly seen in general outpatients in the developing countries (Kleinman, 1988).

Somatization, a Professional Transcultural Reinterpretation

The WHO Collaborative Study on Strategies for Extending Mental Health Care (Harding et al., 1983b) can be considered a landmark in the development of professional mental health care in the developing countries. The study was conducted in primary care populations in pilot study areas in Cali, Colombia; near Chandigarh, India; in Niakhar, Senegal; near Khartoum, Sudan; in Manila, the Philippines; in Fayoum, Egypt; and in Porto Alegre, Brazil. The study was designed to test the feasibility and effectiveness of a set of simple steps taken to provide effective care for selected priority conditions in each of the areas. It included making comparisons between baseline observations carried out before the interventions and repeat observations carried out after the interventions had been introduced.

Before the intervention program began, health staff were largely unable to diagnose mental disorders, either alone or in combination with physical disorders. The actual rate of mental disorder among adult patients in primary health care in the areas where the study was completed, found with a screening procedure that included a Self-Reporting Questionnaire and the Present State Examination, ranged from 10.6 percent to 17.7 percent. Health staff in the areas failed to detect about two-thirds of the psychiatric cases during the base-line observations. The five commonest reasons for attendance quoted by the patients were headache, abdominal pain, cough, genito-urinary symptoms, and fever (Harding et al., 1980). Psychological symptoms, such as anxiety, depression, and sleep disturbance, were quoted very infrequently as reasons for attendance. Most patients with mental disorders, gave a physical symptom as the reason. The majority of such cases missed by the primary health workers were among patients complaining of headache, abdominal pain, cough, back pain, and weakness. Patients quoting three or more reasons for attendance were twice as likely to be suffering from mental disorder (30 percent) than patients quoting one reason only (15 percent). So far, it may be concluded that patients in the study areas had a tendency to somatize their psychosocial problems, while health workers apparently did not pick up the psychological cues that the self-reporting questionnaire did.

After the training component of the intervention program had been introduced, diagnostic sensitivity of the primary health workers against the Self-Reporting Questionnaire improved considerably, except in the Indian area where the research team had decided beforehand that minor health problems were not their concern. They felt that the modern psychiatrist had little to offer, either in theory or in practice, over and above traditional forms of healing and support.

Central to the whole study concerning adults was the Self-Reporting Questionnaire, an inventory of twenty-four items selected from other such instruments (e.g. the GHQ), which was translated and back-translated, and validated and calibrated in each study area (Harding et al., 1983a). Since a majority of patients attending the clinics were illiterate, research workers were trained to read the questions to all subjects. Written instructions were provided, and training programs had been prepared in which clear criteria were given for recording positive or negative responses. In the training program, the SRQ was used to reorient the primary health worker toward a different category of disease, and ultimately their patients toward a different category of illness. Here illness refers to the patient's perception, experience, expression, and pattern of coping with symptoms, while disease refers to the way practitioners recast illness in terms of their theoretical models of pathology (Kleinman, 1988).

How valid was this procedure? According to Kleinman "assuring the validity of psychiatric diagnoses should involve a conceptual tacking back and forth between the psychiatrist's diagnostic system and its rules of classification, alternative taxonomies, his clinical experience, and that of the patient, which includes the patient's interpretation." This applies in particular to a transcultural exercise like the WHO Collaborative Study, which aimed at reorienting patients and their health workers towards psychologization of their distress. This is justified as long as it concerns treatable conditions. In the following sections we will look at somatization as a transculturally valid category and at the ethnocentric qualities of an instrument such as the SRQ. Finally, the chapter will conclude with a discussion of the diagnosis and management of more persistently somatizing patients in primary care in a developing country.

Somatization in a Transcultural Perspective

In the industrialized world we are inclined to consider, for example, immigrants from North Africa as people who somatize their distress. It is likely that every sociocultural environment has its own way of facilitating the expression of distress with the more or less conscious objective of mobilizing support. The result is a process of negotiation which may reveal conflicts between the basic perceptions and values of sufferer and healer (Kirmayer, 1984). The very use of the word "somatization" expresses this conflict because it tells us that the patient is not performing according to the expectations of the health professional. By this we mean the expectations of the Western doctor: psychiatrists from the Indian subcontinent and the Far East complain about the "overloading of a few emotions (anxiety and depression) only and the tendency to psychologize in Western societies" (Wig et al., 1985).

Kirmayer (1984), in a recent review of the literature on culture, affect, and somatization, has listed various definitions of somatization: the presentation of physical symptoms in the absence of organic pathology, or the amplification of physical complaints accompanying organic disease beyond what can be accounted for by physiology; the presentation of somatic symptoms in place of personal or social problems; or the hypothetical mechanisms by which emotions can give rise to somatic signs and symptoms of illness. The latter include the vegetative manifestations of depression and anxiety, conversion symptoms, and psychophysiological disorders.

Somatization always involves a discrepancy between where the observer believes a problem is located or how he expects it to be expressed and the subject's experience and expression of it in the body. Kirmayer emphasizes that to understand somatization we must understand the observer's frame of reference as well as the patient's. On the basis of his extensive review of the literature, Kirmayer is convinced that "somatization has been found wherever it has been sought and, worldwide, somatic symptoms are more common than emotional complaints as a way of presenting psychosocial distress. Viewing somatization as an anomaly or pathological process seems hard to sustain in the face of its widespread prevalence. Instead, it is the more exotic phenomenon of 'psychologization,' occurring among an educated Western urban minority, that may require special explanation."

From his survey he concluded that somatic symptoms are a common type of presentation to both Western-style physician and traditional healer, even when emotional and interpersonal conflict seem obvious to all concerned. In addition, there is a tendency for somatic and psychological symptoms to occur together in the same people and under similar circumstances. According to Kirmayer, this challenges any simple dichotomy of symptoms.

This view is supported by several studies conducted in the Western world. For example, Ginsberg and Brown (1982) found that severely depressed mothers in a London suburb tended to visit their general practitioner for minor or non-specific somatic complaints in their children, i.e., they somatized by proxy. Likewise, Mechanic (1980) studied what differentiates the determinants of physical and psychological complaining. His assumption is that the two major determinants are actual experience with symptoms and illness on the one hand, and cultural influences on the definition of illness on the other. He found that reporting physical symptoms is culturally more neutral, whereas reporting psychological symptoms is more dependent on social acceptability. In this research in Wisconsin, the social desirability response bias was significantly associated with reporting psychological symptoms but not with reporting physical symptoms. Mechanic suggests "that even the reporting of relatively specific physical symptoms constitutes part of an illness behavior and response pattern that transcends a narrow view of physical illness"; and "such symptom reports are in part dependent on psychological state and may reflect to some extent an extrasensitivity to bodily sensations as a result of situational stress or prior learning."

The above implies that ratings on an instrument such as the Self-

Reporting Questionnaire may differ considerably in meaning from one cultural environment to another, indicating more of physical illness in one, situational distress in another, or socially established attitudes towards the self in a third. This, in turn, has implications for the interventions planned for the kind of "cases" detected with the Self-Reporting Questionnaire. The significance of meaning or interpretation to the interventions will be discussed in the final sections of this chapter.

The Transcultural Reinterpretation of Meaning

Applying instruments like the Self-Reporting Questionnaire transculturally amounts to a dual process of reinterpretation. On the one hand, it involves the health workers in a process of reorientation from common physical symptoms to underlying psychological distress, on the other, it is a first step in trying to detect what the patients' illness behavior might mean to themselves. Kortmann (1987) focused on the latter, using the SRQ with three groups of Ethiopians: psychiatric outpatients, patients from various other outpatient clinics, and residents of Addis Ababa who were not undergoing any form of treatment.

First, the English version of the SRQ was translated, backtranslated, tried out, revised, once more backtranslated, and then finalized. Just as in the WHO *Collaborative Study on Strategies for Extending Mental Health*, the questionnaire was read to the patients, many of whom were illiterate. However, the procedure thereafter was different. While the questionnaire was being administered, the investigator kept notes on questions that had to be repeated and on the patient's spontaneous comments accompanying the requested "yes" or "no." Next, the list of twenty-four questions was run through a second time to obtain more detailed information on all positive responses and on those that had drawn comments from the respondent. Finally, on the basis of this clarification the investigator judged whether it did or did not confirm the presence of psychopathology, as implied in each question. Comparing the original with the revised responses, Kortmann could distinguish three kinds of problems in communication which appeared to invalidate some of the originally positive responses. They had to do with language (7 percent), motivation (7 percent) and conceptualization (26 percent). The four psychotic items in the SRQ induced problems of communication more often (respectively 14, 5, and 48 percent), than did the nonpsychotic items (6, 8 and 23 percent). The language in which some questions were couched proved too difficult or circumstantial to be understood by a number of respondents without being repeated or clarified. The explanations of other respondents showed that their positive responses did not reflect truly what they experienced, but indicated simulation or exaggeration in order to escape from an unpleasant employment situation or from military service. Conceptual difficulties were more numerous. For example, "poor appetite" led often to misunderstanding in those respondents who lacked sufficient food. "Sleeping badly" was frequently connected with nightmares and sleep-walking only, and not so much with falling and staying asleep. "Unhappiness" and "crying more than usual" were automatically linked to the loss of a relative (commonly of a violent nature at that time), and particularly to the crying which is culturally more or less obligatory at a funeral. Questions regarding the "difficulty of making decisions" and "playing a useful part in life" had strong political overtones in a culture in which freedom of expression had always been limited.

Kortmann questioned the validity of the SRQ also because of the "large discrepancies between terms used spontaneously by Ethiopians to express their feelings of being sick when they were seeking help, and the concepts to which the SRQ questions refer. Seventy percent of the psychiatric group sought help for complaints such as burning sensations in the head, or the feeling that worms were crawling and biting in their brain. What Kortmann failed to appreciate here is the purpose of the SRQ as an instrument of reinterpretation, from "somatization" on the part of the patient towards "psychologization" as required by the mental health professionals. That the latter was quite successful is evident from his own finding that in psychiatric outpatients the SRQ had a sensitivity of 90 percent and a specificity of 44 percent at a cut-off point of 8/9 against the psychiatrist's assessment when applying DSM-IIIR criteria (Kortmann, 1986); in the group of normal respondents sensitivity was 100 percent and specificity 86 percent at a cut-off point of 4/5. It is interesting to note that amongst the patients of other (somatic) clinics, sensitivity was 63 percent and specificity 68 percent at a cut-off point of 8/9. Kortmann supposed that the SRQ-scores reflect illness behavior in general, in addition to psychiatric illness.

Orley and Wing (1979) had similar problems of communication when they used the PSE in a community survey in two Ugandan villages. They suggest that it is better not to bother with direct translations of the original questions but to start instead with formulating the concepts behind the questions in the desired language, or translating the glossary of definitions first and then matching the PSE translation to the glossary. They gave pertinent examples of the fallacy of direct translations without due consideration of meaning. For example, unless "Can people read your thoughts?" is translated into "Can strangers know your thoughts?" the interpretation by the respondent involves reading books, and therefore does not make sense. Another example is that of defining the period of time to be reviewed. In Lugandan, a direct translation of "last month" would refer to the previous period from one new moon to the next. Furthermore, the authors also found marked differences in the attitudes of respondents towards the interviewer and his curiosity. Questions implying comparison with others would be responded to by returning the question: "How can I know about others?." This may also reflect differences in the interpretation of meaning regarding a health questionnaire between a community sample with little interest in illness behavior at the time of the survey and patients displaying illness behavior in reaction to distress. In the final sections of this chapter it will become clear that attitudes play a key role in defining interventions to deal with somatization.

Diagnosing the Persistently Somatizing Patient

A sad-looking young man of eighteen years, having exhausted the medical resources of his home town, Debre Markos, is referred to a psychiatric clinic in Addis Ababa, some 300 miles away. There he complains of burning sensations in the head, as if something is crawling under his skin. The almost continuous feeling of heaviness in his head changes occasionally into a stabbing pain, particularly when he moves his head. In addition he has a troublesome itch inside his throat, which he tends to study in the mirror. There is also a tight feeling over the right chest. Not counting his gastritis, which was diagnosed years ago, these complaints have worried him almost daily for about two years, especially when he is outside in the sharp light of the sun. He was the eldest child in a family of six, but a few years ago his parents died and the family broke up. Seven years ago he started attending a church school near his village. After his parents died, he moved on to Debre Markos to attend a more advanced church school. His two brothers had to find employment as shepherds in order to survive. His sister married a poor farmer. They have all had a hard time. At this point in the interview the patient starts to cry. Although his own position has improved slightly since he became a deacon, he feels absolutely helpless to support his relatives, which he considers his duty as the eldest of the siblings. The patient denies strongly any relationship between his worries and his vague complaints for which no physical cause can be found.

This is the kind of case detected with the help of the SRQ. However, the WHO Collaborative Study on Strategies for Extending Mental Health Care was quite ambiguous about such patients. The participants were aware that it is common for such patients to shop around or be referred fruitlessly from one clinic to another. Yet, they also knew that reorienting primary health workers so they would try to get patients to reinterpret their complaints is no easy job, particularly in a developing country with other pressing problems in primary care. It was therefore decided that the objective of training should merely be the identification of such cases in order at least to prevent unnecessary referral (Giel and Workneh, 1980).

Because physical examination usually results in normal or, at most, dubious findings, the identification of this type of problem rests almost exclusively on the verbal and non-verbal behavior of the patient. In general, information provided by a patient has two distinct aspects: that of its actual content, for example, on the duration or location of his complaints, and that determining his relationship with the doctor, for example, how seriously the information is to be taken by the doctor or the extent to which the patient wants to influence the doctor's actions. Awareness of the relationship the patient is trying to establish is extremely important. The following characteristics determine the actual content of the complaint:

(1) one vague physical complaint only, which remains hard to grasp and is totally unsymptomatic of any known physical condition, e.g. crawling under the skin or heat in the head or body; (2) a multitude of physical complaints which, on further questioning, again lead to nothing specific, for example, coldness, numbness, tightness, itching, choking, heaviness, blurred vision. (3) complaints which, although specific to physical conditions, are expressed in an exaggerated manner, with too much suffering implied; (4) more specific psychological complaints such as insomnia, lack of concentration, irritability, anxiety, worry, and sexual inadequacy.

The verbal and nonverbal behavior of the patient establishing his relationship with the doctor and the health services has the following features: (1) contrary to local custom, most adult patients appear unaccompanied by concerned relatives, whose patience has already been exhausted; (2) their explanations will be lengthy, worried, difficult to interrupt, and not in the form of clear responses to pointed questions; (3) if patients are literate they are likely to carry a list of their symptoms with them to ensure that they do not overlook anything; (4) they may mention that, elsewhere, gastritis and amoebiasis have, of course, already been diagnosed; (5) depending on whether the patients are seen in an urban or rural clinic, their attendance will be one in a long series of visits to a variety of medical institutions and traditional healers, none of whom has been able to alleviate their suffering; (6) without being asked, they may produce a sheaf of papers, prescriptions, and laboratory findings, indicating the failure of others to satisfy their needs; and, finally, (7) they may put a row of medicine bottles on the doctor's desk.

The doctor's contribution to the non-verbal part of the interaction are signs of irritation, based on his own mounting apprehension of impending failure to provide relief for so much suffering, and his groping for the prescription pad and the right kind of tranquilizer or placebo.

The complaints and suffering of these patients should not be taken as simulated or as conscious malingering. On the contrary, they are often unhappy people, full of worries about the possible causes of their illness and, even more so, about its future development and harmful consequences for vital bodily and mental functions. Worries about the latter, for example, the brain will ultimately be affected and rot away, overshadow by far the actual complaint.

The complaints probably originate in anxiety which may result from a recent threatening life experience such as loss of a relative, divorce, illness, or separation in the family etc., and with which the patient is unable to cope properly, either because of unfavorable circumstances or due to a lack of inner resources. Alternatively, anxiety may be more deeply rooted and based on early neurotic conflicts which were reactivated for unknown reasons. In both cases, the sufferers' anxiety is accompanied by anger and depression about their own helplessness to change this situation and, as these feelings threaten this self-esteem, they have to be repressed. Turning to bodily sensations (somatization) is a way of coping with the original anxiety. This explains why it is so difficult to deal with such symptoms. Their removal, for example by giving the patient some insight into his condition (reinterpretation through psychologization), would reactivate the underlying and disturbing anxiety, anger, and depression. Kleinman (1988) gives a beautiful example of a woman with the diagnosis of neurasthenia, which is acceptable in Chinese culture, whose social situation was, nevertheless, clearly unpalatable. Yet, recognition of this fact (the psychologization of neurasthenia) would place her in a culturally unacceptable position. Complaining was, therefore, patient's inadequate way of coping with a difficult situation or with life in general.

While the mechanism described above sets the process of somatization in motion, another factor, i.e., secondary illness gain, favors its continuation. The sick role offers certain additional advantages to patients, such as the concern of their entourage and exemption from a number of tasks at home or at work. Even though these benefits may be quite dubious and not really acceptable, at least not for a prolonged period of time, they tend to perpetuate the sick role. It is difficult for the patients' relatives to object openly, since they are obviously sick and seeing a doctor. The same applies to the sanctioning of a situation by the traditional healer who uncovers a bad spirit possession his client.

Management of the Somatizing Patient in a Developing Country

Once the primary worker in a developing country has been induced to diagnose and reinterpret somatization in this way, he is left with the unhappy task of deciding what to do next, to improve, for example, on the successes of the traditional healer. Management of such patients depends on which level of care in the network of health services is involved. The primary health worker in his health station or the medical assistant in a health center at the next level of care may do little more than proceed with the first tentative steps in the total management of such cases. All will have the following spontaneous responses in common: (1) they will feel overwhelmed by vague and multiple complaints which challenge their professional responsibility not to miss a serious physical illness; (2) they will be under pressure of time in their busy outpatient clinic; (3) they will get frustrated by their failure to come to grips with the symptoms; (4) they will tend to defer a decision by referring the patients for further examinations; (5) if they do suspect an emotional basis for the complaint, they will not dare to touch it—either because they consider a person's emotions his private property or because they are afraid to be confronted with socially unacceptable emotions, such as that of a divorced woman.

If health-workers are not aware of this complementary relationship with the patient, and respond only to the content of the complaint, escalation is likely. Disqualification of one complaint as not indicative of any significant physical condition will force the patient to come forward with yet another. Referral for specialist or laboratory examination will only justify the complaint and will firmly establish the patient in his complaining attitude. Confirming the complaint as symptomatic of a physical condition, for example, by linking it to some dubious X-ray or laboratory finding, will not relieve the patient's worries and leads to unjustified medical attention to his problem. Therefore, it is the relationship which has to be managed rather than the content of the complaint.

It is clear that this kind of reinterpretation of physical symptoms required of the health-worker poses considerable problems. In the context of the WHO *Collaborative Study on Strategies for Extending Mental Health Care*, this led to formulation of the following sequence of steps in the management:

Step 1. While taking the history of the patient, health workers should recognize the above listed features of the complaint and relationship as indicative of their emotional background. Such recognition should not follow only after all possible physical causes have been excluded.

Step. 2. A physical examination, strictly within the limitations of the clinic and the capabilities of the health worker, should be made to show patients that their suffering is taken seriously and not considered as simulated or malingering.

Step 3. Next, the patients should be firmly confronted with the negative findings and comforted with regard to the content of their worries. If examination reveals a physical condition, not coinciding with their complaints, patients should be told of this discrepancy, while their physical condition is treated. Depending on the training, time, and interest of the health worker, management of the case can stop here, with an explanation that this is as far as they can go.

Step 4. Health workers with more interest, time, or training may, at this stage, explore the patient's life situation for a recent more or less threatening experience. They may also venture to suggest a solution or refer the patient to community agents for advice and assistance. If no such events can be detected and a neurotic conflict is suspected, the health worker may decide to close the case.

Step 5. This step brings the health worker, without undue effort and with a possibility of success, into the realm of psychiatry, because it involves giving patients insight into how their worrying attitude is more crippling than the content of the complaint itself. More difficult is to show patients how their illness behavior and dependent attitude are influencing their relationships, and the extent to what they provide them with a self-defeating protection. Here the main problem for health workers will be that they will immediately be confirmed more strongly in the complementary relationship with the danger of an escalation of medicalization on their part and of further somatization on that of the patient. In this case, health workers will have to focus on this relationship with the patient. It is essential for this step for health workers to set a limit on the number of contacts with the patient. This will prevent false conclusions on both sides or the continuation of a relationship which no longer serves a useful purpose. If the health worker remains unsuccessful, referral to a mental health service can be considered, but it should be noted that, in most neurotic' cases, the psychiatrist does little more than has been described under Steps 4 and 5.

Medication can be introduced, in the form of benzodiazepines, at each step but their prescription needs very careful consideration because they may lead to dependency or become part of the escalation as prescription also carries a message to the patient. It is first necessary to ask what drugs have already been used, for how long, and in what dosage? The chances are that the patient has already exhausted the list, because they are among the most widely distributed drugs in the Third World. If medication is unavoidable, it should aim at a clearly indicated symptom or complex of symptoms, and the drug should be prescribed for a limited period of only two or three weeks. If the drugs do not help they should be discontinued with an explanation that they are obviously not the answer to patient's problem.

Escalation of medication takes two forms. Either patients want endless continuation of a prescription because it worked and they fear recurrence of their anxiety, or they demand other and stronger prescriptions because the previous one was ineffective. Requests for medication can become instrumental in manipulating the doctor-patient relationship, with a tendency on the part of health-workers to yield too easily to compensate for this sense of failure.

So far, this discussion of the management or reinterpretation of somatization shows that for most health workers it is more a matter of what not to do.

Conclusion

In this chapter some recent developments in transcultural psychiatry have been discussed. They have to do with the interpretation or rather the reinterpretation of psychiatric reality. Describing taxons is an attempt at a professional reinterpretation, which illustrates that some of the diagnostic categories of DSM-IIIR are perhaps interpretations of reality, i.e., culture-bound syndromes instead of universal classes of disease. Anorexia nervosa is an example, and perhaps also the recategorization of neurasthenia (Kleinman, 1988), which lingers on in China, but seems to have reappeared as dysthymia in DSM-IIIR.

The discussion of an important transcultural study coordinated by WHO reveals the magnitude of the problem that results from the decision to reinterpret common physical complaints in primary care in developing countries.

References

Baasher, T., El Hakim, A.S.E.D., El Fawal, K., Giel, R., Harding, T.W., and Wankirii R.N. (1983) On vagrancy and psychosis. *Community Mental Health Journal* 19, 27–41.

Bloom, J.D. and Gelardin, R.D. (1985) Uqamairineq and Uqumanigianiq: Eskimo sleep paralysis. In: Simons and Hughes *The Culture-Bound Syndromes.* pp 117–122. Reidel, Dordrecht.

Giel, R., Gezahegn, Y., and van Luijk, J.N. (1968) Faith-healing and spirit-possession in Ghion, Ethiopia. *Social Science and Medicine* 2, 63–79.

Giel, R., Kitaw, Y., Workneh, F., and Mesfin, R. (1974) Ticket to heaven: Psychiatric illness in a religious community in Ethiopia. *Social Science and Medicine*, 8, 549–556.

Giel, R. and Workneh, F. (1980) Coping with outpatients who cannot cope: management of persistent complainers in an African country. *Transactions of the Royal Society of Tropical Medicine and Hygiene*, 74, 475–478.

Ginsberg, S. and Brown, G.W. (1982) No time for depression: a study of help-seeking among mothers of pre-school children. In: D. Mechanic, *Symptoms, Illness Behavior, and Help-Seeking*. Watson, New York.

Harding, T.W., de Arango, M.V., Baltazar, J., Climent, C.E., Ibrahin, H.H.A., Ladrido-Ignacio, L., Murthy, R.S.., and Wig, N.N. (1980) Mental disorders in primary health care; a study of their frequency and diagnosis in four developing countries. *Psychological Medicine* 10, 231–241.

Harding, T.W., Climent, C.E., Diop, Mb., Giel, R., Ibrahim, H.H.A., Strinivasa Murthy, R., Suleiman, M.A., and Wig, N.N. (1983a) The WHO Collaborative Study on Strategies for Extending Mental Health Care, II: The Development of New Methods, *American Journal of Psychiatry*, 140, 1474–1480.

Harding, T.W., d'Arrigo Busnello, E., Climent, C.A., Dio, Mb., El Hakim, H., Giel, R., Ibrahim, H.H.A., Ladrido-Ignacio, L., and Wig, N.N. (1983b) The WHO Collaborative Study on Strategies for Extending Mental Health Care, III: Evaluative Design and Illustrative Results. *American Journal of Psychiatry* 140, 1481–1485.

Hughes, C.C. (1985) Culture-bound or construct-bound? The syndromes and DSM-III. In: Simons and Hughes. *The Culture-Bound Syndromes*. pp 3–24. Reidel, Dordrecht.

Kapur, R.L. (1987) Commentary on culture-bound syndromes and international disease classification, *Culture, Medicine, and Psychiatry* 11, 43–48.

Kahane, Y. (1984) The Zar spirits, a category of magic in the system of mental health care in Ethiopia. Research report of the Institute of Desert Investigation. Ben Gurion University, Israel.

Kirmayer, L.J. (1984) Culture, affect and somatization: Part I. *Transcultural Psychiatric Research Review* 21, 159–188.

Kirmayer, L.J. (1984) Culture, affect and somatization: Part II. *Transcultural Psychiatric Research Review* 21, 237–262.

Kleinman, A. (1988) *Rethinking Psychiatry: from Cultural Category to Personal Experience*. Free Press, New York.

Kortmann, F. (1986) Problemen in transculturele communicatie: de Self-Reporting Questionnaire en de psychiatrie in Ethiopië. van Gorcum, Assen.

Kortmann, F. (1987) Problems in transcultural communication in transcultural psychiatry. *Acts Psychiatria Scandinavica* 75, 563–570.

Kroll, J. (1988) Cross-cultural psychiatry, culture-bound syndromes and DSM-III, *Current Opinion in Psychiatry*, 1, 46–52.

Lishman, W.A. (1987) *Organic Psychiatry; the Psychological Consequences of Cerebral Disorder*. Blackwell, London.

Mechanic, D. (1980) The experience and reporting of common physical complaints. *Journal of Health and Social Behavior* 21, 146–155.

Ness, R.C. (1985) The Old Hag phenomenon as sleep paralysis: a biocultural interpretation. In: Simons and Hughes. *The Culture-Bound Syndromes*. pp 123–145. Reidel, Dordrecht.

Orley, J. and Wing, J.K. (1979) Psychiatric disorders in two African villages. *Archives of General Psychiatry* 36, 513–520.

Simons, R.C. and Hughes, C.C. (1985) *The Culture-Bound Syndromes; Folk Illnesses of Psychiatric and Anthropological Interest*. Reidel, Dordrecht.

Simons, R.C. (1985) Sorting the culture-bound syndromes. In: Simons and Hughes. *The Culture-Bound Syndromes*. pp. 25–38. Reidel. Dordrecht.

WHO (1978) ICD, Mental Disorders: Glossary and guide to their classification in accordance with the ninth revision of the International Classification of Diseases, Geneva.

Wig, N.N., Kusmanto Setyonegoro, R., Shen, Yu-Cum, and Sell, H. (1985) Problems of psychiatric diagnosis and classification in the Third World. In: *Mental Disorders; Alcohol- and Drug-Related Problems. International Perspectives on their Diagnosis and Classification.* Excerpta Medica, Amsterdam.

12

The Relevance of Psychosocial Risk Factors for Treatment and Prevention

Julian Leff

Introduction

The medical model of disease is quite often incorrectly identified with a strictly biological view of aetiology and pathology. It is in fact a model that postulates the existence of disease entities that are harmful in a variety of ways to the individual sufferer. It stands in contrast to social models which postulate that the individuals who are perceived by society as threatening are designated as sick. The morbid process, in this kind of thinking, lies in the relationship between the individual and society and is not located within the individual. The medical model asserts that the individual would suffer from an illness regardless of society's attitude towards him/her, although the course of the illness might well be influenced by the attitudes of people in the sufferer's social milieu. Social models maintain that the "illness" would disappear if society's attitude changed from rejection to acceptance of the individual. In a nutshell, social models cast the individual in the role of a victim of society, whereas the medical model views him/her as the victim of a disease process. The medical model does *not* exclude social factors and processes but views them as operating on a disturbance of the individual's bodily structure and/or function. The term "bodily" includes the brain, the integrity of which is essential for the normal functioning of mental processes.

The contrast between the models is brought into sharp focus by a consideration of schizophrenia. The medical model conceptualizes this condition as a disease of the brain which has its basis in morbid structural and functional changes in that organ. Until recently, that remained a working hypothesis with very little supportive evidence. However, in the past decade the development of brain imaging techniques has revealed structural abnormalities in the brains of a proportion of schizophrenic patients (e.g., Smith et al., 1988). It is consequently more difficult to sustain social models that state that schizophrenia is a pejorative label applied by psychiatrists to people who are in conflict with society. This view was prevalent in the 1960s and was promulgated by Laing (Laing and Esterson, 1964). It received a boost from the Russian practice of diagnosing political dissidents as schizophrenic, although the international community of psychiatrists vigorously opposed this as an abuse of psychiatry (Bloch and Reddaway, 1984).

Research on schizophrenia within the Social Psychiatry Unit has always been firmly based on the medical model. The assumption has been that schizophrenia is a disease of the brain that renders the sufferer particularly susceptible to stresses arising from the social environment. The thrust of the research has been directed at identifying and measuring the relevant stresses, examining their interaction, determining whether they are specifically linked to schizophrenia, and studying their effects on measures of biological function. Each of these aspects will be reviewed here with a main focus on schizophrenia, but with consideration given to other psychiatric and non-psychiatric conditions where these are illuminating.

Measuring Social Stress

The concept of stress has passed into public usage, and most people harbor an amorphous notion that it is harmful, without being able to specify in what way. The situation in psychiatry in the fifties was not much better. There was a wide range of theoretical models of the ways in which stress might operate to cause disease, but very little was available in the way of measurement. The concept of stress remained global and hence virtually undefinable. A major advance was achieved by the development of measures of acute stress, in the form of life events, and chronic stress, as represented by relatives' Expressed Emotion (EE).

Life Events

The initial approach to research in this area was either to study prospectively the onset of illnesses following a particular event, such as bereavement or induction into the army (Steinberg and Durell, 1968), or to use an inventory of possible events to enquire retrospectively into the period before the onset of an episode of illness (Dohrenwend, 1975). The issue of the relative psychological impact of a particular event was tackled by asking a panel of judges to rank the list of events in order of increasing stress. A consensus list was compiled, at the top of which was death of spouse. There are a number of problems with this approach.

Firstly, it relies on the individual to check off from the list any events that have occurred in the relevant time period, without any prompting of memory. Secondly, the timing of the event is supplied by the respondent without any cross-checking. Thirdly, the psychological impact of any event on a specific individual may vary enormously according to the circumstances. For instance, the effect of a death in the family must depend on the age of the deceased, whether or not it could be anticipated, and the quality of the relationship between the subject and the deceased. Brown effectively tackled the problems by developing an interview technique to elicit life events—the Life Events and Difficulties Schedule (LEDS), and by pioneering a method of assessing the emotional impact of each event on an individual by taking the context into account (Brown and Harris, 1978).

Research based on this technique firmly established that life events clustered in the three months before the onset of depressive episodes in women but that their impact depended on the presence of certain vulnerability factors: loss of mother before the subject was age 11, the absence of a confiding relationship, the presence of three or more children under age 15, and the lack of a job (Brown and Harris, 1978). Furthermore, it was established that only events that represented a significant loss were followed by depression.

Subsequent work by others has confirmed some, but not all of these findings, while Brown and his colleagues have discovered that the vulnerability factors vary according to the social class and cultural milieu of the subject. However, the model that is supported by these results remains a seminal one for the field and is clearly applicable to other psychiatric disorders. It is a model that has been proposed in a general form by others (e.g., Zubin and Spring, 1977), but specifies interactions between the factors involved in considerably more detail. It postulates that only people who are vulnerable will respond to an event involving a severe or moderate loss with a depressive illness. Vulnerability can be estimated by the degree of the subject's self-esteem. This may be lowered by the experience of poor mothering during childhood, and additionally by the lack of a supportive current relationship. A job outside the home may raise self-esteem by providing the experience of competence in an extraneous activity. The emotional demands stemming from three or more children at home under 15 years of age are self-evident, but it should be noted that middle-class women can buy-in help to ease the burden, while this may be beyond the reach of working-class women, particularly if they lack the income from a part-time or full-time job. Genetic factors can be incorporated in the model as conferring an additional risk of depression, but there is still controversy over their role in the aetiology of depressions in the neurotic range of the spectrum.

It is worth stressing that the great bulk of research has focused exclusively on women and that it is uncertain that this model would apply to depression in men. The model has value in suggesting further research, particularly into the postulated links between early experience of mothering and current level of self-esteem. It is of course possible that women who have experienced poor parenting in childhood choose marital partners who are incapable of providing adequate emotional support (Harris et al., 1987). The association between depression and a poor marital relationship, as confirmed by the work on relatives' EE (Vaughn and Leff, 1976b; Hooley et al., 1986), might then be a product of an enduring personality factor in the patient. One way of exploring this possibility would be to employ techniques of assessing attributional style (Brewin and Furnham, 1986). Individuals who attribute misfortune to global, stable, and internal factors, even after a depressive episode has resolved, may turn out to have a predilection for critical partners.

Determination of the direction of cause and effect between the factors in this model is a very complex matter, which will be discussed below. It is timely, now, to consider the specificity of the association between life events and episodes of depression. Before embarking on his research into depression, Brown studied the social environment of schizophrenic patients, including the occurrence of life events (Brown and Birley, 1968; Birley and Brown, 1970). Life events that were independent of the patient's behavior occurred in the three weeks before onset of an episode of schizophrenia to 46 percent of patients compared with 14 percent of healthy controls (p<0.001). This finding indicates that life events are not specific stressors for any particular psychiatric illness. Indeed subsequent studies have shown that life events are also associated with the onset of non-psychiatric conditions including myocardial infarction (Connolly, 1976), acute abdominal pain with a healthy appendix (Creed, 1981), and other painful gastrointestinal disorders (Craig and Brown, 1984). However, Brown and Birley's (1968) study of schizophrenia suggested that life events operate over a shorter time period in precipitating episodes of this condition than in the case of depression: three weeks instead of three months. The association between life events and the onset of schizophrenia and the short time period of their influence have both received substantial confirmation in a recent study by the World Health Organisation (Day et al., 1987). This collaborative study involved nine different centers located in developing and developed countries and employed a slightly extended version of the life events schedule used currently by Brown and his colleagues. In two of the centers insufficient cases were collected to justify analysis, while in the Ibadan center very few life events were recorded during any time period preceding onset of schizophrenia. In the other six centers, there was a highly significant concentration of life events in the three weeks before episodes of schizophrenia.

Another approach to specificity concerns the contextual ratings of impact discussed above. This technique for measuring the degree of threat posed by an event was developed after the study of schizophrenia was completed. However, Brown and his colleagues (1973) applied it retrospectively to the data collected in the original study (Brown and Birley, 1968) and found that more than 70 percent of all events reported by schizophrenic subjects were of little or no threat. If confirmed, this would represent a striking difference from depression, episodes of which are mostly preceded by moderately or severely threatening events. In fact, Leff and Vaughn (1980) in a study to be described below, failed to support this finding, although they employed a somewhat different measure of the desirability of events. They found that 64 percent of events experienced by schizophrenic patients were judged to be undesirable compared with 67 percent of those experienced by depressed patients. The WHO study used a measure of impact closer to Brown's contextual threat rating and found that 61 percent of events reported for the schizophrenic patients were of moderate or severe impact. Hence these two studies are in close agreement and conflict with Brown's retrospective analysis of his earlier data. Further studies are needed to resolve this issue, but as it stands, the role of life events in precipitating episodes of schizophrenia and depression cannot be differentiated on the basis of the degree of threat they pose.

Relatives' Expressed Emotion

This measure of the relatives' emotional attitudes towards the patient was developed initially by Brown and Rutter (1966) and later modified by Vaughn and Leff (1976a). The early work was concerned with schizophrenia, but has subsequently broadened to include a wide range of psychiatric and nonpsychiatric conditions. The research on schizophrenia has consistently found a significant relationship between three elements of EE, critical comments, hostility, and overinvolvement, and the course of positive symptoms (Brown et al., 1972; Vaughn and Leff, 1976b; Vaughn et al., 1984; Moline et al., 1985; Jenkins et al., 1986; Neuchterlein et al., 1986; Leff et al., 1987; Tarrier et al., 1988). Failure to replicate this association by some workers can be explained on the basis of methodologciencies (Dulz and Hand, 1986; MacMillan et al., 1986), but in one study the lack of an association between EE and the outcome of ophrenia cannot be ascribed to problems with design or technique ker et al., 1988). The majority of studies, however, support the original ding, and these are displayed in Table 12.1.

The Camberwell Family Interview (CFI) from which EE ratings are made, is generally conducted at the time of the patient's admission to hospital. It was always assumed that the way the relative responded in the interview was representative of his or her behavior towards the patient in the home. However, evidence on this point was not sought until recent years, during which a number of studies of direct interaction between relative and patient have been conducted (Miklowitz et al., 1984; Strachan et al., 1986; Szmuckler et al., 1987). These have demonstrated that there is a close correspondence between ratings of critical comments in the CFI and in direct interactions. The same is not true of overinvolvement, possibly because this rating can be made on the basis of behavior reported by the relative of a kind that may be difficult to observe in an hour or less of interaction in an experimental setting, for example, excessive self-sacrifice.

Critical comments are by no means confined to the relatives of schizophrenia patients and were found by Vaughn and Leff (1976b) to be as common in the relatives of individuals with depressive neurosis. However, the prediction of relapse in these depressed patients was not achieved using a threshold of six critical comments, which was a powerful predictor of the outcome of schizophrenia. Instead, Vaughn and Leff found it necessary to lower the threshold to two critical comments to achieve a significant prediction of depressive relapse. This finding was treated with

TABLE 12.1
Relatives EE and Schizophrenic Relapse over 9 months–1 year

			RELAPSE RATES %	
Study	**City**	**Ethnic Group**	**High EE**	**Low EE**
Brown et al 1972	London	British	58	16
Vaughn & Leff 1976	London	British	50	12
Vaughn et al 1984	Los Angeles	Anglophone	56	17
Moline et al 1985*	Chicago	White & Black	91	31
Karno et al 1986	Los Angeles	Mexican	58	26
Tarrier et al 1988	Salford	British	53	22
Neuchterlein et al† 1986	Los Angeles	Anglophone	37	0
Leff et al 1987†	Chandigarh	Indian	31	9

*Threshold of 9 critical comments
†First onset or recent cases only

caution but has recently been replicated by Hooley et al. (1986). The data from these two studies suggest that patients with schizophrenia have a differential sensitivity to relatives' critical attitudes compared with those suffering from depression. However a study of obese women by Fisch-mann-Havstad and Marston (1984) revealed that they were as sensitive to their spouses' criticism as depressed patients; a threshold of two critical comments predicted whether they would maintain a weight loss achieved by dieting.

Recent research on patients with Parkinson's disease has identified relatives' critical comments as a determinant of the course of their symptoms; not the motor disturbances, but the dementia (McCarthy, personal communication). As with schizophrenia, the threshold for prediction of outcome was six critical comments. Thus, although there is some diagnostic specificity in the predictive thresholds, it is by no means absolute.

Relatives' EE has been measured in a number of current studies involving patients with anorexia nervosa (Szmuckler et al., 1985), childhood epilepsy, diabetes, and inflammatory bowel disease. The outcome of this research has yet to be reported, but is certain to throw light on the predictive thresholds of the component scales of EE.

Relationships between Life Events and Relatives' Expressed Emotion

We have seen that the time period during which events cluster has some specificity for schizophrenia, whereas the degree of threat implicit in events is non-specific, as is the stress occasioned by relatives' EE. Perhaps diagnostic specificity lies in the ways in which these acute and chronic stresses interact. This possibility was explored by Leff and Vaughn (1980). In their comparative study of patients with schizophrenia and depressive neurosis (Vaughn and Leff, 1976b), they had included measures both of life events and of relatives' EE. This made it possible to examine the relationship between these two forms of stress in each diagnostic group.

When they divided the schizophrenic patients into high EE and low EE groups, they found a significant difference in the experience of life events during the three *months* before onset of an episode of illness. Out of the twenty-one high EE patients, six had experienced an event compared with eleven of the sixteen low EE patients (exact p=0.02). This difference became even more pronounced when the three *weeks* before onset were examined, the rates being one out of twenty-one (5 percent) high EE patients compared with nine out of sixteen (56 percent) low EE patients (exact p=0.001). By contrast, the depressed patient with high and low criticism relatives (threshold of two critical comments) showed no difference in their experience of life events in the three *weeks* before onset, but a significant difference during three *months*. These data confirm the findings from other studies of the different time periods over which events exert their effects on depression and schizophrenia. Furthermore, among the depressed patients, life events were more frequent in high criticism than in low criticism homes (76 percent vs. 33 percent, exact p = 0.04). This is the reverse of the interaction seen in schizophrenic patients between these two forms of stress. The findings for depressed patients lend some support to Brown's model, since they indicate that, in the greater proportion (70 percent in this study) of depressed neurotic patients, life events operate in conjunction with a vulnerability factor. In this instance, the factor measured—critical comments made by a relative—almost certainly represents another aspect of a poor supportive relationship that Brown measured through intimacy.

From these data, we might conclude that life events and relatives' EE rarely act in conjunction to bring about episodes of schizophrenia. This would be premature, since a consideration of the role of prophylactic antipsychotic medication alters the picture. In Leff and Vaughn's (1980) study, only six of the schizophrenic patients were found to be receiving regular medication, and all lived in high EE homes. In a subsequent paper, Leff et al. (1983) added data on high EE patients on regular medication who had either relapsed or remained well during a follow-up period after discharge. The number was rather small, totalling fourteen, of whom six had relapsed. Five of these six had experienced a threatening life event in the three weeks before relapse compared with two of the eight patients who remained well (exact p = 0.049). Thus it appears that life events are important precipitants of relapse in high EE patients who take regular prophylactic medication.

These relationships can be formulated in the following statements: schizophrenic patients who are unprotected by medication are vulnerable to acute stress in the form of life events and chronic stress represented by life with a high EE relative. Patients exposed to the continuous stress of a high EE home relapse in response to everyday interactions. Patients in low EE homes can manage the ordinary routines of life but can be provoked into a relapse by the occurrence of a life event. Patients in high EE homes who are on regular medication are also protected against the stress of interactions with their relatives, but the medication is insufficient to cope with the additional stress of a life event. Patients in low EE homes on medication are sufficiently protected against life events and rarely relapse. In fact, of fifteen such patients followed up for two years by Leff and his colleagues, only a single individual relapsed. Thus it appears that neuroleptic medication can protect schizophrenic patients against either a life event or the stress of high EE home but not against the combination of the two.

Antidepressant medication is not as potent a prophylaxis as antipsychotic medication, which may explain why it has not been incorporated in Brown's model in an analogous way to the above statements concerning schizophrenia. This formulation generates testable hypotheses, in particular that lowering the EE level of the home should reduce the relapse rate of schizophrenic patients on neuroleptic medication. A number of studies that test this hypothesis have been conducted, but before considering them we will discuss the role of social contact between patients and relatives.

Face-to-Face Contact

It is logical to assume that high EE attitudes exert an effect on the patient during the course of social interaction with the relative. To check this assumption, one would like ideally to measure the amount of social interaction that occurs in the home. Short of setting up a recording apparatus in the home, it is necessary to find an indirect measure of interaction. Brown and his colleagues (1972) achieved this by constructing a time budget of a typical week from accounts by the patient and relative. They were then able to calculate the number of hours per week that patient and relative spent together in the same room. This figure excluded time occupied by sleep and was assumed to reflect the amount of social contact that occurred. The measure was named face-to-face contact, and an arbitrary threshold of thirty-five hours per week was established to distinguish between high and low contact.

In the earliest piece of research on relatives' attitudes and schizophrenia, social distance from the relative was found to protect patients in high EE homes from relapse (Brown et al., 1962). In the second study, in which more refined measures were employed, the amount of face-to-face contact made no difference to the relapse rate of patients in low EE homes (Brown et al., 1972). However, as in the earlier study, low face-to-face contact appeared to confer some degree of protection on patients living with high EE relatives. The relapse rate was 19 percent for patients spending less than thirty-five hours per week with high EE relatives compared with 79 percent for those in high contact, a highly significant difference (p<0.01). Very similar findings emerged from Vaughn and Leff's (1976b) replication, the relapse rates being 29 percent and 57 percent for low contact and high contact respectively. Once again, contact did not exert a significant effect in low EE homes. Given the consistency of these findings, it is surprising that in no study outside the Social Psychiatry Unit has face-to-face contact been identified as a significant predictor of relapse for schizophrenic patients. This discrepancy is unlikely to be due to technical problems with the measure, although it is not always easy to determine accurately, particularly when informants are vague about their weekly activities. Nor is it feasible to ascribe it to cultural differences in patterns of socialization, since studies conducted in London (MacMillan et al., 1986) and Salford (Tarrier et al., 1988) have also failed to replicate this result. We cannot explain this difference between research within and outside the Unit, and face-to-face contact continues to be viewed as a significant factor in Unit work.

One study has examined the role of face-to-face contact in a non-schizophrenic illness, namely depressive neurosis (Vaughn and Leff, 1976b). It was found that the amount of face-to-face contact between patients and relatives did not relate to relapse patterns. However this factor was associated with the number of initial comments made by relatives. Depressed patients whose relatives made two or more critical comments had significantly less contact with them than did patients whose relatives were low on criticism (exact p = 0.024). Thus face-to-face contact has quite a different significance in depression compared with schizophrenia. Instead of representing a protective factor, it is associated with the relative's expression of criticism. Virtually all the relatives of depressed patients in this study were spouses. Consideration of individual case histories suggested that low contact with a spouse at the time of admission to hospital was indicative of a poor relationship between patient and spouse that antedated the depressive illness. It seems likely that low contact and high criticism are both indicators of a poor marriage, and that it is the poor quality of the marriage that predicts relapse of depression. Once more this interpretation echoes the findings of Brown and Harris (1978).

Studies of Therapeutic Intervention in Families

As we stated above, the model of schizophrenia formulated on the basis of naturalistic studies can be tested by experimentally manipulating the family environment and looking for changes in the patients' relapse rate. A number of studies of this type have now been completed, although not all of them were designed specifically to test a model of this kind. The two studies conducted in the Unit were of this nature, and represent a logical progression of the series of naturalistic studies carried out over fifteen years or so. At the time the first study was being planned, in 1976, there was no published study demonstrating the success of a family intervention for schizophrenia. There was a large body of work on abnormalities in the parents of schizophrenic patients which was stimulated by theories of family causation of the illness. However, an extensive review of these studies by Hirsch and Leff (1975), failed to identify any feature that was specific to the parents of schizophrenic patients. There was a relevant study of family intervention in progress, but we were unaware of it until it was published two years later (Goldstein et al., 1978) when our own trial was already under way.

Under these circumstances we were impelled to construct our own program of therapeutic intervention aimed at reducing relatives' EE and/ or face-to-face contact. We included in the trial patients who were in high contact with high EE relatives since they would be expected to have a high relapse rate even when on regular prophylactic medication—about 50 percent over nine months. If the model derived from the naturalistic studies was correct, either lowering EE or face-to-face contact below the threshold would be expected to reduce the relapse rate to about 15 percent over nine months. Knowledge of the anticipated relapse rates gave us a fairly precise idea of the number of patients that should be entered in the trial: in fact, twenty-four did so.

The package of interventions we designed included an education component, a relatives group, and family sessions in the home. The education program consisted of two lectures on the aetiology of schizophrenia, the symptoms, course, and treatment and management of the condition. They were delivered in the home, relatives were allowed unlimited time to ask questions, and we left with them a booklet incorporating the substance of the lectures. This has subsequently been published by the National Schizophrenia Fellowship. We did not include the patient in the education program, which was often carried out while he or she was still in hospital. We left it up to the relatives' discretion whether or not to give the patient the booklet to read.

We chose to give the lectures in the home because we thought that relatives would absorb the information more readily when at ease on their own territory. A test of their knowledge before and after the education revealed that more relatives knew that the diagnosis was schizophrenia (hardly surprising!) and that they had become more optimistic about the future (Berkowitz et al., 1984). As part of the information on aetiology, we strongly emphasized that there was no evidence that relatives cause the disease. We felt this was very important both to assuage the guilt that most relatives experience, and to indicate that we did not hold them responsible. As it turned out, making the effort to come to their homes and bringing them something they valued—information—helped to engage relatives in the intervention program.

The relatives group, to which patients were not invited, was intended to help relatives with the everyday problems of living with a sufferer from schizophrenia. It served other functions, including a safety valve for emotions such as anger and anxiety, support for isolated relatives and a forum for peer pressure on individuals to change. The group was run once a fortnight by two professionals, but each relative attended on average once a month. The group was open, and new relatives joined when patients entered the study.

Family sessions were held in the home in parallel with the group and had similar functions, except that patients were included. This gave the professional involved the opportunity for direct observation of patient-relative interaction. It also allowed them greater flexibility, for example they could choose to see the parents together without the patient present, to see the patient with his or her sibling, or any other combination. The average number of family sessions was six, with a range of one to twenty-five, though only one family was seen on more than ten occasions.

Once a patient was inducted into the study, the family was randomly assigned to the package of interventions or to routine treatment. The latter meant in practice that the relatives were offered little or no professional assistance. Virtually all the patients were maintained on depot neuroleptics to eliminate non-compliance as a confounding factor. Relapse was defined as either a return of psychotic symptoms in patients who were free of them on discharge or as an exacerbation in patients with a persistent level of florid symptoms. Clinical assessment was conducted with the Present State Examination (PSE) (Wing et al., 1974), which includes items covering the negative symptoms of schizophrenia, although these did not contribute to the judgment of relapse.

The interventions were offered to the experimental families on a regular basis for nine months after the patient's discharge. Thereafter they were continued at an attenuated level until the two year point. Repeat EE and PSE assessments were conducted at nine months, but only the patients' clinical state was assayed at two years.

The experimental and control relatives did not differ in their levels of critical comments or overinvolvement initially. By nine months there had been no significant change in either EE scale for the control relatives, but a significant reduction in critical comments expressed by the experimental relatives from a mean of 16.7 to 6.5 ($p<0.005$). As a consequence, six of the 12 experimental families underwent a reduction from high to low EE. Face-to-face contact had fallen below thirty-five hours per week for five experimental families, but there was an overlap in some instances with reduction in EE. The aim of the intervention, a reduction in either EE or contact, was achieved in nine of the twelve experimental families. Was this matched by a fall in the patients' relapse rate? In fact the relapse rate in the control group was exactly as predicted, 50 percent while that in the experimental group was even lower than predicted, 8 percent rather than 15 percent. The difference between the experimental and control groups was significant (exact p = 0.032). Furthermore, the one experimental relapse that did occur was in a family in which neither aim of the intervention was achieved (Leff et al., 1982).

These findings not only supported one of the chief postulates of the model but indicated that a form of social treatment could augment the effectiveness of drug treatment in keeping patients free from schizophrenic relapse. We had a number of reservations about this study: the small number of families involved, the ineffectiveness of the interventions in reducing overinvolvement over nine months, and the two year results. By two years the relapse rate in control patients who remained on drugs had risen to 78 percent, while that for experimental patients was 20 percent. The latter figure however, does not represent their morbidity adequately, since two experimental patients committed suicide. There were no successful suicides in the control group, raising the worrying possibility that the intervention might have negative as well as positive effects. However, both suicides occurred in families which failed to show a reduction in either EE or face-to-face contact by nine months, and there were serious problems other than the patient's illness in both families, as described by Leff et al. (1985). When the suicides are added to the relapses, the morbidity in the experimental group becomes 40 percent, which is not significantly different from that in the control group.

In families in which the aims of the intervention were met by nine months and where the patient remained on medication, the two year relapse rate was 14 percent, which is significantly different from the 78 percent rate in the control group (exact p = 0.01). This finding adds further support to the hypothesis that ameliorating the family environment will reduce the relapse rate.

The success of this novel intervention in changing the majority of experimental families in the desired direction stimulated us to ask which component of the package might be responsible for its effectiveness. We therefore mounted another study of the same population, namely high EE, high contact patients. We were already convinced that the education component was an important introduction to the intervention but was insufficient by itself to produce major changes in families. This impression was later confirmed by a study by Tarrier et al., (1988) which evaluated education separately from other interventions. Consequently, we decided to compare education plus a relatives group with education plus family therapy. The differences between the two therapeutic streams are firstly that patients are excluded from the first, but included in the second, and secondly that the resource implications of the second are much greater than of the first. Two therapists running a group can deal with up to six families at a time, whereas family sessions involve two therapists in regular visits to each patient's home.

In the event, offering relatives a place in the group without conducting any family sessions proved problematic, since only five of the eleven relatives in this stream attended the group even once. It was much more difficult for families to refuse home visits, and this occurred in only one case, in which the patient declined further visits after four months. The changes in EE at the nine months follow-up were very similar to the first trial. There was a highly significant reduction in critical comments in both streams but no significant change in overinvolvement. One difference from the first trial was that in the second a significant *increase* in warmth was observed. This is noteworthy since in the naturalistic studies high warmth in the absence of the high EE negative emotions was associated with a low relapse rate (Brown et al., 1972; Vaughn and Leff, 1976b). The finding indicates that the interactions did not simply neutralize negative emotions but also increased the relatives' support for the patient (Leff et al., 1989).

The relapse rates at nine months were different, but not significantly so. One out of twelve patients (8 percent) relapsed in the family therapy stream compared with four out of eleven (36 percent) in the relatives group stream. Thus the outcome of education plus family therapy was identical with that of the whole intervention package in the first trial. The outcome of the relatives group stream looks worse but is confounded by the non-attenders of the group. Three of the relapses occurred in non-attending families and only one in the six families who attended. This suggests that if relatives can be persuaded to come to the group, the outcome for patients is comparable with that produced by family sessions in the home. In the first trial in which family sessions were employed in conjunction with the group, attendance at the group was good, with only a single family failing to come at least once. This led us to recommend that relatives groups are set up, but that at least one family session is held in the home initially, to engage relatives in the intervention. Some additional family sessions may be required to boost flagging group attendance, and for some families who refuse to come to the group at all, it will be essential to provide regular sessions in the home.

These practical recommendations are, in one sense, the end product of a consistent line of research pursued in the Unit over 30 years. Research by other groups has produced convergent findings, although not necessarily based on measures of life events and relatives' EE. There have now been seven studies published of a form of family intervention combined with maintenance neuroleptics for schizophrenic patients. Six of these have produced consistent results in favour of family intervention as displayed in Table 12.2 The only discrepant study (Dulz and Hand, 1986) utilized a form of psychoanalytic group therapy for the families which differs in intention and practice from the approach in the other six studies. The weight of evidence is strongly in favor of incorporating family intervention for schizophrenia in routine clinical practice. However, judging from past experience, there is likely to be a considerable delay before this happens. In an attempt to cut short this delay, we are intending to initiate a study of the capacity of psychiatric nurses to be trained in the relevant family and group intervention techniques and to put them into practice. Hopefully, the demonstration that the interventions can be effectively delivered by nurses, as opposed to research psychiatrists and psychologists, will influence clinical teams working in non-academic settings.

The stages of research that have been completed, or remain to be tackled, can be summarized as follows: (1) establish an association between one or more psychosocial factors and the outcome of the medical condition under study; (2) devise an intervention designed to modify the significant psychosocial factors and subject it to a controlled trial, in which the course of the medical condition is the independent variable; (3) demonstrate that the intervention can be utilized in a practical way in an ordinary clinical setting.

Stages 1 and 2 have been achieved with respect to schizophrenia, and we are on the verge of embarking on stage 3. This same sequence of research strategies can be applied to any medical condition: depressive neurosis is an obvious choice, as stage 1 has already been completed and has given rise to models of the action of psychosocial factors in depression which are ripe for testing with trials of interventions. This fruitful approach, which has developed in the Unit over a long period of time, is as applicable to non-psychiatric as to psychiatric conditions. If the current

TABLE 12.2
Outcome of Family Treatment Trials for Schizophrenia

Study	Relapse rates over 6–12 Months (%)	
	Control	Experimental
Goldstein et al (1978)	48	0
Falloon et al (1982)	44	6
Leff et al (1982)	50	8
Hogarty et al (1986)	41	0
Tarrier et al (1987)	53	12
Leff et al (1989)		8*
		17†

* Family therapy
† Relatives group attenders

work on ulcerative colitis and Crohn's disease has a positive outcome and progresses beyond stage 1, a vista would open up of psychosocial treatments for the so-called psychosomatic diseases.

References

Berkowitz, R., Eberlein-Fries, R., Kuipers, L. and Leff, J. (1984). Educating relatives about schizophrenia. *Schizophrenia Bulletin, 10*, 418–429

Birley, J.L.T. and Brown, G.W. (1970). Crises and life changes preceding the onset or relapse of acute schizophrenia: clinical aspects. *British Journal of Psychiatry*, 116, 327–33.

Bloch, S. and Reddaway, P. (1984). *Soviet Psychiatric Abuse: The Shadow Over World Psychiatry*. London: Victor Gollancz.

Brewin, C.R. and Furnham, A. (1986). Attributional versus preattributional variables in self-esteem and depression: A Comparison and test of learned helplessness theory. *Journal of Personality and Social Psychology, 50*, 1013–1020.

Brown, G.W. and Birley, J.L.T. (1968). Crises and life changes and the onset of schizophrenia. *Journal of Health and Social Behaviour, 9*, 203–214.

Brown, G.W., Birley, J.L.T. and Wing, J.K. (1972). Influence of family life on the course of schizophrenic disorders: a replication. *British Journal of Psychiatry, 121*, 241–258.

Brown, G.W. and Harris, T. (1978). *The Social Origins of Depression*. London: Tavistock.

Brown, G.W., Harris, T. and Peto, J. (1973). Life events and psychiatric disorders, 1: Some methodological issues. *Psychological Medicine, 3*, 74–87.

Brown, G.W., Monck, E.M., Carstairs, G.M. and Wing, J.K. (1962). Influence of family life on the course of schizophrenic illness. *British Journal of Preventive and Social Medicine, 16*, 55–68.

Brown, G.W. and Rutter, M. (1966). The measurement of family activities and relationships: a methodological study. *Human Relations, 19*, 241–263.

Connolly, J. (1976). Life events before myocardial infarction. *Journal of Human Stress, 2*, 3–17.

Craig, T.K.J. and Brown, G.W. (1984). Goal frustration and life events in the aetiology of painful gastrointestinal disorder. *Journal of Psychosomatic Research, 28*, 411–421.

Creed, F. (1981). Life events and appendectomy. *Lancet, 1*, 1381–1385.

Day, A., Neilsen, J.A., Korten, A., Ernberg, G., Dube, K.C., Gebhart, J., Jablensky, A., Leon, C., Marsella, A., Olatawura, M., Sartorius, N., Stromgren, E., Takahashi, R., Wig, N. and Wynne, L.C. (1987). Stressful life events preceding the acute onset of schizophrenia: A cross-national study from the World Health Organization. *Culture, Medicine and Psychiatry, 2*, 123–206.

Dohrenwend, B.P. (1975). Sociocultural and sociopsychological factors in the genesis of mental disorders. *Journal of Health and Social Behavior, 16*, 365–392.

Dulz, B. and Hand. I. (1986). Short-term relapse in young schizophrenics. In (eds. M.J. Goldstein, I. Hand and K. Hahlweg). *Treatment of Schizophrenia*. Berlin: Springer-Verlag.

Falloon, I.R.H., Boyd, J.L., McGill, C.W., Razani, J., Moss, H.B. and Gilderman,

A.M. (1982). Family management in the prevention of exacerbations of schizo-phrenia. *New England Journal of Medicine*, *306*, 1437–1440.

Fischmann-Havstad, L. and Marston, A.R. (1984). Weight loss maintenance as an aspect of family emotion and process. *British Journal of Clinical Psychology*, *23*, 265–271.

Goldstein, M.J., Rodnick, E.H., Evans, J.R., May, P.R.A. and Steinberg, M.R. (1978). Drug and family therapy in the aftercare treatment of acute schizophre-nia. *Archives of General Psychiatry*, *35*, 169–177.

Harris, T.O., Brown, G.W. and Bifulco, A. (1970). Loss of parent in childhood and adult psychiatric disorder: The Walthamstow Study, 2. The role of inadequate substitute care. *Psychological Medicine*, *17*, 163–183.

Hirsch S.R. and Leff J.P. (1975). *Abnormalities in the Parents of Schizophrenics*. Maudsley Monograph No. 22. Oxford. Oxford University Press.

Hogarty, G.E., Anderson, C.M., Reiss, D.J., Kornblith, S.J., Greenwald, D.P., Javna, C.D. and Madonia, M.J. (1986). Family psychoeducation, social skills training, and maintenance chemotherapy in the aftercare treatment of schizo-phrenia. I. One-year effects of a controlled study on relapse and Expressed Emotion. *Archives of General Psychiatry*, *43*, 633–642.

Hooley, J.M., Orley, J. and Teasdale, J.D. (1986). Levels of Expressed Emotion and relapse in depressed patients. *British Journal of Psychiatry*, *148*, 642–647.

Karno, M., Jenkins, J.H., de la Selva, A., Santana, F., Telles, C., Lopes, S. and Mintz, J. (1987). Expressed emotion and schizophrenic outcome among Mexi-can-American families. *Journal of Nervous and Mental Disease*, *175*, 143–151.

Laing, R.D. and Esterson, D. (1964). *Sanity, Madness and the Family*, London: Tavistock.

Leff, J., Berkowitz, R., Shavit, N., Strachan, A., Glass, I. and Vaughn, C. (1989). A trial of family therapy v. a relatives group for schizophrenia. *British Journal of Psychiatry*, *154*, 58–66.

Leff, J.P., Kuipers, L., Berkowitz, R., Eberlein-Fries, R. and Sturgeon, D. (1982). A controlled trial of social intervention in schizophrenic families. *British Journal of Psychiatry*, *141*, 121–134.

Leff, J.P., Kuipers, L., Berkowitz, R. and Sturgeon, D. (1985). A controlled trial of social intervention in the families of schizophrenic patients: two year follow up. *British Journal of Psychiatry*, *146*, 594–600.

Leff, J.P., Kuipers, L., Berkowitz, R., Vaughn, C.E. and Sturgeon, D. (1983). Life events, relatives' Expressed Emotion and maintenance neuroleptics in schizo-phrenic relapse. *Psychological Medicine*, *13*, 799–806.

Leff, J.P. and Vaughn, C.E. (1980). The interaction of life events and relative's Expressed Emotion in schizophrenia and depressive neurosis. *British Journal of Psychiatry*, *136*, 146–53.

Leff, J.P., Wig, N., Ghosh, A., Bedi, H., Menon, D.K., Kuipers, L., Korten, A., Ernberg, G., Day, R., Sartorius, N. and Jablensky, A. (1987). Influence of relatives' Expressed Emotion on the course of schizophrenia in Chandigarh. *British Journal of Psychiatry*, *151*, 166–173.

MacMillan, J.F., Gold, A., Crow, T.J., Johnson, A.L. and Johnstone, E.C. (1986). Expressed Emotion and relapse. *British Journal of Psychiatry*, *148*, 133–144.

Miklowitz, D.J., Goldstein, M.J., Falloon, I.R.H. and Doane, J.A. (1984). Interac-tional correlates of Expressed Emotion in the families of schizophrenics. *British Journal of Psychiatry*, *144*, 482–487.

Moline, R.A., Singh, S., Morris, A. and Meltzer, H. (1985). Family expressed emotion and relapse in schizophrenia in 24 urban American patients. *American Journal of Psychiatry*, *142*, 1078–1081.

Neuchterlein, K.H., Snyder, K.S., Dawson, M.E., Rappe, S., Gitlin, M. and Fogelson, D. (1986). Expressed emotion, fixed dose fluphemazine decanoate maintenance and relapse in recent-onset schizophrenia. *Psychopharmacology Bulletin*, *22*, 633–639.

Parker, G., Johnston, P. and Hayward, L. (1988). Parental 'Expressed Emotion' as a predictor of schizophrenic relapse. *Archives of General Psychiatry*, *45*, 806–813.

Smith, G.N., Iacono, W.G., Moreau, M., Tallman, K., Baser, M. and Flak, B. (1988). Choice of comparison group and findings of computerised tomography in schizophrenia. *British Journal of Psychiatry*, *153*, 667–674.

Steinberg, H. and Durell, J. (1968). A stressful social situation as a precipitant of schizophrenic symptoms: An epidemiological study. *British Journal of Psychiatry*, *114*, 1097–1105.

Strachan, A.M., Leff, J.P., Goldstein, M.J., Doane, J. and Burtt, C. (1986). Emotional attitudes and direct communication in the families of schizophrenics: A cross-national replication. *British Journal of Psychiatry*, *149*, 279–287.

Szmuckler, G.I., Berkowitz, R., Eisler, I., Leff, J. and Dare, C. (1987). Expressed Emotion in individual and family settings: a comparative study. *British Journal of Psychiatry*, *151*, 174–178.

Szmuckler, G.I., Eisler, I., Russell, G.F.M. and Dare, C. (1985). Anorexia nervosa, parental 'expressed emotion' and dropping out of treatment. *British Journal of Psychiatry*, *147*, 265–271.

Tarrier, N., Barrowclough, C., Vaughn, C., Bamrah, J.S., Porceddu, K., Watts, S. and Freeman, H. (1988). The community management of schizophrenia: a controlled trial of a behavioural intervention with families to reduce relapse. *British Journal of Psychiatry*, *153*, 532–542.

Vaughn, C.E., Snyder, K.S., Jones, S., Freeman, W.B. and Falloon, I.R.H. (1984). Family factors in schizophrenic relapse: a California replication of the British research on expressed emotion. *Archives of General Psychiatry*, *41*, 1169–1177.

Vaughn, C.E. and Leff, J.P. (1976a). The measurement of expressed emotion in the families of psychiatric patients. *British Journal of Clinical and Social Psychology*, *15*, 157–165.

Vaughn, C. and Leff, J.P. (1976b). The influence of family and social factors on the course of psychiatric illness: a comparison of schizophrenic and depressed neurotic patients. *British Journal of Psychiatry*, *129*, 125–137.

Wing, J.K., Cooper, J.E. and Sartorius, N. (1974). *The Measurement and Classification of Psychiatric Symptoms*. Cambridge University Press: Cambridge.

Zubin, J. and Spring, B. (1977). Vulnerability: a new view of schizophrenia. *Journal of Abnormal Psychology*, *86*, 103–126.

13

The Epidemiology of Affective Disorders

Paul E. Bebbington

Introduction

Traditionally, psychiatry has been a branch of medicine, with which it shares a particular scientific approach. This lies essentially in the use of disease theories; syndromes, once demarcated, can be used to test theories of causation and treatment. If syndromes turn out not to be useful they can be abandoned and the clinical phenomena regrouped in other ways. This procedure is a powerful technique for extending knowledge (Wing, 1977). There are, of course, other strategies for organizing the subject matter of mental aberration, but this approach has been very influential from the time psychiatry emerged as a separate discipline. It is this use of disease categories that permits the application of the epidemiological method to the psychiatric field.

Epidemiology is the study of the distribution of disorders in populations, with the aim of discovering possible causes or of throwing light on the way that public and private agencies serve to identify, prevent, or alleviate the disorders. In studying any particular disorder, the epidemiologist is faced with three major problems: enumerating the size and characteristics of the population under review, defining the disorder sufficiently precisely to be able to count its frequency, and specifying which subgroups of the population will be likely to yield disproportionate numbers of cases (MacMahon and Pugh, 1970).

Epidemiology, therefore, depends on the establishment of various types of "rate"—incidence, prevalence, morbid risk and so on. This has two universal components—identifying "cases" in the numerator, and the "population" in the denominator. Specifying these and identifying subgroups of the population with differing rates comprise the *epidemiological method*. Its application to "depression" raises problems common to the study of any disorder lacking an objective standard and agreed criteria for definition.

Case-finding depends on agreement over classification. Over the last two decades or so, the subclassification of affective disorders has attracted much interest but no overall consensus. Distinctions have been made between bipolar and unipolar, delusional and non-delusional, type A and type B, endogenous and reactive, psychotic and neurotic depressions, between pure depressive disease and depressive spectrum disorder, and, among the chronic depressions, between characterological disorder and "subaffective dysthymia." These categories often make good clinical sense, but they have been validated in terms of symptom clusters, course, psychobiological correlates, and family history. They have not been used in social or epidemiological studies, and findings concerning the social origins of affective disorder cannot therefore be related to them.

In the study of affective disorders, problems of interpretation have been increased by the frequency of affective symptoms in the community at large. Cases coming to the attention of psychiatrists may not therefore be typical of all affective disorders, and their sociodemographic characteristics may merely reflect the influences bringing the patient to treatment, rather than those that precipitate onset. The identification of social groups at high risk for affective disorder must in consequence be corroborated in unreferred samples, and good techniques of case-finding become even more essential (Bebbington et al., 1980).

The presentation of epidemiological findings in terms of sociodemographic variables implies at any rate the possibility of some kind of social theory of these disorders. Variations in incidence or prevalence of disorders by social class or by sex may be interpreted in terms of differential exposure to some biological factor, but it is equally plausible that they may result from psychosocial influences. The basic rule of interpretation in epidemiology—that any associations found can only provide clues or hypotheses as to the direction of cause and effect—applies particularly to the study of affective disorder.

In this chapter, I will summarize evidence about the frequency of affective disorders and the extent to which social attributes can be used to define groups at high risk. The impact of psychosocial adversity on affective disorders will be evaluated, along with the factors that determine individual susceptibility to such stresses. The possibility of distinguishing mild depressions from the more severe "endogenous" forms in terms of their social correlates will be assessed. The role of social support in protecting the individual from affective disorders will be outlined. Finally, the scanty literature on the social epidemiology of bipolar disorder and of anxiety states will be reviewed.

Areas not covered include the interaction between social and biological variables, reviewed by Bebbington and McGuffin (1989), the presentation of affective disorders in primary care (Blacker and Clare, 1988) and the social outcome of affective disorder (Bebbington, 1982; Lee and Murray, 1988; Kiloh et al, 1988).

The Frequency of Depressive Disorders

In Western countries, rates of depressive disorders can be established from data routinely collected about patients contacting psychiatric clinics. Statistics based on hospital admissions are subject to undefined selection factors. Case registers are more satisfactory because contacts with day hospitals and non-hospital day centers, ambulatory clinics, and various forms of non-hospital residential unit are recorded as well as admissions to hospital. Record linkage allows the computation of rates of "first-ever" contact with one of these services. Values for the incidence of affective disorders culled from published statistics of this sort are displayed in Table 13.1. Sturt and her colleagues (1984) have calculated that the lifetime risk of contacting psychiatric services in Camberwell, South London, for treatment of an affective disorder is 11 percent for men and 20 percent for women.

As noted above, there are good grounds for extending studies into the area of non-treated incidence and prevalence. The methodological difficulties here are just as great, but of a different kind. The most severe disorders are relatively rare, and it is beyond the scope of most investigators to screen a large enough population to examine rates within all the subgroups that would be desirable. Compliance is much lower in population surveys—it is not uncommon for a third of the sample to be lost if there is a two-stage design (a first screen followed by a more intensive interview). Techniques of interview suitable for referred patients may not be appropriate for a household survey, and the threshold at which minimal "mental ill-health" becomes severe enough to be counted as a "case" is hard to specify. Determining the onset of relatively mild disorders is likewise often difficult (Duncan-Jones, 1981). Most population surveys are therefore restricted to measuring prevalence rather than incidence, and inferences concerning causes must be appropriately cautious.

There are now a number of sample population surveys, mainly from North America and Europe, that are based on the use of standardized instruments for establishing the case status of individuals. The results

TABLE 13.1

Incidence of Depression Based on Register Data

Reference	Place	Base Population	Disorder Type	Sex	Rate per 10[5]
Adelstein et al. (1968)	Salford, England	>15 years	Depressive Psychosis	Both	97
				M	65
				F	123
Baldwin (1971)	NE Scotland	All	Manic depressive reactions	M	25
				F	52
			All Depressions	M	87
				F	201
Pederson et al. (1972)	Monroe Co., N.Y.	>15 years	Psychotic Depression	Both	33
				M	27
				F	37
Der & Bebbington (1987)	Camberwell, England	>15 years	Severe Depression	M	29
				F	52
			All Depressions	M	144
				F	270

TABLE 13.2
Prevalence of CATEGO Depressive Classes (%)

Site	N	Male	Female	Total
Uganda (Orley & Wing 1979)	206	17.0	21.0	18.9
Canberra (Henderson et al, 1979)	756(157)	2.6	6.7	4.8
Camberwell (Bebbington et al, 1981)	800(310)	4.8	9.0	7.0
Edinburgh (Surtees et al, 1983)	576		6.9	
Athens (Mavreas et al, 1986)	489	4.3	10.1	7.4
Nijmegen (Hodiamont et al, 1987)	3232(486)[1]			5.5
Santander (Vazquez-Barquero et al, 1987)	1223(452)[1]	4.5	7.8	6.2
Camberwell (Cypriot) (Mavreas and Bebbington 1987)	307	4.2	7.1	5.6
Finland[2] (Lehtinen et al, 1990)	742	2.4	6.5	4.6

Note: Studies that do not give a breakdown in terms of CATEGO classes are not included.
[1]Two-stage survey—numbers given PSE at 2nd stage in brackets. Prevalences weighted to represent original population.
[2]Age adjusted figures.

show a considerable degree of convergence. Table 13.2 includes studies using the PSE. The Ugandan figures are really very high, but those apart, the range of values for men is from 2.4 to 4.8 percent, and for women from 5.9 percent to 10.1 percent. These variations are of the order that could plausibly be explained by the effects of different local circumstances: it is entirely reasonable that Camberwell, an inner city area in South London, should have around twice the rates seen in the affluent planned Australian city of Canberra. The Ugandan values might represent over-rating of PSE items, the insecurity of the rural Third World at the time of Amin's excesses, the prevalence of alcohol-related symptoms, or the unavailability of treatment.

Table 13.3 lists results from studies using the DIS for the six-month prevalence of the category Major Depressive Disorder, which represents a fairly high threshold. Values for most sites are remarkably consistent. The

TABLE 13.3
Six Month Prevalence of Major Depressive Episode (%)

Site	N	Male	Female	Total
Baltimore (Myers et al., 1984)	3481	1.3	3.0	2.2
New Haven (Myers et al., 1984)	3058	2.2	4.6	3.5
St. Louis (Myers et al., 1984)	3004	1.7	4.5	3.2
Piedmont (Blazer et al., 1985)	3921†			1.7
Los Angeles (Burnham et al., 1987)	3125			3.1
Puerto Rico (Canino et al., 1987)	1551	2.4	3.3	3.0
Edmonton (Bland et al., 1988)	3258	2.5	3.9	3.2
Taiwan‡ (Hwu et al., 1989)				
Taipei	5004			0.6
Small town	3005			1.1
Rural	2995			0.8

Note: Detailed one year prevalence data for the five ECA sits are provided by Weissman et al., 1988.
†weighted to take account of deliberate over sampling of the elderly.
‡One year prevalence.

overall one-month prevalence of Major Depressive Disorder varies from 1.7 to 2.6 percent. Six-month prevalences are available for more sites, and overall prevalence varies from 1.7 to 5.3 percent (males 1.3–3.4 percent, females 3.0–7.1 percent).

As with the PSE community surveys, those using the DIS display fairly close agreement, especially when it is considered that the populations are not standardized for demographic differences like age. The low rate in Taiwan may represent a real difference or some local oddity in the administration of the DIS. They are unlikely to be explained solely in terms of simple demographic factors such as the age structure of the population. The tendency of the Chinese to express depression in neurasthenic terms (Kleinman, 1986) would be minimized by the use of a standard instrument, and the rate for somatization disorder in Taiwan does not seem to be raised, as might be expected if the subjects were indeed expressing depressed mood in somatic terms (Hwu et al., 1989).

There is dispute about how much of the prevalence of affective disorders is due to chronic conditions (Sashidharan et al., 1988; Murphy et al., 1989; Bebbington et al., 1989a), and therefore about whether high prevalence is translated into a very high morbid risk. Bebbington and his colleagues found that many of the conditions uncovered in their population survey were transient, and this was reflected in an extremely high rate of disorder before the age of sixty-five (49 percent for men, 70 percent for women). Murphy and her colleagues (1989) found much more chronicity and their lifetime risk was correspondingly less. This issue requires to be resolved by an epidemiological study specifically designed to establish morbid risk, as this is crucial for genetic studies.

None of the studies so far published provides data of sufficient accuracy and stability over a number of years to allow conclusions concerning changes in incidence or prevalence with time. Klerman (1978, 1988) and Schwab and colleagues (1979) speculate that depression is becoming more common. Hagnell and colleagues (1982), using data collected in 1947, 1957, and 1972 in a Swedish rural community, suggest that the incidence of severe depression is decreasing, but that depression of mild to moderate severity is increasing, particularly in young adult males (who have a high rate of unemployment).

Recently, data from family studies of affective disorder have been used to analyze the age-specific incidence for successive cohorts of subjects (Klerman et al., 1985: Gershon et al., 1987; Lavori et al., 1987). These suggest that as the twentieth century proceeds, the population is becoming increasingly prone to depression, and that this emerges at a younger age (Klerman, 1988). However, such studies have to answer the charge that all they are revealing is selective forgetting on the part of older subjects (Bromet et al., 1986), or even a failure to recognize symptoms as psychological (Hasin and Link, 1988).

Macrosocial Factors—Gender, Marital Status, Family Responsibility, Parity, Social Class, Employment

The most robust finding, perhaps in all psychiatric epidemiology, is that depressive disorders, however defined, whatever the sample, and irrespective of the instrument used for identification, are commoner in women than in men (Adelstein et al., 1968; Pederson et al., 1970; Rosenfield 1980; Bebbington et al., 1981a; von Zerssen and Weyerer 1982; Bebbington, 1988). Some authors (Paykel and Rowan, 1979; Weissman and Klerman, 1977; Weissman et al., 1984) consider that the marital role involves more stress for women than for men. There is certainly good evidence that being married is in this respect much less protective for women than for men

(Bebbington et al., 1981a; Bebbington, 1987a; Der and Bebbington, 1987; Bebbington and Tansella, 1989), although not everyone has found this (e.g., Gebhardt and Klimitz, 1986). Many other studies have found that young married women looking after small children are particularly at risk (Grad de Alarcon et al., 1975; Baldwin, 1971; Bebbington et al., 1981a; Brown and Harris, 1978; Moss and Plewis, 1977; Richman, 1974, 1977). Recently, it has been suggested that the excess of affective disorders in women is entirely accounted for by those who have borne children, irrespective of whether they were still engaged in looking after them (Gater et al., 1989). This suggests that marital status and childcare effects might be mere reflections of some biological process implicit in female parity. This may be so for the more severe affective disorders, but it seems that an effect of marital role still provides a better explanation in moderate disorders (Bebbington et al., 1991a). This is given support by the finding that marital status has different associations with minor affective disorder in different cultures. For instance, married women are at low risk of disorder in Mediterranean countries (Mavreas et al., 1986; Vazquez-Barquero et al., 1987), and in rural New Zealand (Romans-Clarkson et al., 1988). If the effect of marital status is culture-bound, it seems unlikely to be related to biological effects.

Another sociodemographic association of affective disorder is that with social class. In general, it is found that if a broad definition of depressive disorders is used, there is an inverse relationship between social prestige and disorder (e.g., Dohrenwend and Dohrenwend, 1969; Brown and Harris, 1978; Comstock and Helsing, 1976, Uhlenhuth et al., 1974, Warheit et al., 1973; Surtees et al., 1983). Although some studies have not confirmed this (e.g., Bebbington et al., 1981a, Blumenthal and Dielman, 1975; Weissman and Myers, 1978; Brown et al., 1977; Hare and Shaw, 1965; Taylor and Chave, 1964) a reasonable consensus is that the prevalence of disorder is indeed increased in the lower social class, albeit perhaps less markedly so than some have claimed. For more severe depressive disorders, the risk is much less affected by social class (Bagley, 1973; Der and Bebbington, 1987; Bebbington, 1988).

Brenner (1973) suggested that higher rates of admission for mental illness were associated with periods of high unemployment, though others have disputed the nature of the relationship (Gravelle et al., 1981). There seems little doubt that at the individual level, becoming unemployed increases the risk of affective disorder (e.g., Finlay-Jones and Eckhardt, 1981; Eales, 1988; Kessler et al., 1987), although most resulting cases are minor (Warr, 1984). Banks and Jackson (1982) concluded from a longitudinal study of young people that unemployment has ill-effects on mental health that are reversed when work is obtained (Jackson et al., 1982). Jenkins and colleagues (1982) found similar effects when employees were threatened with redundancy, effects that were neutralized if the threat was removed. In addition, Fagin (1981) showed that the mental and physical health of families deteriorated when the chief wage earner became unemployed.

Many workers in the field of unemployment research have been influenced by Jahoda's emphasis on the "latent functions" of employment. She lists six such functions: time structure, social contact, activity, status, purposefulness, and sense of control (Jahoda, 1982). These aspects of employment are plainly important, and the effects of unemployment must include consequences related to them. So, for instance, Eales (1988) and Bolton and Oatley (1987) argue that the continuing availability of social support modifies the risk. However, unemployment itself causes changes in the individual's social network (Jackson, 1988). Fryer (1988) has argued that this has sometimes operated to the exclusion of considerations relating to the manifest function of employment, viz., earning a living. In this context, Kessler and his colleagues (1987) studied three possible sources of strain: financial, marital, and that due to constriction of "affiliative interaction." Their longitudinal study suggested that the most important and direct was financial, and that financial hardship increased the impact of any supervening misfortunes. The importance of financial difficulties also emerged from the study of Frese and Mohr (1987).

Like unemployment, work means different things to different folk. For women, work has a particular set of possible meanings that lie behind the general finding that women at work have low levels of psychiatric disorder. The extent of any financial difficulty and of other commitments and burdens, and the availability of social support are crucial. So are interest and involvement. Warr and Parry (1982) concluded that most evidence pointed to a protective effect of employment in working class but not in middle class women. Parry (1986; Parry and Shapiro, 1986) suggests that the important factor is whether work provides extra social support. If it does not, it may actually increase the burdens on women.

Psychosocial Stress

Psychosocial stress is the organizing concept that lies behind theories of the social aetiology of psychiatric disorders. It arises from the subjects' perception of their social world, hence "psychosocial," and is to be distinguished from other types of stress, for instance, physiological stress. Many of the social correlates of depressive disorders can be conceptualized as environmental stress factors: low occupational status, unemployment (particularly if it arrives suddenly, in the form or redundancy), and the burdens of family (e.g., having to care for small children). Although there are many varieties of psychosocial stress, the sort that is easiest to research, and has therefore been most studied, takes the form of life events and chronic difficulties. Life events are relatively sudden changes in the subject's social world. It can be imagined that a lack of change might be equally stressful, for instance, circumstances of unremitting hardship, so another major component of current adversity is in the form of chronic problems. Chronic problems and life events are not as independent as they might seem, since life events can occur repeatedly and also initiate chronic problems, and since chronic problems can have acute exacerbations. However, most studies have for convenience considered them separately.

It must be emphasized that life events and difficulties form only part of the stresses human beings must face. However, it is only by restricting themselves to defined and definable categories that researchers in social psychiatry can start to investigate the idea that psychosocial stress has an important bearing on the onset of psychiatric disorders.

The first requirement for research of this type is to obtain a history of life events. Merely quizzing the subject is unreliable, and two methods have been developed to get around this problem. The first is the "inventory" approach (Dohrenwend et al., 1978; Holmes and Rahe, 1967; Paykel et al., 1971; Sarason et al., 1978; Tennant and Andrews, 1976). The researchers construct an a priori list of happenings that they are prepared to accept as significant events (divorce, childbirth, deaths in the family, job changes, and so on). This list is then presented to subjects, either in an interview or as a printed schedule, and they are asked to indicate whether they have themselves experienced any item on the list. This procedure is an advance, but has three main disadvantages: happenings important to the subject cannot be counted if they are not on the list; the events on the list are really event categories, and the subject must often decide if their experiences fit the category; and the procedure is not in any case very reliable.

The second method was developed by Brown (1974) in response to the deficiencies of the first. This imposes structure on history taking by enquiring about possible happenings in the different role areas of the subject's life—as parent, householder, employee, etc. Events and difficulties are not defined beforehand, rather the interviewer records details of all likely candidates, which are then evaluated by a rating panel.

Clearly, not every event is of equal impact. It might be supposed that subjects experiencing events would be in a position to give a good account of their impact, but, particularly for research purposes, this account may be dangerously distorted (Tennant et al., 1981a). People try to make sense of their predicament, and this may lead them to assess too highly the impact of an event that has been followed by a change in mental state (the "search after meaning": Brown, 1974). In addition, depressed people take a gloomy view of their experiences and might also tend to exaggerate their misfortunes ("black spectacles"). Researchers have tried to get round this problem by obtaining independent ratings.

Potentially there are many dimensions along which life events might be evaluated. Most authorities have chosen to concentrate on the amount of *change* or the amount of *stress* involved in the event. The degree of stressfulness appears to be the best predictor of psychiatric disorder (Mueller et al., 1977; Tennant and Andrews, 1978).

Each method of taking a history of life events is associated with a particular way of assessing their impact. Because the events in inventories are pre-defined, they can be pre-rated. This is done by using a rating sample (e.g., Paykel et al., 1976a). Subjects in this sample, ideally but rarely representative of the population to be studied, are asked to rate events on a scale defined by anchor points. For instance, they may be told "death of a child" is defined as 1000, "marriage" as 500. Fortunately, subjects make rather similar ratings when asked to do this. The average values of their ratings for each event are then taken to be the definitive score of that event. The advantage of this method is that it give a sort of default evaluation of the events: the impact the event might make on the person in the street. The disadvantage is that it takes no account of variation in individual circumstances.

The interview technique clearly cannot rely on predetermined ratings, as events are not pre-defined. This has resulted in the development of rating by a panel of independent raters (Brown and Harris, 1978; Brown, 1989). The interviewer presents a vignette of the event to the panel, giving details of its social context, but omitting any account of the subject's mental state or actual reaction to the event. Only events with significant impact are used in analysis, so the rating procedure is also part of the procedure of event definition. This method, while retaining objectivity of rating, does permit variations of individual circumstances to be incorporated.

Although these judgments are more meaningful and can be more reliable than is the case with the inventory technique (Mendels and Weinstein, 1972; Parry et al., 1981; Tennant et al., 1979; Neilson et al., 1988), they do not wholly overcome the problem of contamination. The respondent provides information about the event, its severity and its date, and also about any disorder that might possibly be reactive, and *its* date. The problem is not overcome by having two interviews or two informants and is only partially overcome by carrying out repeated interviews. The further question of whether depressed people are more likely to recall events than others has not yet been resolved (Brown et al., 1973; Bebbington et al., 1981b).

Another advantage of the interview over the inventory technique is that there is probably less decrement in memory over time and less need for another informant (Bebbington et al., 1981b; Brown et al., 1973, 1977; Jenkins et al., 1979; Schless and Mendels, 1978; Uhlenhuth et al., 1977; Yager et al., 1981). On the whole, therefore, in spite of some continuing disadvantages, it seems the better technique.

Brown and Harris (1978; Harris and Brown, 1989) devised, in addition, a method of categorizing events as "logically independent," "possibly independent," and "dependent," the last category containing events that probably arose because a disorder was already present or developing.

Virtually every study of affective disorder, whether set in the general population or in the clinic, has shown an excess of stressful life events before onset, and it is now generally accepted that the relationship is causal (Bebbington et al., 1981b; Brown and Harris, 1978; Cadoret et al., 1972; Cooke, 1981; Costello, 1982; Fava et al., 1981; Henderson et al., 1981; Markush and Favero, 1974; Myers et al., 1974; Paykel et al., 1969; Surtees et al., 1986; Thompson and Hendrie, 1972). Nevertheless, many interesting questions remain about the nature of this relationship.

Variations in Susceptibility

Clearly not everyone who experiences a severe life event becomes psychiatrically ill. People vary in their susceptibility to stress. The concept of vulnerability involves an assumption that some prior condition or event has sensitized an individual to react adversely to a subsequent stressor. Vulnerability may be genetic, but most theories have concerned possible social-psychological antecedents. One major theme involves early loss events, such as separation from or loss of one or both parents when a child. This makes a lot of theoretical sense, but earlier reviews came to negative conclusions (Granville-Grossman, 1968; Tennant et al., 1981b). The current state of the evidence is reviewed at length by Tennant in Chapter 14.

Brown and Harris (1978) used early loss as a component of their "vulnerability model" of depression. They argued that Camberwell women were more likely to become depressed in response to life events or difficulties if they were subject to certain vulnerability factors, alone or in combination. These vulnerability factors would not, by themselves, precipitate a disorder. They comprised loss of mother before age eleven, not being in paid employment, being involved in child care, and lacking a confiding relationship. Independent replication studies have not provided much support for this model, except for the last-named factor, which will be discussed below.

Vulnerability due to social circumstances is likely to be closely bound to the local culture. Psychological vulnerability is now being intensively studied with the favored variables including self-esteem and the attitudinal characteristics derived from the current cognitive models of depression put forward by Beck (1976, 1983), Abramson and her colleagues (1978), and others (Bebbington, 1985; Nezu and Ronan, 1985; Olinger et al., 1987; Brewin, 1989). These cognitive models of depression receive support from the replicated finding that neurotically depressed patients are especially sensitive to an adverse family environment, and break down easily, even at the mildest levels of stress (Vaughn and Leff, 1976; Hooley et al., 1986). However, the relationship between cognitive vulnerability and depression may be complex. In a prospective study, Ingham and his colleagues (1987) found that low self-esteem was predictive only in women who had experienced prior episodes of depression, and may indeed have been a marker of incomplete recovery. Teasdale and Dent provide further evidence for this view (Teasdale and Dent, 1987; Teasdale, 1988; Dent and Teasdale, 1988), and the study of Lewinsohn and his colleagues (1988) can be similarly interpreted.

A possible determinant of psychological vulnerability is the experience of inadequate parenting (Parker, 1988). Parker and his colleagues (1979) have developed the Parental Bonding Instrument (PBI), which requires subjects to score their parents' attributes during the first 16 years of the subjects' lives. The scale has good psychometric properties (Parker, 1983). The central problem of such an instrument is the extent to which it recapitulates the real world of childhood. Surprisingly, there is good agreement between subjects and their siblings about parental attitudes towards the former, even when their relationships with their parents was remarkably different, and scores are not much affected by current depressed mood (Parker, 1983; Gotlib et al., 1988).

The PBI has two subscales, "care" and "protection." Low scores on "care" and high scores on "protection" are both associated with an increase in depressive symptoms. Low care may be more damaging than over-protection, and the worst combination may be over-protection and a low care score (Parker, 1988; Gotlib et al., 1988). The association with poor parenting is probably restricted to the less severe depressions (Parker et al., 1987). Poor parenting may well be the mechanism that lies behind the association of adult depression with childhood separation from parents.

The establishment of an interrelationship between various levels of vulnerability is a continuing topic of research with clear clinical significance.

Precipitation and Symptom Pattern

It is generally agreed that depressive disorders referred for specialist advice and treatment tend to be more severe, and probably to have a different symptom pattern (e.g., more delusions and hallucinations, more guilt, more retardation, more negative disturbance, and more likelihood of being associated with mania) than those found among non-referred samples (Wing et al., 1981; Dew et al., 1988). Whether the more severe disorders are really clinically distinct from the less severe is still controversial. The question of whether they are also less likely to be precipitated by *environmental adversity*, that is, are less *reactive*, deserves further examination.

Underlying these issues is the further problem of how to define *normality*. In common-sense terms, a reaction of *distress* should be proportional to the severity of adversity. Similar issues are raised by other conditions defined by reference to events, such as post-traumatic stress disorder (Horowitz et al., 1980). Distress not amounting to a depressive disorder, the transient situational reaction of DSMIII, (APA, 1980), has been particularly thoroughly described by using follow-up interviews with people who have suffered bereavement or trauma. There is some disagreement as to the extent to which these reactions can be called pathological (Clayton et al., 1972, 1975; Parkes, 1965, 1975). To draw the line between normal and pathological reactions, i.e., to define deviance, is not at the moment possible using objective measures. Symptomatically, the conditions overlap to a considerable degree.

Research reports bearing on the proposition that certain symptoms of depression are not associated with adversity show a curious schism. On one hand, multivariate studies almost invariably find that a lack of antecedent adversity discriminates endogenous from reactive cases as powerfully as any of the "endogenous" symptoms (Carney et al., 1965; Feinberg and Carrol, 1982; Garside et al., 1971; Hamilton and White, 1959; Kay et al., 1969; Kiloh and Garside 1963; Mendels and Cochrane, 1968; Rosenthal and Gudeman, 1967; Rosenthal and Klerman, 1966). However, the results might be confounded by age; depression in older people is more likely to be of an endogenous type, and life events are rarer in older subjects. Paykel (1971) reported findings similar to those quoted above, but when he controlled for age the discriminant power of adversity was lost, suggesting that the effect of age might indeed account for the results of the other multivariate studies.

The results of these multivariate studies stand in contrast to those specifically designed to test the association of adversity with different symptom patterns in depression. Even without controlling for age, the experience of preceding adversity in endogenous and reactive groups is usually similar (e.g., Thompson and Hendrie, 1972; Hudgens et al., 1967; Leff et al., 1970; Brown and Harris, 1978, p213; Benjaminsen, 1981; Katschnig et al., 1981, 1986; Katschnig, 1984; Brugha and Conroy, 1985; Bebbington et al., 1988). Some more recent studies do provide support for a particular association of adversity with a neurotic symptom picture (Paykel et al., 1984; Roy et al., 1985; Zimmerman et al., 1986). Approaching the problem from a slightly different direction, Nelson and Charney (1980) showed that depressive states reactive to social stresses were much less likely to fulfill the criteria for primary affective disorder. Finally, Tennant and his colleagues (1981c) found an association between life events that neutralize the effect of previous threatening events and improvement in depressive symptoms, but only in "non-endogenous" conditions.

The contrasting results described above could arise from various differences of method (Katschnig et al., 1986). A further artifact might account for the findings of the multivariate studies: clinical psychiatrists make the distinction between endogenous and reactive depression on grounds both of characteristic symptoms and of the relationship with potential psychosocial stressors (Katschnig et al., 1981). Since clinician's judgments are used as the basis for validating the multivariate functions, or in claiming that the psychosocial history is relevant to onset, it is not surprising that the relationship with preceding adversity appears highly significant. In some studies, the discriminant function actually included the clinician's judgment of whether there had been significant social precipitants.

On the other hand, many of the direct comparison studies have used periods of analysis for preceding life events which may have been too long. The period which seems to be important if events are to lead to "normal" affective responses is limited to two or three months before onset (Brown and Harris, 1978; Bebbington et al., 1981b). Comparison on the basis of longer preceding periods may obscure differences between groups. However, Katschnig (1984) conducted analyses identical to those of Bebbington and his colleagues (1981b), but failed to find differences in the history of adversity between symptomatic groups.

The data from our own most recent study (Bebbington et al., 1988) do not support a difference in relation to psychosocial adversity between the categories of endogenous and neurotic depression, and the temporal distribution of events is very suggestive of a causal role in both types. The actual number of events shortly before onset was far greater than expected even in the fairly eventful lives of the local population. This study used methods closely similar to those of our earlier Camberwell Community Survey (Bebbington et al., 1981a), and we are unable to offer a convincing explanation for the widely discrepant results, except that the neurotic conditions seen in the clinic are more severe than those seen in the community, and might therefore be less strongly related to adversity.

The criteria for the distinction between "endogenous" and "neurotic" symptom patterns vary between studies, and might cause discrepancies in their results. Katschnig and his colleagues (1986) argue for a "polydiagnostic" approach, in which several standard distinctions between forms of depression are applied. When these workers used this with their own data, no classification corresponded to differences in psychosocial reactivity (Katschnig et al., 1981).

To conclude, many studies show slight differences between endogenous and reactive depressions in the frequency of antecedent adversity. These differences are rarely statistically significant, but the consistency of the finding might reflect a type 2 error. However, if the differences are indeed genuine, they are also small, suggesting only minor changes in relative risk with symptom picture.

The distinction between endogenous and reactive symptom pictures cannot therefore be validated to a telling extent in this way. Can other epidemiological correlates do better?

Other Epidemiological Distinctions Between Subtypes of Affective Disorder

There is some suggestion that the female-to-male sex ratio for depressive disorders is less for the more severe disorders. Although the recent and enormous ECA studies from the United States display a ratio on the low side (Regier et al., 1988), the ratio tends to be higher in the community than in patient series (Bebbington, 1988). Moreover, in all referred series of patients where results are quoted separately for affective psychosis and for depressive neurosis, the ratio is greater in the latter (e.g., Baldwin, 1971; Weeke et al., 1975; Der and Bebbington, 1987). The effect is consistent but not major. One possible explanation is that part of the female preponderance is accounted for by social rather than biological factors, these operating most noticeably on the milder disorders and therefore most noticeably in the general population.

A more marked pattern is that provided by age-specific incidence rates. The variation in prevalence in community surveys is inconsistent (Comstock and Helsing, 1976; Bebbington et al., 1981a; Henderson et al., 1981). The recent ECA surveys showed a definite peak, both for major depressive disorder and for dysthymia, between ages twenty-five and forty-four (Regier et al., 1988), although major depressive disorder in the community is still a relatively mild condition. However, when we turn to referred series, the results are quite consistent. The peak age of first psychiatric admission or contact for depressive psychosis is in late middle or early old age, while that for neurotic depression is much earlier, especially for women (Shepherd, 1957; Norris, 1959; Jaco, 1960; Silverman, 1968; Baldwin 1971; Gardiner et al., 1974; Der and Bebbington, 1987). This seems unlikely to arise because older subjects with neurotic disorder are less frequently referred (Bebbington, 1988).

These findings in the community make it unlikely that the increase in the incidence of severe disorder with age arises from the influence of the adverse social factors that undoubtedly bear on the elderly in many areas of the developed world. If so, an increase in the milder disorders, at least *pari passu* and possibly preferentially, would also be expected, but we have seen that this is not the case.

However, there are instances where the age effect is reversed by factors, in particular, marital status, that are readily interpreted only in social terms. In those who are divorced, widowed, or separated, the early peak for neurotic depression becomes exaggerated, whereas the increasing incidence with age is actually reversed for depressive psychosis (Carstairs, 1985; Bebbington, 1987, 1988; Der and Bebbington, 1987).

My own speculation is that this distinction between moderate and severe depression is valid, that the age effect in the former arises because of social influences, and that aging exerts a releasing effect on severe depressions. This releasing effect is probably biological, although the contribution of the neurobiology of aging to the susceptibility to depression is as yet ambiguous (Veith and Raskind, 1988). The age effect in severe depressions thus looks like a default option, open to reversal, but only by social factors of the most adverse character.

Another line of investigation has produced relevant data. Kendell and Di Scipio (1968) found that patients with "endogenous" depressions were less neurotic and less introverted following recovery than patients with "neurotic" depressions. Other workers reporting similar results are Benjaminsen (1981), Kerr and colleagues (1970), Paykel and colleagues (1976) and Perris (1971). Patients with bipolar depression are especially unlikely to show introverted and neurotic traits (Hirschfeld and Klerman, 1978), and personality disorders are apparently much less common in *melancholia* (severe "endogenous" depression) than in other depressive disorders (Charney et al., 1981). All these authors agree that "non-endogenous" depression is frequently precipitated by adverse environmental circumstances operating on someone whose personality is already somehow vulnerable.

Finally, Parker and his colleagues (1987) suggest that the association of the experience of poor parenting is apparent in neurotic depressives, but not in endogenous forms of the disorder. The distinction between endogenous and neurotic depression still clings to its claims of usefulness, despite failures to corroborate it in many areas.

Adversity and the Sociodemographic Correlates of Depression

If it is accepted that life events are causally related to depressive illness, it may be asked if the association explains that of other sociodemographic variables with depression. It has been argued that psychosocial factors lie behind the high rates of depression in women (Paykel and Rowan, 1979; Weissman and Klerman, 1977). Are life events and chronic difficulties candidates for an explanation of this type? For the experience of adversity to offer, on its own, an explanation of high rates of depression in women, it would have to be demonstrated that they experience more, or more upsetting, life events than men. This was indeed shown by Bebbington and his colleagues (1981a, 1991b) and by Brown and Birley (1968), but other workers have found that women do not tend to experience more life event stress than men (Thoits, 1982a; Uhlenhuth and Paykel 1973a and b; Uhlenhuth et al., 1974). Women may be exposed to more chronic problems than men (Pearlin and Johnson, 1977; Pearlin and Lieberman, 1977; Radloff, 1975). Bebbington and his colleagues (1991b) have recently conducted a study of this issue, using loglinear analysis. Although adversity was indeed commoner in women, such experiences were unable to account for their excessive frequency of minor affective disorder.

It is possible that women respond badly to the life events they do experience, being more likely to develop depression as a result. This obviously implies some special susceptibility in women requiring explanation. Two lines of evidence can be used to assess this. First, it appears that women do not assess events as being more stressful (Paykel et al., 1971). However, there is evidence of some increase in the relative risk and attributable risk of depression in response to life events in women (Bebbington et al., 1981b; Cooke and Hole, 1983). This may be largely due to certain subgroups of women who are especially prone to depression in response to life events, the issue of sociodemographic vulnerability described above. If the index of attributable risk is used, the data both of Brown and Harris (1978) and Bebbington and his colleagues (1984) reveal that the risk of depression attributable to life events was considerably increased in working class women at home with young children.

A further possibility is that the stress women experience arises in ways that cannot be categorized as discrete life events, or even as chronic difficulties. In particular, there may be attributes of women's status in society and the roles available to them that miss the net in this way (Parry, 1987).

The other obvious sociodemographic association of disorder that might be explicable in terms of adversity is that with social class. It would after all be reasonable to suggest that persons of lower social class experience more adversity (Faris and Dunham, 1939; Langner and Michael, 1963). A number of studies confirm this (Bell et al., 1982; Brown and Birley, 1968; Dohrenwend, 1970, 1973; Dohrenwend and Dohrenwend, 1969; Kessler and Cleary, 1980; Myers et al., 1974; Pearlin and Lieberman, 1977; Thoits, 1982; Bebbington et al., 1991b). However, this excess of adversity is rarely sufficient to account for class differences in risk of affective disorder. For example, Brown and Harris (1978) found approximately four times as much disorder in working class as in middle class women, and also showed that life events were somewhat commoner in the working class group. However within this group, those most likely to experience adversity did not have the greatest probability of disorder. Bebbington and his colleagues (1991b) have provided complex analyses of this issue. Although the association of disorder with lower social class in their sample was neither large nor significant, it was indeed eliminated by controlling for adversity. This suggests that the association could have arisen *because* working class people experience more hardship. However, in the data both of Brown and Harris (1978) and of Bebbington and his colleagues (1986), class itself meets the requirements for a conditional effect on life events. In other words, class operates as a vulnerability factor: some of the prevalence of disorder in the working class is accounted for by their susceptibility to the adversity they do experience. This issue remains an open one.

There is some evidence to suggest that unemployment is associated with an increased rate of life events (Catalano and Dooley, 1977; Bebbington et al., 1991b). However, this does not account for the adverse effects of unemployment discussed above (Bebbington et al., 1991b). Unemployment, like class, may operate as a vulnerability factor (Brown and Harris, 1978; Kessler et al., 1987).

Bebbington and his colleagues (1991b) have also examined the complex associations of marital status, childcare, and parity with gender and disorder in terms of exposure to psychosocial adversity. In all cases, the subgroups with high risk of minor psychiatric disorder had also experienced more adversity, but in no case was this an adequate explanation for the macrosocial distribution of disorder.

It is clear from this review of the issue that most high risk groups still require explanation in psychosocial terms, and that, with the possible exception of the association with social class, high rates of psychosocial adversity (at least as measured) do not provide this.

Social Support

In recent years, the topic of social support has attracted considerable interest from those engaged in the study of psychiatric disorders. The area as a whole has been well reviewed by Broadhead and his colleagues (1983), Turner (1983), Henderson (1984), and in the volume edited by Cohen and Syme (1985), especially the chapter by Kessler and MacLeod (1985).

The concept has many sources, including Durkheim's development of the idea of *anomie* (Durkheim, trans. 1951), Cooley's concept of the *primary group* (1909) and Bowlby's ideas on *attachment* (1971). Social relationships extend from the intimacies of lovers to the relatively impersonal qualities of a commercial transaction, so there is a real problem in deciding on the qualities of social support relevant to mental health research. Psychologists have defined the behavioral, affective and cognitive aspects of the concept (Hinde, 1979), sociologists have focussed more on the function of social support for the individual and the structures within which it is offered (Mitchell, 1969; Weiss, 1974). These viewpoints are not easy to integrate, and this is one reason for the variety of measures used.

The idea of the *primary group* takes account both of the structure and of the function of social relationships. Primary group membership involves people in intimate association and cooperation (i.e., behavior), but such groups are primary particularly because they help form the social nature and ideals of the individual. People also interact with those who are not members of their primary group, and the totality of those with whom a person interacts forms his or her *social network* (Mitchell, 1969).

Both the structure and function of social networks might affect the risk of psychiatric disorder. Structure includes such items as size of primary group, size of secondary group, whether other members of the network know and interact with each other, whether members of the primary group are members also of the subject's household, and so on. The potential functions of social relationships are many (Weiss, 1974; Kahn and Antonucci, 1980), but several workers agree on the usefulness of distinguishing between practical help and emotional support (Dean and Lin, 1977; Kaplan et al., 1977; Thoits, 1982b; Parry and Shapiro, 1986).

Although a number of workers have reported deficiencies in the size of the social networks of patients (Brugha et al., 1982, Cohen and Sokolovsky, 1978; Henderson et al., 1978; Sokolovsky et al., 1978; Tolsdorf, 1976), most research has concentrated on the perceived function of relationships, even though there are much greater problems of measuring this than their structural characteristics. As these conceptual problems have not been overcome, there is no generally accepted measure of social support, or of networks, despite a number of hopeful developments (e.g., Brown and Bifulco, 1985; Brugha et al., 1987; Dean and Ensel, 1982; Henderson et al., 1978, 1981; Lin and Dean, 1984; McCallister and Fischer, 1978; O'Connor and Brown, 1984; Sarason et al., 1982, 1983). Most researchers, however, have thought up a few questions of their own, albeit of face validity, as the basis of their ratings. This immediately casts doubt on most reports in the literature, and certainly makes comparisons between studies difficult.

There is now a considerable body of research addressed to the "buffer theory" of social support, although most studies have been of minor affective disorder (Alloway and Bebbington, 1987). It expresses the intuitively acceptable idea that being able to turn to people for support mitigates the effects of misfortunes and attenuates the development of psychiatric disorder. The buffer theory has been used to account both for the *onset* of psychiatric disorder and for its *exacerbation*.

In the research on the buffer theory, workers have chosen to focus on practical or emotional support or both. In most cases, researchers have decided intuitively that it is the *emotional* support of *close* relationships that is likely to be important in preserving psychological well-being and staving off the effects of misfortune.

Until very recently, researchers have examined the effect of *routine* social support. However, it is likely that if social support has an effect in moderating the impact of acute psychosocial stress, it is because it is available and drawn on at the time of crisis. The assessment of crisis social support in the context of specific life events is recent, although one such study has now been published (Brown et al., 1986). Crisis support is very difficult to measure except retrospectively.

There are now many studies of social support and psychiatric disorder. Alloway and Bebbington (1987) reviewed twenty three cross-sectional and twelve longitudinal studies. Their conclusion was that there was almost certainly a direct association of minor psychiatric disorder with impaired social support, but the claim that this operated by increasing the subject's response to psychosocial adversity was less well founded. Moreover, it has not been ruled out that these results are spurious or the consequence of contamination.

The sophisticated longitudinal study of Henderson and his colleagues (1981) suggests one possible interpretation of the relationship between support and disorder. Among other measures of support were Availability of Attachment and Perceived Adequacy of Attachment. The buffer theory was corroborated only if the Perceived Adequacy measure was used. As Availability is a more objective measure, Henderson and his colleagues (1981) were thrown back on an alternative explanation, namely that Perceived Adequacy was acting as a reflection more of personality than of the actual state of relationships.

One of the most interesting studies is that of Brown and his colleagues (1986). This involved a follow-up study of women in Islington, North London. At the first interview, the sample was divided into cases and noncases. Noncases were followed up after one year. The authors present results separately for wives and for the single women. Among wives, they found that the existence of a confiding relationship at the first interview was not associated with a lower risk of depression in the succeeding year, nor did it interact with life events in the way predicted by the vulnerability model. In contrast, single mothers were less likely to become depressed after the first interview if they had access to socially supportive relationships, although the authors do not report on any interaction with life events in this group.

This design is a powerful one, and it is disquieting that it offers relatively little confirmation of the role of social support. Brown and his colleagues (1986) argue persuasively that the discrepancy in findings between the wives and the single mothers arises because in the former social support at the first interview was a poor reflection of the actual ("crisis") support obtained in the face of life events. This could be so, but it does mean that the role of social support has been salvaged by interpreting the negative prospective finding in the light of an assessment made retrospectively, and thus open to all the objections to retrospective measures.

The Epidemiology of Bipolar Disorder

Relatively little has been published on the epidemiology of bipolar affective disorder. However, it is clear that risk factors are different from those in unipolar depression.

Boyd and Weissman (1982) quote a number of studies giving a range for the morbid risk of bipolar disorder between 0.6% and 0.9%. This is a little lower than the morbid risk for schizophrenia. These authors also report incidence values between 7 and 32 per 10^5 per year. Our own values from the Camberwell register for the incidence of mania are less, between 4 and 5 per 10^5 per year for each sex.

The sex ratio is much closer to unity than for any form of unipolar depression, and the age-specific incidence is also different. In our own

Camberwell data, there was little variation in the incidence of mania with age (Der and Bebbington, 1987), and Boyd and Weissman (1982) suggest that, if there is any association, the peak incidence is rather earlier than that of severe unipolar depression.

Finally, the association of bipolar illness with social class may be different. Some studies suggest increased incidence in the higher social classes (Odegaard, 1956; Noreik and Odegaard, 1966). Bagley (1973), using early data from the Camberwell register, suggested that there was little relationship between occupational class and affective disorders, with the exception that bipolar cases tended to cluster in the higher classes. From the early study by Stern-Piper (1925) comes a suggestion that the social class correlates of manic depressive illness and moderate depressions are different, with the former clustering at the higher end, and the later at the lower end, of the social spectrum. Similar findings emerge from more recent reports (Woodruff et al., 1971; Monnelly et al., 1974).

Although the macrosocial correlates of bipolar disorder help to distinguish it from schizophrenia, the influence of psychosocial stress in the two conditions may be similar, serving to contrast them with unipolar and minor depressive disorder. There are relatively few studies of life events in mania, and all are beset with methodological failings (Ambelas, 1979, 1987; Dunner et al., 1979; Kennedy et al., 1983; Glassner and Haldipur, 1983). The results are nevertheless suggestive of an association. Events preceding episodes of mania seem to occur in very close proximity to the onset, as they appear to in schizophrenia (Brown et al., 1973; Day et al., 1987). It is possible that the events are more associated with first rather than subsequent episodes of mania (Ambelas, 1987), and this again may show similarities with schizophrenia (Al Khani et al., 1986). This raises the possibility that an initial stress both reveals a diathesis and lowers the threshold to subsequent stress.

Another form of psychosocial stress that has been linked to relapse in bipolar disorder is that detected by the Expressed Emotion measure (Miklowitz et al., 1988). The threshold appears similar to that in schizophrenia, and differs from that in neurotic depression (Kuipers and Bebbington, 1988).

Epidemiology of Anxiety Disorders

Once again, in comparison to unipolar depressive disorders the epidemiology of anxiety has not received the attention it merits. Problems of definition abound, particularly with the fairly recent American separation of panic disorder from the body of anxiety disorders. Marks (1986) has summarized the relatively few community surveys of prevalence. Apart from the outlying finding of Vaisanen (1975), most gave values for anxiety *disorders* of all types of a few percent (2.9 to 8.4). Female preponderance is greatest for agoraphobia, least for social phobia. *Symptoms*, particularly phobic symptoms, are much commoner, and are frequently present in those with diagnoses other than anxiety. Recent results from studies using the Present State Examination are given in Table 13.4. The results from the ECA studies have not been presented in a coherent manner: it is not possible to give overall rates for anxiety states, as the combined categories provided include obsessional disorders and somatization disorders, but leave out Generalized Anxiety Disorder, a class which was unavailable in the earlier studies. Moreover, because it is easy to meet the criteria of more than one condition it is not possible to calculate rates which might be more useful for the current purpose. The reader is therefore referred to the original sources referenced in Table 13.3.

It is clear that, like depression, symptoms of anxiety are frequent wherever they are sought. It is possible that depressive disorders are more common than anxiety states in Northern Europe, but that the reverse is true in Mediterranean cultures and the United States (Bebbington et al., 1981; Hodiamont et al., 1987; Mavreas et al., 1986; Mavreas and Bebbington, 1987; Ozturk et al., 1980; Surtees et al., 1983; Surtees and Sashidaran, 1986; Vazquez-Barquero et al., 1987). The results from the ECA studies (Regier et al., 1988) do suggest that anxiety disorders, especially phobic states, may be commoner in the black community: this may account for the very high prevalence of such disorders in Baltimore and the Piedmont, both areas with a considerable black population in their samples.

Most of the phobic symptoms in the community are specific, cause little disability, and rarely lead the sufferer to the primary care physician or psychiatrist. Agoraphobia is relatively rare in the community, but, being

TABLE 13.4
Prevalence of CATEGO anxiety classes (%)

Site	Male	Female	Total
Uganda (Orley & Wing 1979)	2.8	4.0	3.4
Canberra (Henderson *et al.* 1979)	4.1	3.0	3.5
Camberwell (Bebbington *et al.* 1981)	1.0	4.5	2.9
Edinburgh (Surtees *et al.* 1983)		2.8	
Athens (Mavreas *et al.* 1986)	3.9	12.1	8.2
Nijmegen (Hodiamont *et al.* 1987)			2.0
Santander (Vazquez-Barquero *et al.* 1987	2.4	6.2	4.5
Camberwell (Cypriot) (Mavreas and Bebbington (1987)	2.7	10.5	6.6
Finland (Lehtinen *et al.* 1990)	0.8	3.0	1.9

Note: Studies that do not give a breakdown in terms of CATEGO classes are not included more disabling, is more frequently represented in referred series (Agras, 1969, Marks, 1969).

Although anxiety is associated with considerable distress in the general population, it appears to be less socially disabling than the minor depressive conditions (Hurry et al., 1983; Hecht & Wittchen, 1988: Fredman et al., 1988). Much anxiety is clearly circumstantial, being related to anticipation of outcomes that are uncertain and possibly adverse. Anticipatory anxiety of this type must be regarded as a normal part of human experience—"exam nerves" and the like. The definition of "anxiety states" carries implications similar to the separation of depressive disorders from normal sadness. The area is conceptually murky in both types of affective disorder (Bebbington, 1987b). However, the relationship of anxiety states to circumstances is probably different and less clearly related to anticipations. An example is the high level of anxiety symptoms in post-traumatic stress disorder (Horowitz et al., 1980), where most of the implications of the precipitatory event are related to the past, although the subjects' view of the world may be affected such that they regard themselves much more clearly as a fragile envelope. There is thus a sense that the anxiety state proper has a certain autonomy from the precipitating circumstance.

There is relatively little research on the relationship between antecedent adversity and the emergence of anxiety states. Some studies assess life events and anxiety symptoms at a point in time, often in non-representative populations—college students, evening class attenders, and the like. With the exception of Flannery (1986), who found an association in women but not in men, all have shown a significant association between life events and symptoms of anxiety (Lauer, 1973; Miller et al., 1976; Sarason et al., 1978). However, such studies are impossible of causal interpretation, as no attempt was made to date onset.

Four studies have sought, and found, an increased frequency of events before the onset of anxiety states (Barrett, 1979; Finlay-Jones and Brown, 1981; Blazer et al., 1987; Eaton and Ritter, 1988). There were some problems of method and interpretation in the first, but it appeared that subjects with anxiety disorders reported more events than a control group, and differed from a depressive group in having fewer "exit" and undesirable events. Finlay-Jones and Brown (1981) found that the events preceding the onset of anxiety states were more likely to be threatening and less likely to be associated with losses than those preceding depressive conditions. Loss events and exit events have similar connotations. Recently, however, using the Baltimore ECA data, Eaton and Ritter (1988) failed to corroborate these findings.

These results therefore require further replication, but they raise once more the issue of what we mean by anxiety states and how we distinguish them from normal anxiety. Certainly the events preceding these so-called anxiety states sound similar to the sorts of circumstance that we associate with the normal experience of anxiety.

Conclusions—Directions for Further Research

This review of the social epidemiology of affective disorders reveals important issues requiring further research. First, although there has been a convergence in the definition of a threshold for recognizing the existence of affective disorder, more needs to be done before we know quite what we mean when we quote values for the prevalence of depressive disorders and anxiety states, and before we can be sure that comparisons between different sites reflect real differences in prevalence rather than differences in criteria or in their application. There is a particular need for a purpose-designed study to establish lifetime prevalence and morbid risk, as without this information, geneticists are unable to estimate the heritability of affective disorders.

Secondly, epidemiology has provided a reasonable consensus in its primary task of identifying high risk groups, but we now need to know the basis of increased risk. This requires detailed study of the attributes both of the subjects and of their circumstances.

Thirdly, the role of psychosocial adversity is known to be important in the genesis of affective disorders, but we have no clear account of variations in individual susceptibility, although we have good leads, and theories of more than adequate complexity.

Next, the literature on social support is now extensive, but serious methodological problems remain to be overcome. It is clear that the social networks of depressive patients are constrained, but it is not clear how this comes about or how it is related to the emergence of depression.

Finally, the epidemiology of severe affective disorders and of anxiety disorders has not been sufficiently studied, and we particularly need corroborated accounts of their social determinants.

References

Abramson, L.Y., Seligman, M.E.P., and Teasdale, J.D. (1978). Learned helplessness in humans: critique and reformulation. *Journal of Abnormal Psychology*, *87*, 49–74.

Adelstein, A.M., Downham, D.Y., Stein, Z., and Susser, M.W. (1968). The epidemiology of mental illness in an English City. *Social Psychiatry*, *3*, 47–59.

Agras, S., Sylvester, D. and Oliveau, D. (1969). The epidemiology of common fears and phobias. *Comprehensive Psychiatry*, *10*, 151–156.

Al Khani M.A.F., Bebbington, P.E., Watson, J., and House, F. (1986). Life events and schizophrenia: A Saudi Arabian Study. *British Journal of Psychiatry, 148,* 12–22.

Alloway, R. and Bebbington, P.E. (1987). The buffer theory of social support: a review of the literture. *Psychological Medicine, 17,* 91–108.

Ambelas, A. (1979). Psychologically stressful events in the precipitation of manic episodes. *British Journal of Psychiatry, 135,* 15–21.

Ambelas, A. (1987). Life events and mania: A special relationship? *British Journal of Psychiatry, 150,* 235–240.

American Psychiatric Association (1980). *Diagnostic And Statistical Manual of Mental Disorders (DSMIII),* 3rd edition, American Psychiatric Association, Washington, D.C.

Bagley, C. (1973). Occupational class and symptoms of depression. *Social Science and Medicine, 7,* 327–339.

Baldwin, J.A. (1971). Five year incidence of reported psychiatric disorder. In: J.A. Baldwin (ed.) *Aspects of the Epidemiology of Mental Illness: Studies in Record Linkage,* Boston, Little Brown & Co.

Banks, M.H. and Jackson, P.R. (1982). Unemployment and risk of minor psychiatric disorders in young people: cross-sectional and longitudinal evidence. *Psychological Medicine, 12,* 789–98.

Barrett, J.E. (1979). The relationship of life events to the onset of neurotic disorders. In: J.E. Barrett (ed.). *Stress and Mental Disorder,* New York, Raven Press.

Bebbington, P.E. (1982). The course and prognosis of affective psychosis. In: *Cambridge Handbook of Psychiatry,* Vol. III. (ed. J.K. Wing). Cambridge University Press.

Bebbington, P.E. (1985a). Psychosocial etiology of schizophrenia and affective disorders. In: R. Michels (ed). *Psychiatry.* Philadelphia, Lippincott.

Bebbington, P.E. (1985b). Three cognitive theories of depression. *Psychological Medicine, 15,* 759–771.

Bebbington, P.E. (1987a). Marital status and depression: a study of English national admission statistics. *Acta Psychiatrica Scandinavica, 75,* 640–650.

Bebbington, P.E. (1987b). Misery and beyond: the pursuit of disease theories of depression. *International Journal of Social Psychiatry, 33,* 13–20.

Bebbington, P.E. (1988). The social epidemiology of clinical depression. In: A.S. Henderson and G. Burrows (eds). *Handbook of Studies in Social Psychiatry,* Amsterdam, Elsevier.

Bebbington, P.E., Hurry, J., and Tennant, C. (1980). Recent advances in the epidemiology of minor affective disorders in the community. *Proceedings of the Royal Society of Medicine, 73,* 315–317.

Bebbington, P., Hurry, J., Tennant, C., Sturt, E., and Wing, J.K. (1981a). The epidemiology of mental disorders in Camberwell. *Psychological Medicine, 11,* 561–80.

Bebbington, P.E., Tennant, C., and Hurry, J. (1981b). Life events and the nature of psychiatric disorder in the community. *Journal of Affective Disorders 3,* 345–66.

Bebbington, P.E., Sturt, E., Tennant, C., and Hurry, J. (1984). Misfortune and resilience: a community study of women. *Psychological Medicine, 14,* 347–364.

Bebbington, P.E., Hurry, J., and Tennant, C. (1986). Adversity and working class vulnerability to minor affective disorder. *Journal of Affective Disorder, 11,* 115–120.

Bebbington, P.E., Hurry, J., and Tennant, C. (1988). Adversity and the symptoms of depression. *International Journal of Social Psychiatry, 34*, 163–171.

Bebbington, P.E., Brugha, T. MacCarthy, B., Potter, J., Sturt, E, Wykes, T., Katz, R., and McGuffin, P. (1988). The Camberwell Collaborative Depression Study. I. Depressed probands: Adversity and the form of depression. *British Journal of Psychiatry, 152*, 754–765.

Bebbington, P.E. and McGuffin, P. (1989). Interactive models of depression: the evidence. In: E.S. Paykel and K. Herbst (eds). *Depression: an Integrative Approach*, London, Heineman Medical.

Bebbington, P.E. and Tansella, M. (1989). Gender, marital status and treated affective disorders in South Verona: a case-register study. *Journal of Affective Disorders, 17*, 83–91.

Bebbington, P.E., Katz, R., McGuffin, P., Tennant, C., and Hurry, J. (1989). The risk of minor depression before age 65: results from a community survey. *Psychological Medicine, 19*, 393–400.

Bebbington, P.E., Dean, C., Der, G., Hurry, J., and Tennant, C. (1991a). Gender, parity and the prevalence of minor affective disorder. *British Journal of Psychiatry* (in press).

Bebbington, P.E., Tennant, C., and Hurry, J. (1991b). Adversity in groups with an increased risk of minor affective disorder. *British Journal of Psychiatry* (in press).

Beck, A.T. (1976). *Cognitive Therapy and the Emotional Disorders*. International Universities Press. New York.

Beck, A.T. (1983). Cognitive therapy of depression: New perspectives. *In Treatment of Depression: Old Controversies and New Approaches* (eds. P.J. Clayton and J.E. Barrett) pp 265–290. Raven Press: New York.

Bell, R.A., LeRoy, J.R., and Stephenson, J.J. (1982). Evaluating the mediating effects of social support upon life events and depressive symptoms. *Journal of Community Psychology, 10*, 325–40.

Benjaminsen, S. (1981). Primary non-endogenous depression and features attributed to reactive depression. *Journal of Affective Disorders, 3*, 245–59.

Blacker, C.V.R. and Clare, A.W. (1987). Depressive disorder in primary care. *British Journal of Psychiatry, 150*, 737–751.

Bland, R.C., Newman, S.C., and Orn, H. (1988). Epidemiology of psychiatric disorders in Edmonton. *Acta Psychiatrica Scandinavica, 77, Supplementum 338*.

Blazer, D., Hughes, D., and George, L.K. (1978). Stressful life events and the onset of a generalized anxiety syndrome. *American Journal of Psychiatry, 144*, 1178–1183.

Blazer, D., George, L.K., Landerman, R., Pennybacker, M., Melville, M.L. Woodbury, M., Manton, K.G., Jordan, K., and Locke, B. (1985). Psychiatric disorders: a rural/urban comparison. *Archives of General Psychiatry, 42*, 651–656.

Blumenthal, M.D. and Dielman, T.E. (1975). Depressive symptomatology and role function in a general population. *Archives of General Psychiatry, 32*, 985–991.

Bolton, W. and Oatley, K. (1987). A longitudinal study of social support and depression in unemployed men. *Psychological Medicine, 17*, 453–460.

Bowlby, J. (1971). *Attachment and Loss: I: Attachment*, Harmondsworth, Penguin.

Boyd, J.H. and Weissman, M.M. (1982). Epidemiology. In: E.S. Paykel (Ed). *Handbook of Affective Disorders*, Edinburgh, Churchill-Livingstone.

Brenner, M.H. (1973). *Mental Illness and the Economy*. Cambridge, Mass. Harvard University Press.

Brewin, C.R. (1989). Cognitive change processes in psychotherapy. *Psychological Review*, *96*, 379–394.

Broadhead, W.E., Kaplan, B.H., James, S.A., Wagner, E.H., Schoenbach, V.J., Grimson, R., Heyden, S., Tibblin, G., and Gehlbach, S.H. (1983). The epidemiologic evidence for a relationship between social support and health. *American Journal of Epidemiology*, *117*, 521–537.

Bromet, E.J., Dunn, L.O., Connell, M.O., Dew, M.A., and Schulberg, H.C. (1986). Long-term reliability of diagnosing lifetime major depression in a community sample. *Archives of General Psychiatry*, *43*, 435–440.

Brown, G.W. and Birley, J.L.T. (1968). Crises and life changes and the onset of schizophrenia. *Journal of Health and Social Behaviour*, *9*, 203–214.

Brown, G.W. (1974). Meaning, measurement and stress of life events. In: B.S. Dohrenwend and B.P. Dohrenwend (eds.). *Stressful Life Events: Their Nature and Effects*. New York, John Wiley.

Brown, G.W., (1989). Life events and measurement. In: G.W. Brown and T.O. Harris (eds.) Life Events and Illness. London, Unwin Hyman.

Brown, G.W., Harris, T.O., and Peto, J. (1973). Life events and psychiatric disorders. Part 2: Nature of causal link. *Psychological Medicine*, *3*, 159–176.

Brown, G.W., Davidson, S., Harris, T., Maclean, U., Pollock, S., and Prudo, R. (1977). Psychiatric disorder in London and North Uist. *Social Science and Medicine*, *11*, 367–377.

Brown, G.W., Harris, T.O., and Copeland, J.R. (1977). Depression and loss. *British Journal of Psychiatry*, *130*, 1–18.

Brown, G.W. and Harris, T.O. (1978). *Social Origins of Depression*, London, Tavistock.

Brown, G.W. and Bifulco, A. (1985). Social support, life events and depression. In: I.G. Sarason and B.R. Sarason (eds.). *Social Support: Theory, Research and Application*, Dordrecht, Martinus Nijhoff.

Brown, G.W., Andrews, B., Bifulco, A., Adler, Z., and Bridge, L. (1986). Social support, self-esteem and depression. *Psychological Medicine*, *16*, 813–832.

Burnham, M.A., Hough, R.L., Escobar, J.I., Karno, M., Timbers, D.M., Telles, C.A., and Locke, B.Z. (1987). Six month prevalence of specific psychiatric disorders among Mexican Americans and non-Hispanic whites in Los Angeles. *Archives of General Psychiatry*, *44*, 687–694.

Cadoret, R.J., Winokur, G., Dorzab, J., and Baker, M. (1972). Depressive disease: Life events and onset of illness. *Archives of General Psychiatry*, *26*, 133–6.

Canino, G.J., Bird, H.R., Shrout, P.E., Rubio-Stipec, M., Bravo, M., Martinez, R., Sesman, M., and Guevara, L.M. (1987). The prevalence of specific psychiatric disorders in Puerto Rico. *Archives of General Psychiatry*, *44*, 727–735.

Carney, M.W.P., Roth, M., and Garside, R.F. (1965). The diagnosis of depressive syndromes and the prediction of ECT response. *British Journal of Psychiatry*, *111*, 659–74.

Carstairs, V. (1985). Marital status and admission to hospital for different categories of mental illness. Presented at WPA Section of Epidemiology and Community Psychiatry meeting: "The Future of Psychiatric Epidemiology." Edinburgh, Scotland, 23–26 Sept.

Catalano, R. and Dooley, C.D. (1977). Economic predictions of depressed mood in a metropolitan community. *Journal of Health and Social Behaviour*, *18*, 292–307.

Charney, D.S., Nelson, J.C., and Quinlan, D.M. (1981). Personality traits and disorder in depression. *American Journal of Psychiatry*, *138*, 1601–4.

Clancy, K. and Gove, W.R. (1974). Sex differences in mental illness: an analysis of response bias in self reports. *American Journal of Sociology*, *80*, 205–16.

Clark, R. (1949). Psychosis, income and occupational prestige. *American Journal of Sociology*, *54*, 433–440.

Clayton, P.J. (1975). The effect of living alone on bereavement symptoms. *American Journal of Psychiatry 132*, 133–7.

Clayton, P.J., Halikas, J.A., and Maurice, W.L. (1972). The depression of widowhood. *British Journal of Psychiatry*, *120*, 71–8.

Cohen, C. and Sokolovsky, J. (1978). Schizophrenia and social networks. *Schizophrenia Bulletin*, *4*, 546–560.

Cohen, S. and Syme, L. (eds.) (1985). *Social Support and Health*, New York, Academic Press.

Comstock, G.W. and Helsing, K.J. (1976). Symptoms of depression in two communities. *Psychological Medicine*, *6*, 551–563.

Cooke, D.J. (1981). Life events and syndromes of depression in the general population. *Social Psychiatry*, *16*, 181–6.

Cooke, D.J. and Hole, D.J. (1983). The importance of stressful life events. *British Journal of Psychiatry*, *143*, 397–400.

Cooley, C.H. (1909). *Social Organisation: a Study of the Larger Mind*. C. Scribner's Sons, New York.

Costello, C.G. (1982). Social factors associated with depression: a retrospective community study. *Psychological Medicine*, *12*, 329–39.

Day, R., Neilsen, J.A., Korten, A., Ernberg, G., Dube, K.C., Gebhart, J., Jablensky, A., Leon, C., Marsella, A., Olatawura, M., Sartorius, N., Stromgren, E., Takahashi, R., Wig, N., and Wynne, L.C. (1987). Stressful life events preceding the acute onset of schizophrenia: a cross-national study from the World Health Organization. *Culture, Medicine and Psychiatry*, *11*, 123–206.

Dean, A. and Ensel, W.M. (1982). Modelling social support, life events, competence and depression in the context of age and sex. *Journal of Community Psychology*, *10*, 392–408.

Dean, A. and Lin, N. (1977). The stress-buffering role of social support: problems and prospects for systematic investigation. *Journal of Nervous and Mental Disease*, *165*, 403–17.

Dent, J. and Teasdale, J.D. (1988). Negative cognition and the persistence of depression. *Journal of Abnormal Psychology*, *97*, 29–34.

Der, G. and Bebbington, P.E. (1987). Depression in inner London: a register study. *Social Psychiatry*, *22*, 73–84.

Dew, M.A., Dunn, L.O., Bromet, E.J., and Schulberg, H.C. (1988). Factors affecting helpseeking during depression in a community sample. *Journal of Affective Disorders*, *14*, 223–234.

Dohrenwend, B.P. and Dohrenwend, B.S. (1969). *Social Status and Psychological Disorder: A Causal Inquiry*. Wiley: New York.

Dohrenwend, B.P. and Dohrenwend, B.S. (1974). Social and cultural influences on psychopathology. *Annual Review of Psychology*, *25*, 417–452.

Dohrenwend, B.S. (1970). Social class and stressful events. In: Hare, E.H. and Wing, J.K. (eds.). *Psychiatric Epidemiology*. New York, Oxford University Press.

Dohrenwend, B.S. (1973). Social status and stressful life events. *Journal of Personality and Social Psychology*, *28*, 225–235.

Dohrenwend, B.S., Krasnoff, L., Askenasy, A.R., and Dohrenwend, B.P. (1978). Exemplification of a method for scaling life events: the PERI life events scale. *Journal of Health and Social Behaviour*, *19*, 205–229.

Duncan-Jones, P. (1981) The natural history of neurosis: Probability models. In: *What is a case? The Problem of Definition in Psychiatric Community Surveys.* (eds. J.K. Wing, P.E. Bebbington and L.N. Robins). London: Grant McIntyre.

Dunner, D.L., Patrick, V., and Fieve, R.R. (1979). Life events at the onset of bipolar affective illness. *American Journal of Psychiatry*, *136*, 508–511.

Durkheim, E. (1951) *Suicide: A Study in Sociology.* Trans. J.A. Spaulding and G. Simpson. New York, Free Press.

Eales, M.J. (1988). Depression and anxiety in unemployed men. *Psychological Medicine*, *18*, 935–945.

Eaton, W.W. and Ritter, C. (1988). Distinguishing anxiety and depression with field survey data. *Psychological Medicine*, *18*, 155–166.

Fagin, L. (1981): *Unemployment and Health in Families.* London. DHSS.

Faris, R.E.L. and Dunham, H.W. (1939). *Mental Disorders in Urban Areas.* New York, Hafner.

Fava, G.A., Munari, F., Pavan, L. and Kellner, R. (1981). Life events and depression: a replication. *Journal of Affective Disorders*, *3*, 159–65.

Feinberg, M. and Carroll, B.J. (1982). Separation of subtypes of depression using discriminant analysis: I Separation of unipolar endogenous depression from non-endogenous depression. *British Journal of Psychiatry*, *140*, 384–91.

Finlay-Jones, R. and Brown, G.W. (1981). Types of stressful life event and the onset of anxiety and depressive disorders. *Psychological Medicine*, *11*, 803–16.

Finlay-Jones, R. and Eckhardt, B. (1981). Psychiatric disorder among the young unemployed. *Australian and New Zealand Journal of Psychiatry*, *15*, 265–270.

Flannery, R.B. (1986). Major life events and daily hassles in predicting health status: methodological inquiry. *Journal of Clinical Psychology*, *42*, 485–487.

Fredman, L., Weissman, M.M., Leaf, P.J., and Bruce, M.L. (1988). Social functioning in community residents with depression and other psychiatric disorders: Results of the New Haven Epidemiologic Catchment Area study. *Journal of Affective Disorders*, *15*, 103–112.

Frese, M. and Mohr, G. (1987). Prolonged unemployment and depression in older workers: a longitudinal study of intervening variables. *Social Science and Medicine*, *25*, 173–178.

Fryers, D. (1988). The experience of unemployment in social context. In: S. Fisher & J. Reason (eds.). *Handbook of Life Stress, Cognition and Health.* London, Wiley.

Gardiner. A.Q., Petersen, J., and Hall, D.J. (1974). Aspects of the treatment of patients prior to referral to psychiatric out-patient services. In: D.J. Hall, N.C. Robertson and R.J. Eason (eds.). *Psychiatric Case Registers*, DHSS Statistical and Research Report Series No. 7, London, HMSO.

Garside, R.F., Kay, D.W.K., Wilson, I.C., Deaton, I.D., and Roth, M. (1971). Depressive syndromes and the classification of patients. *Psychological Medicine*, *1*, 333–8.

Gater, R.A., Dean, C., and Morris, J. (1989). The contribution of child bearing to the sex difference in first admission rates for unipolar affective psychosis. In press: *Psychological Medicine*, *19*, 719–724.

Gershon, E., Hamovit, J.H., Guroff, J.J., and Nurnberger, J.I. (1987). Birth cohort changes in manic and depressive disorders in relatives of bipolar and schizoaffective patients. *Archives of General Psychiatry*, *44*, 314–9.

Glassner, B. and Haldipur, C.V. (1983). Life events and early and late onset of bipolar disorder. *American Journal of Psychiatry*, *140*, 215–217.

Gotlib, I.H., Mount, J.H., Cordy, N.I., and Whiffen, V.E. (1988). Depression and perceptions of early parenting: A longitudinal study. *British Journal of Psychiatry*, *152*, 24–27.

Grad de Alarcon, J., Sainsbury, P., and Costain, W.R. (1975). Incidence of referred mental illness in Chichester and Salisbury. *Psychological Medicine*, *5*, 32–54.

Granville-Grossman, K.L. (1968). The early environment in affective disorder. In: Coppen, A. and Walk, A. (eds.). *Recent Developments in Affective Disorders*, Ashford, Kent, Headley Brothers.

Gravelle, H.S.E., Hutchinson, G., and Stern, J. (1981). Mortality and unemployment: a critique of Brenner's time series analysis. *Lancet*, *ii*, 675–9.

Hagnell, O., Lanke, J., Rorsman, B. and Öjesjö L. (1982). Are we entering an age of melancholy? Depressive illness in a prospective epidemiological study over 25 years: the Lundby Study, Sweden. *Psychological Medicine*, *12*, 279–89.

Hall, D.J. (1971). Social class and psychiatric referral of economically active males. In: J.A. Baldwin (ed.). *Aspects of the Epidemiology of Mental Illness: Studies in Record Linkage*, Boston, Little, Brown & Co.

Hamilton, M. and White, J.M. (1959). Clinical syndromes in depressive states. *Journal of Mental Science*, *105*, 985–98.

Hare, E.H. and Shaw, G.K. (1965). *Mental Health on a New Housing Estate: A Comparative Study of Health in two Districts in Croydon*. Maudsley Monograph No. 12. London, Oxford University Press.

Harris, T.O. and Brown, G.W. (1989). The LEDS findings in the context of other research: an overview. In: G.W. Brown and T.O. Harris (eds.). Life events and Illness. London, Unwin Hyman.

Hasin, D. and Link, B. (1988). Age and recognition of depression: Implications for a cohort effect in major depression. *Psychological Medicine*, *18*, 683–688.

Hecht, H. and Wittchen, H-U (1988). The frequency of social dysfunction in a general population sample and in patients with mental disorders. A comparison using the Social Interview Schedule. *Social Psychiatry and Psychiatric Epidemiology*, *23*, 17–29.

Henderson, A.S. (1984). Interpreting the evidence on social support. *Social Psychiatry*, *19*, 49–52.

Henderson, A.S., Duncan-Jones, P., McAuley, H., and Ritchie, K. (1978). The patient's primary group. *British Journal of Psychiatry*, *132*, 74–86.

Henderson, S., Duncan-Jones, P., Byrne, D.G., Scott, R., and Adcock, S. (1979). Psychiatric disorders in Canberra: a standardized study of prevalence. *Acta Psychiatrica Scandinavica*, *60*, 355–374.

Henderson, A.S., Byrne, D.G., and Duncan-Jones, P. (1981). *Neurosis and the Social Environment*, Sydney, Academic Press.

Hinde, R.A. (1979). *Towards Understanding Relationships*, London, Academic Press. Hirschfeld, R.M.A. and Klerman, G.L. (1979). Personality attributes and affective disorders. *American Journal of Psychiatry*, *136*, 67–70.

Hodiamont, P., Peer, N. and Syben, N. (1986). Epidemiological aspects of psychiatric disorder in a Dutch Health Area. *Psychological Medicine*, 495–506.

Holmes, T.H. and Rahe, R.H. (1967). The Social Readjustment Rating Scale. *Journal of Psychosomatic Research*, *11*, 213–18.

Hooley, J.M., Orley, J., and Teasdale, J. (1986). Levels of Expressed Emotion and relapse in depressed patients. *British Journal of Psychiatry*, *148*, 642–647.

Horowitz, M.J., Wilner, N., Kaltreider, N., and Alvarez, W. (1980). Signs and symptoms of post-traumatic stress disorder. *Archives of General Psychiatry*, *37*, 85–92.

Hudgens, R.W., Morrison, J.R., and Barchka, R. (1967). Life events and onset of primary affective disorders. A study of 40 hospitalised patients and 40 controls. *Archives of General Psychiatry*, *16*, 134–145.

Hurry, J., Tennant, C., and Bebbington, P.E. (1980). Selective factors leading to psychiatric referral. *Acta Psychiatrica*, Supplementum *285*, 315–323.

Hurry, J., Sturt, E., Bebbington, P., and Tennant, C. (1983). Sociodemographic association with social disablement in a community sample. *Social Psychiatry*, *18*, 113–21.

Hwu, H.-G., Yeh, E.-K., and Chang, L.-Y. (1989). Prevalence of psychiatric disorders in Taiwan defined by the Chinese Diagnostic Interview Schedule. *Acta Psychiatrica Scandinavica*, *79*, 136–147.

Ingham, J.G., Kreitman, N.B., Miller, P.McC., Sashidharan, S.P., and Surtees, P.G. (1987). Self appraisal, anxiety and depression in women: a prospective enquiry. *British Journal of Psychiatry*, *151*, 643–51.

Jaco, E.G. (1960). *The Social Epidemiology of Mental Disorders*, New York, Russell Sage Foundation.

Jackson, P.R., Stafford, E.M., Banks M.H., and Warr, P.B. (1982). Work involvement and employment status as influences on mental health: a test of an interactional model. SAPU Memo 404. University of Sheffield.

Jackson, P.R. (1988). Personal networks, support mobilization and employment. *Psychological Medicine*, *18*, 397–404.

Jahoda, M. (1982). *Employment and Unemployment*. Cambridge, Cambridge University Press.

Jenkins, C.D., Hurst, M.W., and Rose, R.M. (1979). Life changes: do people really remember? *Archives of General Psychiatry*, *36*, 379–84.

Jenkins, R., MacDonald, A., Murray, J., and Strathdee, G. (1982). Minor psychiatric morbidity and the threat of redundancy in a professional group. *Psychological Medicine*, *12*, 799–807.

Kahn, R.L. and Antonucci, T.C. (1980). Convoys over the life course: attachment, roles and social support. In: P.B. Baltes and O.G. Brim (eds.). *Life Span Development and Behaviour. Vol. 3*, New York, Academic Press.

Kaplan, B.H., Cassel, J.C., and Gore, S. (1977). Social support and health. *Medical Care*, *15*, 47–58.

Katschnig, H. (1984). Commentary to Paul Bebbington, Inferring causes: some constraints in the social psychiatry of depressive disorders. *Integrative Psychiatry*, *2*, 77–9.

Katschnig, H., Brandl-Nebehay, A., Fuchs-Robetin, G., Seelig, P., Eichberger, G., Strobl, R., and Sint, P.P. (1981). *Lebensverändernde Ereignisse, Psychoziale Dispositionen und Depressive Verstimmungszustände*. Wien, Abteilung für Sozialpsychiatrie und Dokumentation. Psychiatrische Universitätsklinik.

Katschnig, H., Pakesh, G., and Egger-Zeidner, E. (1986). Life stress and subtypes of depression. In: H. Katschnig (ed.). *Life Events and Psychiatric Disorders: Controversial Issues*, Cambridge, CUP.

Kay, D.W.K., Garside, R.F., Beasmish, P., and Roy, J.R. (1969). Endogenous and neurotic syndromes of depression—a factor analytic study of 104 cases. Clinical features. *British Journal of Psychiatry*, *115*, 377–88.

Kendell, R.E. and di Scipio, W.J. (1968). Eysenck Personality Scores of patients with depressive illnesses. *British Journal of Psychiatry*, *114*, 767–70.

Kennedy, S., Thompson, R., Stancer, H.C., Roy, A., and Persad, E. (1983). Life events precipitating mania. *British Journal of Psychiatry*, *142*, 398–403.

Kerr, T.A., Shapira, K., Roth, M., and Garside, R.F. (1970). The relationship between the Maudsley Personality Inventory and the course of affective disorders. *British Journal of Psychiatry*, *116*, 11–19.

Kessler, R.C. and Cleary, P.D. (1980). Social class and psychological distress. *American Sociological Review*, *45*, 463–78.

Kessler, R.C. and MacLeod, J. (1985). Social support and mental health in community samples. In S. Cohen and L. Syme (eds.) *Social Support and Health*, New York Academic Press.

Kessler, R.C., Turner, J.B., and House, J.S. (1987). Intervening processes in the relationship between unemployment and health. *Psychological Medicine*, *17*, 949–962.

Kiloh, L.G. and Garside, R.F. (1963). The independence of neurotic depression and endogenous depression. *British Journal of Psychiatry*, *109*, 451–63.

Kiloh, L.G., Andrews, G., and Neilson, M. (1988). The long-term outcome of depressive illness. *British Journal of Psychiatry*, *152*, 752–7.

Klerman, G.L. (1978). Affective disorders: In: Armand, M. and Nicholi, M.D. (eds.): *The Harvard Guide to Modern Psychiatry*. Cambridge, Mass., Belknap Press.

Klerman, G.L. (1988). The current age of youthful melancholia: evidence for increase in depression among adolescents and young adults. *British Journal of Psychiatry*, *152*, 4–14.

Klerman, G.L., Lavori, P.W., Rice, J., Reich, T., Endicott, J., Andreason, N.C., Keller, M.B. and Hirschfeld, R.M.A. (1985). Birth-cohort trends in rates of major depressive disorder among relatives of patients with affective disorder. *Archives of General Psychiatry*, *421*, 689–93.

Kuipers, L. and Bebbington, P.E. (1988). Expressed Emotion research in schizophrenia: theoretical and clinical implications. *Psychological Medicine*, *18*, 893–910.

Langner, T.S. and Michael, S.T. (1963). *Life Stress and Mental Health*: The Midtown Manhattan Study. London, Collier/MacMillan Ltd.

Lauer, R.H. (1983). The Social Readjustment Scale and anxiety: a crosscultural study. *Journal of Psychosomatic Research*, *17*, 171–174.

Lavori, P.W., Klerman, G.L., Keller, M.B. Reich, T., Rice, J., and Endicott, J. (1987). Age-period-cohort analysis of secular trends in onset of major depression: Findings in siblings of patients with major affective disorder. *Journal of Psychiatric Research*, *21*, 23–35.

Lee, A.S. and Murray, R.M. (1988). The long-term outcome of Maudsley depressives. *British Journal of Psychiatry*, *153*, 741–751.

Leff, M.H., Roach, J.F., and Bunney, W.E. (1970). Environmental factors preceeding the onsets of severe depressions. *Psychiatry*, *33*, 293–311.

Lehtinen, V., Lindholm, T., Veijola, J., and Vaisanen, E. (1990). The prevalence of PSE-CATEGO disorders in a Finnish adult population cohort. *Social Psychiatry and Psychiatric Epidemiology*, *25*, 187–192.

Lewinsohn, P.M., Hoberman, H.M. and Rosenbaum, M. (1988). A prospective study of risk factors for depression. *Journal of Abnormal Psychology*, *97*, 251–264.

Lin, N. and Dean, A. (1984). Social support and depression: a panel study. *Social Psychiatry*, *19*, 83–91.

McCallister, L. and Fischer, C.S. (1978). A procedure for surveying personal social networks. *Sociological Methods and Research, 7*, 131–148.

MacMahon, B. and Pugh, T.F. (1970). *Epidemiology: Principles and Methods.* Boston, Little, Brown.

Marks, I.M. (1969). Fears and Phobias. New York, Academic Press.

Marks, I.M. (1986). Epidemiology of anxiety. *Social Psychiatry, 21*, 167–171.

Markush, R.E. and Favero, R.V. (1974). Epidemiological assessment of stressful life events, depressed mood and psychophysiological symptoms: a preliminary report. In: Dohrenwend B.S. and Dohrenwend B.P. (eds.). *Stressful Life Events: Their Nature and Effects.* New York, John Wiley.

Mavreas, V.G., Beis, A., Mouyias, A., Rigoni, F. and Lyketsos, G.C. (1986). Prevalence of psychiatric disorder in Athens: a community study. *Social Psychiatry, 21*, 172–181.

Mavreas, V. and Bebbington, P.E. (1987). Psychiatric morbidity in London's Greek Cypriot community. I. Association with sociodemographic variables. *Social Psychiatry, 22*, 150–159.

Mendels, J. and Cochrane, C. (1968). The nosology of depression—the endogenous-reactive concept. *American Journal of Psychiatry, 124*, Supplement 1–11.

Mendels, J. and Weinstein, N. (1972). The Schedule of Recent Experiences: a reliability study. *Psychosomatic Medicine, 34*, 527–531.

Miklowitz, D.J., Goldstein, M.J., Nuechterlein, K.H., Snyder, K.S., and Mintz, J., (1988). Family factors and the course of bipolar affective disorder. *Archives of General Psychiatry, 45*, 225–221.

Miller, P. McC. and Ingham, J.G. (1976). Friends, confidants and symptoms. *Social Psychiatry, 11*, 51–8.

Mitchell, J.C. (1969). (ed.). *Social Networks in Urban Situations.* Manchester, Manchester University Press.

Monnelly, E.P., Woodruff, R.A., and Robins, L.N. (1974). Manic depressive illness and social achievement in a public hospital sample. *Acra Psychiatrica Scandinavica, 50*, 318–325.

Moss, P. and Plewis, I. (1977). Mental distress in mothers of pre-school children in Inner London. *Psychological Medicine, 7*, 641–52.

Mueller, D.P., Edwards, D.W., and Yarvis, R.M. (1977). Stressful life events and psychiatric symptomatology: change or undesirability. *Journal of Health and Social Behaviour, 18*, 307–17.

Murphy, J.M., Sobol, A.M., Oliver, D.C. Monson, R.R., Leighton, A.H., and Pratt, L.A. (1989). Prodromes of depression and anxiety. The Stirling County Study. *British Journal of Psychiatry* (in press).

Myers, J., Lindenthal, J., and Pepper, M. (1974). Social class, life events and psychiatric symptoms: a longitudinal study. In: B.S. Dohrenwend and B.P. Dohrenwend (eds.). *Stressful Life Events: Their Nature and Effects.* New York, John Wiley.

Myers, J.K., Weissman, M.M., Tischler, G.L., Holzer, C.E., Leaf, P.J., Orvaschel, H., Anthony, J.C., Boyd, J.H., Burke, J.D., Kramer, M., and Stolzman, R. (1984). Six month prevalence of psychiatric disorders in three communities: 1980–1982. *Archives of General Psychiatry, 42*, 959–67.

Nelson, C.J. and Charney, D.S. (1980). Primary affective disorder criteria and the endogenous-reactive distinction. *Archives of General Psychiatry, 37*, 787–93.

Nezu, A.M. and Ronan, G.F. (1985). Life stress, current problems, problem solving and depressive symptoms: An integrative model. *Journal of Consulting and Clinical Psychology, 53*, 693–697.

Noreik, K. and Odegaard, O. (1966). Psychosis in Norweigians with a background of higher education. *British Journal of Psychiatry*, *112*, 43–55.

Norris, V. (1959). *Mental Illness in London*, Maudsley Monograph No. 6. London, OUP.

O'Connor, P. and Brown, G.W. (1984). Supportive relationships: fact or fantasy? *Journal of Social and Personal Relationships*, *1*, 159–175.

Odegaard, O. (1956). The incidence of psychosis in various occupations. *International Journal of Social Psychiatry*, *2*, 85–104.

Olinger, L.J., Kuiper, N.A., and Shaw, B.F. 91987). Dysfunctional attiutes and stressful life events: an interactive model of depression. *Cognitive Therapy and Research*, *11*, 25–40.

Orley J. and Wing J.K. (1979). Psychiatric disorders in two African villages. *Archives of General Psychiatry*, *36*, 513–520.

Ozturk, O.M., Atakan, Z., and Demirez, E. (1980). An epidemiological study of psychiatric symptoms in a semi-rural area in Turkey. Paper presented at the Mediterranean Social Psychiatry Conference, Dubrovnik, 1980.

Parkes, C.M. (1965). Bereavement and mental illness. Part 1. A clinical study of the grief of bereaved psychiatric patients. *British Journal of Medical Psychology*, *38*, 1–26.

Parkes, C.M. (1975). Determinants of outcome following bereavement. *Omega 6*, 303–323.

Parker, G. (1983). *Parental Overprotection: A Risk Factor in Psychosocial Development*, New York, Grune & Stratton.

Parker, G. (1988). Parental style and parental loss. In: A.S. Henderson & G.D. Burrows (eds.). *Handbook of Social Psychiatry*, Amsterdam, Elsevier.

Parker, G., Kiloh, L. and Mayward, L. (1987). Parental representations of neurotic and endogenous depressives. *Journal of Affective Disorders*, *13*, 75–82.

Parker, G. Tupling, M. and Brown, L.B. (1979). A parental bonding instrument. *British Journal of Psychiatry*, *52*, 1–10.

Parry, G. (1986). Paid employment, life events, social support and mental health in working class mothers. *Journal of Health and Social Behaviour*, *27*, 193–208.

Parry, G. (1987). Sex-role beliefs, work attitudes and mental health in employed and non-employed mothers. *British Journal of Social Psychology*, *26*, 47–58.

Parry, G. and Shapiro, D.A. and Davies, L. (1981). Reliability of life-event ratings: an independent replication. *British Journal of Clinical Psychology*, *20*, 133–4.

Parry, G. and Shapiro, D.A. (1986). Social support and life events in working class women. *Archives of General Psychiatry*, *43*, 315–23.

Paykel, E.S. (1971). Classification of depressed patients: a cluster analysis derived grouping. *British Journal of Psychiatry*, *118*, 275–88.

Paykel, E.S., Myers, J.K., Dienelt, M.N. Klerman, G.L., Lindenthal, J.J., and Pepper, M.P. (1969). Life events and depression: a controlled study. *Archives of General Psychiatry*, *21*, 753–760.

Paykel, E.S., Prusoff, B.A. and Uhlenhuth, E.H. (1971). Scaling of life events. *Archives of General Psychiatry*, *25*, 340–347.

Paykel, E.S., Klerman, G.L., and Prusoff, B.A. (1976). Personality and symptom pattern in depression. *British Journal of Psychiatry*, *129*, 327–34.

Paykel, E.S. and Rowan, P. (1979). Recent advances in research on affective disorders. In: *Recent Advances in Clinical Psychiatry*. Edinburgh, Churchill Livingstone.

Paykel, E.S., Rao, B.M., and Taylor, C.N. (1984). Life stress and symptom pattern in out-patient depression. *Psychological Medicine*, *14*, 559–568.

Pearlin, L.I. and Johnson, J.S. (1977). Marital status, life strains and depression. *American Sociological Review*, *42*, 704–715.

Pearlin, L.I. and Lieberman, M.A. (1977). Social sources of emotional distress. In: R. Simmons (ed.). *Research in Community and Mental Health*. Greenwich, Connecticut. JAI Press.

Pederson, A.M., Barry, D.J., and Babigian, H.M. (1972). Epidemiological considerations of psychotic depression. *Archives of General Psychiatry*, *27*, 193–197.

Perris, C. (1971). Personality patterns in patients with affective disorders. *Acta Psychiatrica Scandinavica*, *47*, *Suppl. 221*, 43–51.

Radloff, L. (1975). Sex differences in depression: the effects of occupation and marital status. *Sex Roles*, *1*, 249–265.

Richman, N. (1974). The effect of housing on pre-school children and their mothers. *Developmental Medicine and Child Neurology*, *16*, 53–8.

Richman, N. (1977). Behaviour problems in preschool children: famiy and social factors. *British Journal of Psychiatry*, *131*, 523–7.

Romans-Clarkson, S.E., Walton, V.A., Herbison, G.P., and Mullen, P.E. (1988). Marriage, motherhood and psychiatric morbidity in New Zealand. *Psychological Medicine*, *18*, 983–990.

Rosenfield, S. (1980). Sex differences in depression: do women always have higher rates. *Journal of Health and Social Behaviour*, *21*, 33–42.

Roy, A., Breier, A., Doran, A.R., and Pickar, D. (1985). Life events and depression: Relation to subtypes. *Journal of Affective Disorders*, *9*, 143–148.

Sarason, I.G., Johnson, J.H., and Siegel, J.M. (1978). Assessing the impact of life changes: development of the Life Experiences Survey. *Journal of Consulting and Clinical Psychology*, *46*, 932–46.

Sarason, I.G. and Sarason, B.R. (1982). Concomitants of social support: attitudes, personality characteristics and life experiences. *Journal of Personality*, *50*, 333–44.

Sarason, I.G. Levine H.M., Bashan, R.B., and Sarason, B.R. (1983). Assessing social support: the Social Support Questionnaire. *Journal of Personality and Social Psychology*, *44*, 127–139.

Sashidharan, S.P., Surtees, P.G., Kreitman, N.B., Ingham, J.G., and Miller, P.McC. (1988). Hospital-treated and general-population morbidity from affective disorders: comparison of prevalence and inception rates. *British Journal of Psychiatry*, *152*, 499–505.

Schless, A.P. and Mendels, J. (1978). The value of interviewing family and friends in assessing life stressors. *Archives of General Psychiatry*, *32*, 565–7.

Schwab, J.J., Bell, R.A., Warheit, G.J., and Schwab, R.B. (1979). *Social Order and Mental Health: the Florida Health Study*. New York, Brunner/Mazel.

Shepherd, M. (1957). *A Study of the Major Psychoses in an English County*, Maudsley Monograph No. 3. London, OUP.

Silverman, C. (1968). *Epidemiology of Depression*, Baltimore, Johns Hopkins Press.

Sokolovsky, J., Cohen, C., Berger, D. and Geiger, J. (1978). Personal networks of ex-mental patients in a Manhattan SRO hotel. *Human Organisation*, *37*, 5–15.

Srole, L., Langner, T., Michael, S.T., Opler, M.K., and Rennie, T.A.C. (1962). *Mental Health in the Metropolis*, New York, McGraw-Hill.

Stern-Piper, L. (1925). Der Psychopathologische Index der Kultur. *Archiv für Psychiatrie* und Nervenkrankheit, *74*, 514–25.

Sturt, E., Bebbington, P.E., Hurry, J., and Tennant, C. (1981). The Present State

Examination used by interviewers from a Survey Agency: Report from the Camberwell Community Survey. *Psychological Medicine, 11*, 185–192.

Sturt, E.S., Kumakura, N., and Der, G. (1984). How depressing life is: lifelong risk of depression in the general population. *Journal of Affective Disorders, 7*, 109–22.

Surtees, P.G., Dean, C., Ingham, J.G., Kreitman, N.B., Miller, P.McC., and Sashidharan, S.P. (1983). Psychiatric disorder in women from an Edinburgh community: associations with demographic factors. *British Journal of Psychiatry, 142*, 238–46.

Surtees, P.G., Miller, P.McC., Ingham, J.G., Kreitman, N.B., Rennie, D., and Sashidharan, S.P. (1986). Life events and the onset of affective disorder: a longitudinal general population study. *Journal of Affective Disorder, 10*, 37–50.

Surtees, P.G. and Sashidharan, S.P. (1986). Psychiatric morbidity in two matched community samples: a comparison of rates and risks in Edinburgh and St. Louis. *Journal of Affective Disorder, 10*, 101–113.

Taylor, Lord and Chave, S. (1964). *Mental Health and Environment*. London, Longman Green.

Teasdale, J.D. (1988). Cognitive vulnerability to depression. *Cognition and Emotion, 2*, 247–274.

Teasdale, J.D. and Dent, J. (1987). Cognitive vulnerability to depression: and investigation of two hypotheses. *British Journal of Clinical Psychology, 26*, 113–126.

Tennant, C. and Andrews, G. (1976). A scale to measure the stress of life events. *Australian and New Zealand Journal of Psychiatry, 10*, 27–33.

Tennant, C. and Andrews, G. (1978). The pathogenic quality of life event stress in neurotic impairment. *Archives of General Psychiatry, 35*, 859–863.

Tennant, C., Smith, A., Bebbington, P.E., and Hurry, J. (1979). The contextual rating of life events: the concept and its reliability. *Psychological Medicine, 9*, 525–528.

Tennant, C., Bebbington, P.E., and Hurry, J. (1980). Parental death in childhood and risk of adult depressive disorders: a review. *Psychological Medicine, 10*, 289–299.

Tennant, C., Bebbington, P.E., and Hurry, J. (1981). The role of life events in depressive illness: Is there a substantial causal relation? *Psychological Medicine, 11*, 379–89.

Tennant, C., Bebbington, P., and Hurry, J. (1981). The short-term outcome of neurotic disorders in the community: the relation of remission to clinical factors and to "neutralising" life events. *British Journal of Psychiatry, 139*, 213–20.

Thoits, P.A. (1982a). Life stress, social support and psychological vulnerability: epidemiological considerations. *Journal of Community Psychology, 10*, 341–62.

Thoits, P.A. (1982b). Conceptual, methodological and theoretical problems in studying social support as a buffer against life stress. *Journal of Health and Social Behaviour, 23*, 145–159.

Thompson, K.C. and Hendrie, H.C. (1972). Environmental stress in primary depressive illness. *Archives of General Psychiatry, 26*, 130–132.

Tolsdorf, C.C. (1976). Social networks, support and coping: an exploratory study. *Family Process, 15*, 407–417.

Turner, R.J. (1983). Social support and psychological distress. In: H.B. Kaplan (ed.). *Psychosocial Stress: Trends in Theory and Practice*, New York, Academic Press.

Uhlenhuth, E.H. and Paykel, E.S. (1973a). Symptom intensity and life events. *Archives of General Psychiatry, 28,* 473–477.

Uhlenhuth, E.H. and Paykel, E.S. (1973b). Symptom configuration and life events. *Archives of General Psychiatry, 28,* 744–748.

Uhlenhuth, E.H., Lipmann, R.S., Balter, M.B., and Stern, M. (1974). Symptom intensity and life stress in the city. *Archives of General Psychiatry, 32,* 759–764.

Uhlenhuth, E., Balter, M.D., Lipman, R.S., and Haberman, S.J. (1977). Remembering life events. In: J.S. Strauss., H.M. Babigian and M. Roff (eds.). *The Origins and Course of Psychopathology.* New York, Plenum Press.

Vaisanen, E. (1975). Psychiatric disorders in Finland. In: T. Andersen, C. Astrup and A. Forsdahl (eds.). Social, Somatic and Psychiatric Studies of Geographically Defined Populations. *Acta Psychiatrica Scandinavica, Supplementum, 263,* 27.

Vaughn, C., and Leff, J.P. (1976). The influence of family and social factors on the course of psychiatric illness: a comparison of schizophrenic and depressed neurotic patients. *British Journal of Psychiatry, 129,* 125–137.

Vazquez-Barquero, J-L., Diez-Manrique, J.F., Pena, C., Aldana, J., Samaniego-Rodriguez, C., Menendez-Arango, J., and Mirapeix, C. (1987). A community mental health survey in Cantabria: a general description of morbidity. *Psychological Medicine, 17,* 227–242.

Veith, R.C. and Raskind, M.A. (1988). The neurobiology of aging: Does it predispose to depression? *Neurobiology of Aging, 9,* 101–118.

Warheit, G.J., Holzer, C.E., and Schwab, J.J. (1973). An analysis of social class and racial differences in depressive symptomatology: a community study. *Journal of Health and Social Behaviour, 14,* 291–295.

Warr, P.B. (1984). Economic recession and mental health: a review of research. *Tijdschrift voor Sociale Gesondheidszorg, 62,* 298–308.

Weeke, A., Bille, M., Videbeck, T., Dupont, A., and Juel-Nielsen, N. (1975). Incidence of depressive syndromes in a Danish county. *Acta Psychiatrica Scandinavica, 51,* 28–41.

Weiss, R. (1974). The provisions of social relationships. In: Z. Rubin (ed.). *Doing Unto Others.* Englewood Cliffs, N.J., Prentice-Hall.

Weissman, M.M. and Klerman, G.L. (1977). Sex differences and the epidemiology of depression. *Archives of General Psychiatry, 34,* 98–112.

Weissman, M.M. and Myers, J. (1978). Rates and risks of depressive symptoms in a United States urban community. *Acta Psychiatrica Scandinavica, 57,* 219–231.

Weissman, M.M., Leaf, P.J., Holzer, C.E., Myers, J.K., and Tischler, G.L. (1984). The epidemiology of depression: an update on sex differences in rates. *Journal of Affective Disorders, 7,* 179–188.

Weissman, M.M., Leaf, P.J., Tischler, G.L., Blazer, D.G., Karno, M. Bruce, M.L., and Florio, M.P. (1988). Affective disorders in five United States communities. *Psychological Medicine, 18,* 141–154.

Wing, J.K. (1977). The limits of standardisation. In: Rakoff, V.M., Stancer, H. and Kedward, H.B. (eds.). *Psychiatric Diagnosis.* New York, Brunner/Mazel.

Wing, J.K., Cooper, J.E. and Sartorius, N. (1974). *The Measurement and Classification of Psychiatric Symptoms.* Cambridge University Press: Cambridge.

Wing, J.K., Bebbington, P.E., Tennant, C., and Hurry, J. (1981). The prevalence in the general population of disorders familiar to psychiatrists in hospital practice. In: What is a "Case"? The Problem of Definition in Psychiatric Community

Surveys. (eds. Wing J.K., Bebbington, P.E., and Robins, L.). London: Grant MacIntyre.

Wing, J.K. and Bebbington, P.E. (1985). The Epidemiology of Depression. In: Beckham, E.E. and Leber, W.R. (eds.). *Depression: Treatment, Assessment and Research*. Dow-Jones-Irwin.

Woodruff, R.A., Robins, L.N., Winokur, G. and Reich, T. (1971). Manic depressive illness and social achievement. *Acta Psychiatrica Scandinavica*, 47, 237–249.

Yager, J., Grant, I., Sweetwood, H.L., and Gerst, M. (1981). Life events reported by psychiatric patients, non-patients and their partners. *Archives of General Psychiatry*, 38, 343–7.

von Zerssen, D. and Weyerer, S. (1982). Sex differences in rates of mental disorders. *International Journal of Mental Health*, 11, 9–45.

Zimmerman, M., Coryell, W., Pfohl, B., and Stangel, D. (1986). The validity of four definitions of endogenous depression: II. Clinical, demographic, familial and psychosocial correlates. *Archives of General Psychiatry*, 43, 234–244.

14

Parental Loss in Childhood: Its Effect in Adult Life

Christopher Tennant

Introduction

For some considerable time the role of parent loss has intrigued mental health workers. Early preoccupations, largely those of psychoanalytically oriented professionals, were on the psychological significance and meaning of the traumatic loss itself and on depression as the outcome. Bowlby (1951) broadened the scope of interest in childhood loss in two ways: first, he suggested a range of outcomes was possible and included depression, anxiety, and antisocial behaviors; and secondly he defined further what he believed to be "toxic" about loss, moving the emphasis away from the meaning of the traumatic event itself to the ongoing disruption in attachment to the parent. Rutter (1972, 1974) took the argument further by concluding, on the basis of the then available evidence, that the loss, be it separation from, or death of a parent, is not the critical factor but that these events may both embrace and subsequently cause a range of other adverse experiences that are more likely to prove pathogenic than the loss itself. Rutter (1985) has pursued this further in postulating a cascade-like effect where early experiences generate a range of other events and experiences which may culminate in psychopathology in later life.

Even though the focus has shifted from the circumscribed event of "loss" to that of loss of attachment of parenting, there may well be other issues that need to be considered, such as complex changes in family dynamics, social relationships, and economic hardship, especially when the loss is by divorce.

Another of the continuing problems of "parent loss" research is the very wide ranging use of the term; greater specification is clearly necessary. First, parental death and parent-child separations should be distinguished. There are many different causes for the latter, but since "loss" usually implies a prolonged or permanent separation, it usually means parent-child separations due to family disharmony. The distinction is important, because parental death and parent-child separations may have quite different effects on the individual as they involve substantially different experiences. They are also likely to differ in their impact on "population" psychopathology: parental death should have far less impact since only 5–8 percent of children experience parental death (Tennant et al., 1981), compared to the 30–40 percent of children who currently face parental divorce in the Western world (Australian Institute of Family Studies, Working Paper 11, 1987). The continuing use of "loss" as a global variable embracing both deaths or permanent separations, by some researchers may lead to inappropriate conclusions and contribute to inconsistency in published findings (Brown and Harris, 1978; Harris et al., 1986; Harris et al., 1987; Bifulco et al., 1987). They are thus treated separately in this discussion.

Parent Death

The effects of parental death on a child may be quite devastating, and there may be a range of severe behavioral and emotional reactions in the immediate aftermath. However, reviews of the long-term effects of parental death seem to indicate that if potential confounding variables are taken into account the long-term psychopathological effect is, in general, nonexistent or negligible (Tennant et al., 1980; Crook and Eliot, 1980). Some studies still use a global "loss" variable (Brown et al., 1978; Harris et al., 1986; Harris et al., 1987; Bifulco et al., 1987; Seligman et al., 1974), but when the data are available to distinguish different types of loss, parent-child separations are associated with morbidity later in life but parental deaths are not. Some studies for instance have assessed parental death alone and show no significant relation to depression, either in patient samples (Perris and Perris, 1978; Perris et al., 1986; Royal et al., 1983; Birtchnell, 1980), or in normal populations (Tennant et al., 1981; Birtchnell, 1980). The last two studies controlled for major confounding variables and, as they were community studies of normal populations, were free of the bias that parental death might predispose to use of psychiatric services rather than causing symptomatic impairment per se. Other studies have assessed deaths and separations in the same sample; separations appear to be related to adult psychopathology, parent deaths do not (Tennant et al.,

1981; Bifulco et al., 1987; Favarelli et al., 1986). The findings in a recent study (Brier et al., 1988) are also consistent with this; the risk of parent death in the depressed and non-depressed groups were not significantly different, at 6.1 percent and 7.6 percent respectively. This conclusion is also confirmed by Roy, who in his earlier studies (Roy, 1978, 1980a,b, 1981a,b,c) used a global "loss" variable and found it predicted adult depression, but when deaths and separations were subsequently examined separately, parent child separations remained a significant predictor of depression (Roy, 1985) while parent deaths did not (Roy, 1983). Thus in those studies where "loss" seemed to predict depression, the effect can largely be attributed to prolonged separations from parents, which is most often due to divorce.

There has been little published evidence concerning the effects of other types of separation experience on adult morbidity. However, in one community study (Tennant et al., 1982) prolonged separations due to marital problems and parental illness were associated with an increased risk of morbidity, whereas the other common causes of separation in this sample (evacuation during World War II, and parent's work or child's schooling), were not. Furthermore, the effect of parental illness was not mediated either by psychiatric illness or by parental death. Hence the evidence remains consistent that prolonged separations due to family discord appear to contribute to adult psychopathology, particularly depression (Tennant et al., 1982).

Family Disharmony and Divorce

In the 1970s, over 30 percent of children in the Western world experienced parental divorce (Australian Institute of Family Studies, Working Paper 11, 1987; Wallerstein and Kelly, 1980). Estimates from the USA indicate that of children born in the early 1980s, some 45 percent will experience parental divorce, 35 percent a subsequent parental remarriage, and 20 percent a second divorce (Wallerstein, 1985a,b). The most dramatic increase in divorce in the USA has been for younger married couples, resulting in children of an increasingly younger age being exposed to divorce and an increasingly prolonged separation from one parent. In nearly half of the children, separation may be "complete," in that contact with the non-custodial parent may cease (Furtstenberg, 1982).

There are as yet no studies of whether this increase in the divorce rate has resulted in the experience being more "normative" for the child, or has led to improved awareness of and catering for the child's needs. Despite the institution of divorce becoming increasingly "normative," most of the child's consequent experiences are not. They include practical problems: there is a decline in family income, they may move to a new house and school and lose friends, mothers may commence work, a new parental partner may appear, and there may be a change in the pattern of contact with other relatives and friends. Continuing parental conflict and loss of contact with the non-custodial parent, usually the father, are not uncommon. Other important consequences include parental emotional distress, loss of a sense of parental competence and impoverished parenting, especially in the early aftermath of the parents' separation. These factors may be reinforced by disruption in the parent's social support network, especially for women. Before reviewing the evidence that separation due to family discord is pathogenic, one needs to be aware of factors which confound most of the studies and may lead to erroneous positive conclusions in some instances.

The first issue, alluded to above, is the various definitions of "divorce." At one extreme, divorce may simply be an official acknowledgement of a change in marital status which appears in the mail. At the other, it is a process embracing the parents' relationship from the time they met, continuing through their relationship even after they are legally divorced, and embracing all the psychological, social, economic, educational, and other effects that this may have on the child. "Divorce" can thus be seen as a complex ongoing process as far as the child is concerned. No studies have been able to address the full complexity of this process, but some inroads into understanding the most important facets of this process have been made, especially in longitudinal studies of divorced families (Heatherington et al., 1982; Wallerstein and Kelly, 1980; Hess and Camara, 1979; Ferguson et al., 1986; Wallerstein 1985a,b). There are many variables potentially confounding the relation between parental divorce and psychopathology in children, but two of the most important (indeed they may be related) are parental psychopathology, which may operate by way of genetic or environmental processes, and disrupted parenting before separation. Parental psychopathology can confound the relationship between divorce and later psychopathology in the child by two means, both of which are dependent on the fact that parental psychopathology can cause marital disharmony and divorce. First is the genetic transmission of psychopathology, most importantly in affective disorders, antisocial personality and alcohol abuse (Cardoret et al., 1985). Secondly, parental psychopathology can have a deleterious effect on the child's social and emotional environment, both before and after separation (Wolkind and Rutter, 1985). Poor parenting undoubtedly causes psychological morbidity both in childhood (Weissman et al., 1987) and in later life (Parker, 1979, 1981, 1983). Both genetic and environmental factors can thus contribute to a spurious relation between childhood separations and subsequent psychopathology. For instance, when parental separations due to parental mental illness are excluded, the apparently greater rate of early losses in depressives than in controls is much reduced (Favarelli et al., 1986). This bias is most marked when "selected" samples are studied, both "volunteers" who may volunteer because of current emotional problems and more pathological separations (Harris et al. 1986) and patient groups selected because of current psychopathology (Perris and Perris, 1978). Hence the most appropriate studies for gauging the strength of any association accurately will be those of unselected community samples.

Selection bias also occurs in other forms. For example, many studies select subjects who have made contact with some helping agency, resulting in a bias towards those most adversely affected psychologically. The use of family court registers also provides some bias, in that some families where permanent parent separation occurs without administrative divorce are not represented. The most useful studies therefore are those based on community samples, such as that of Douglas (1970). However, the problem in these studies is the relatively small number of divorced families included and thus the reduction of statistical power in more detailed analyses of divorce.

Another bias can occur in the psychological and behavioral assessment of the participants in divorce since it is usually not possible for interviewers to be blind to the marital status of the subjects.

It is also crucial to control for the confounding effect of preseparation parenting when assessing the mediating effect of experiences following divorce, especially the post-divorce relationship between child and parents. The relative importance of pre-divorce parent child relationships is highlighted in a study in which pre-separation parenting predicted adult depression but post-separation parenting did not (Kennard and Birtchnell, 1982). The failure to assess the separate effects of both pre-and post-separation parenting confounds most studies (Brier et al., 1988; Harris et al., 1986; Bifulco et al., 1987).

Finally it is worth considering whether there may be a continuity of pathology from childhood to adult life, given that psychological problems in children are common in the aftermath of divorce. This is of importance for two reasons with conflicting implications for the issue of the long term impact of parental divorce. On one hand it might be argued that if there is substantial morbidity immediately following parental divorce, this simply might continue in some form through later years and be observed in adult life. In other words, this continuity of pathology explains why divorce may have long term effects into later life. On the other hand, if there is continuity of disturbance through childhood and into adult life this may simply reflect that children who were disturbed following divorce and who show problems in adult life were also disturbed before divorce, for a variety of non-divorce reasons. In other words, adult psychopathology was not due to divorce but to other possibly unrelated antecedent factors. A decision between these possibilities can only be definitely made if there is adequate assessment of the child and parenting long before divorce actually occurs, as well as in its aftermath. No study has achieved this objective. There is, however, indirect evidence which lends support to the second of the two propositions, and this derives from the type of disorders likely to show continuity between childhood and adult life. Rutter (1984a) in his review assesses four disorders: schizophrenia, manic depressive illness, emotional disorder (neuroses), and anti-social personality. For schizophrenia, he indicates there are cognitive, neurodevelopmental, and interpersonal problems which can be identified in children who subsequently become schizophrenic. Given that there is no evidence to support the fact that divorce predisposes to schizophrenia, and that the disturbances seen in childhood are likely simply to reflect the underlying genetic susceptibility to the disorder, any continuity for disturbances occurring in schizophrenic subjects has no bearing on the possible effects of divorce on schizophrenia. For manic depressive disorder, Rutter (1984a) concludes that there is little continuity, in that those who develop this disorder have not usually had identifiable precursors in childhood. This discontinuity thus supports neither proposition. The third disorder reviewed is that of "emotional" (neurotic) disorders; any continuity of these conditions (given the slender genetic basis for neurosis) might support the first proposition, namely that divorce causes emotional distress which continues into later life. It seems however, that the consistency of neuroses over time is generally quite low (Moss and Sussman, 1980) and that most emotional disturbances in childhood tend to improve or remit completely over time (Kohlberg et al., 1972). Given that these conditions are those most commonly occurring in the aftermath of divorce, and given the largely discontinuous, indeed transient, nature of these disorders (Rutter 1984a), the proposition that neurotic conditions caused by divorce are continuous into adult life is not well supported by this data. The final disorder reviewed is that of anti-social personality which Rutter (1984a) concludes is continuous through childhood and adult life. While it is increasingly evident that there is genetic transmission of anti-social personality (Cadoret et al., 1985), Rutter (1984a) finds that an adverse environment also plays some role, but concludes that an interaction between genes and environment is quite likely (Rutter 1983). In another review Rutter (1984b) examines the process by which environmental factors contribute to personality development. In essence, this includes the finding that one adverse experience is associated with others and indeed with chronic adverse environments;

the latter rather than the former exacts some psychopathological effect. Furthermore, he argues that with conduct disorders in childhood there is a self-perpetuating process, perhaps mediated by the fact that such behaviour adversely affects parenting. (Rutter 1984b). In addition, it appears that chronic adversity affects other variables, such as adaptability, resilience, coping, and self-esteem (Rutter 1982b) which may lead to symptomatic emotional sequalae which are delayed. If divorce does exert long term effects on neurotic illness, this seems to be the most likely process by which it occurs.

In relation to divorce and personality development and related variables, there are a number of coexisting possibilities. First, childhood personality factors preceding divorce may act as confounders by virtue both of genetic effects and of family environmental influences preceding divorce. Secondly, it is possible that childhood personality problems or psychopathology may strain the parents' marriage and contribute to their divorce, a causal relationship not in the direction generally proposed by most researchers. Finally, there is the likelihood that divorce and its sequalae have some influence on later personality psychopathology in children.

Divorce: the Evidence

Included in the following review are those studies of divorce and those which assess loss, defined globally but largely attributable to family discord or divorce and not to parental death (Brier et al., 1988; Harris et al., 1986; Harris et al., 1987; Bifulco et al., 1987). Recent evidence will be highlighted and the studies discussed according to the nature of the sample studied because of different methodological problems.

"Volunteers" with and without Loss

In studies where the response rate is low, the sample will be biased toward "volunteers." Selection bias may then occur in both the "loss" and "no loss" groups. In one such study (Harris et al., 1986; Harris et al., 1987) where the response rate was effectively only 68 percent, the one year period prevalence of depression in "no loss" controls was only 4 percent, remarkably low considering point prevalence rates of approximately 15 percent in comparable normal communities (Brown and Harris, 1978; Bebbington et al., 1981b). This disparity may be due to a "healthy volunteer" effect. In the "loss" group, nearly one third had experienced "aberrant" separations which involved child abuse or gross neglect; this too may reflect selection bias, those with the most aberrant separations being more likely to "volunteer." Such severe losses are more likely to be associated with the confounding factors discussed earlier, namely, parental psychopathology, gross parenting problems, and other social deprivations preceding separation. Volunteer effects may therefore explain why 50 percent of this group was depressed in adult life and the apparent differences in psychological morbidity in the "loss" and "no loss" groups were substantial. Few would argue that gross parental deprivation contributes to adult psychopathology, as seems to be demonstrated by these data. In such circumstances, parent-child separation, far from being toxic, may be positively beneficial. Some researchers thus fail to make an adequate delineation between parent "loss" and parental deprivations preceding loss.

Similar problems are found in another study (Bifulco et al., 1987) where a significant proportion of a working-class sample of women was selected specifically because they were unmarried mothers. Loss of mother by separation but not by death predicted depression; loss of father from either cause did not. Such a sample is also more likely to have experienced social and personal deprivations preceding any parental loss and a range of other more contemporary social stressors after loss, any of which may have contributed more to depression than parental loss itself. Selection of subjects with other problems in this way results in a sample which may be depressed for reasons other than the presumptive causal factor, namely parental loss.

Depressed Adult Patients

The study of depressed patient samples continues to be the most widely used method for assessing the impact of loss (Roy, 1978; 1980a,b; 1981a,b,c; 1985). Where there is greater specification of loss, parent child separations were specifically associated with depression in hospitalized samples (Roy, 1985) but not parental death (Roy, 1983a). Hospitalized depressed subjects have parents with greater psychopathology by way of genetic effects than is the case for normal controls. Parental psychopathology may cause a spurious relation between separations due to family discord and later depression in their offspring, as discussed previously.

Random Community Based Studies

While random community studies avoid some of the biases discussed, they have two other potential limitations. First, the low frequency in the population of both the independent (separation) and dependent variables (depression) could result in a false negative result, merely reflecting inadequate statistical power; large samples however can effectively deal with this problem (Tennant et al., 1982; Kennard and Birtchnell, 1982). Secondly, it could be argued that the dependent variable (depression as it occurs in the community) is inappropriate, being much less severe than in patient groups. However this common "neurotic" depression may in fact be more likely to be caused by environmental stressors than more severe "endogenous" disorders. (Bebbington et al., 1981b).

One of three population studies (Kennard and Birtchnell, 1982) found no increased risk of adult psychopathology in women who had been separated from their mothers. However, the subgroup with maternal separations reflecting "unsatisfactory family circumstances" had more depressive symptoms. This further exemplifies the importance of preceding family disturbance compared to the "loss" itself.

Two other studies report more positive findings. Maternal loss in women was a significant "vulnerability" factor in one London study (Brown and Harris 1978). In the other, which attempted to replicate these findings in the same community, and further refine the loss variable (Tennant et al., 1982) it was found that separations due to marital discord and those due to parental physical illness both predicted adult psychopathology in the offspring, depression, in particular. These studies provide the best and most unbiased evidence that parental separations, particularly due to marital discord, may predispose to adult depression.

Longitudinal Studies of Children of Divorced Parents

Theoretically these studies could provide the strongest evidence that parent-child separations (most usually from father) are pathogenic, but they too have limitations. Frequently the follow-up period is relatively short; any pathology identified may therefore bear little relation to disorders in adult life (Rutter and Cox, 1985). In two studies (Hetherington et al., 1982, Hess and Camara, 1979) emotional disturbance immediately following divorce was initially substantial but diminished over two years. Problems were most marked in boys, with aggressive behavior being prominent. This may be explained by the fact that most separations were from fathers, and parenting problems were greatest for mothers in dealing with their sons. In the second study (Hess and Camara, 1979) there was interestingly, considerable overlap in parental disharmony in divorced and in intact families: in multivariate analyses, parental disharmony predicted the child's emotional disturbance whereas divorce, per se, did not. In a longer six-year follow-up of a birth cohort (Fergusson et al., 1986) findings from multivariate analyses showed yet again that divorce per se did not predict the child's subsequent emotional problems, when social class, economic factors, other life events and marital discord were controlled.

Substantially similar findings are reported from the early years of a ten year longitudinal study (Wallerstein and Kelly, 1980; Wallerstein, 1985a,b). The findings are difficult to interpret since there was no control group and the sample comprised families sufficiently disturbed to have been referred to a counselling clinic at the time. However, by the fifth year of follow up, one third were still judged to be depressed and by 10 years, when most were young adults, some 30 percent had engaged in moderately serious illegal activities, and many had shown educational or occupational decline from their earlier middle class family status (Wallerstein, 1985a).

Thus with all these studies, those in the community excepted, the nature of the criterion and control sample is all important. It could be argued for example that normal, presumably happy, families do not constitute appropriate controls; a case control study of families in turmoil, comparing those who divorce with those who do not, might permit a more accurate assessment of the impact of divorce per se. However, pre-divorce parenting and other variables would need to be controlled. Another approach is to use a cohort in which divorced and intact families are followed over time, with parenting and other variables assessed regularly. The effects of both pre-divorce and post-divorce factors could then be independently assessed.

Thus, despite the plethora of studies appearing to show parent "loss" in childhood causes adult psychopathology, especially depression, the evidence is somewhat fragile. When one distinguishes for instance between parent death and parent child separations, there is no good evidence to suggest that parent death has any significant impact on adult depressive disorders. With parent-child separations, only those occurring in relation to family discord, such as divorce, appear to have any long term impact.

Even these data are brittle when one considers that crucial confounding variables, such as parental psychopathology and the family and social environment before separation, have not been adequately controlled. The failure adequately to control for such factors also limits any assessment of the magnitude of effect of this loss on subsequent adult morbidity even where this might theoretically be possible. Such an assessment is, for instance, not possible in studies of patient samples and normal controls since these studies do not provide data necessary to calculate relative and attributable risk. Random community studies do allow such calculations. However, of the three community studies, one showed no significant effect for maternal separations (Kennard and Birtchnell, 1982), while the other two, both carried out in the same London community, showed some effect of parental loss (Brown and Harris, 1978; Tennant et al., 1981). In the first study of women, the risk of depression in those experiencing maternal loss (deaths and separations) and in the remainder was 23 percent and 8 percent respectively, the relative risk thus being 2.9, while the risk of depression attributable to this loss was 15 percent. Confounding variables were not however, controlled. In the second study of both men and women (Tennant et al., 1982a,b) multiple regression analysis of all childhood loss experiences indicated that only 5 percent of the variance in depression was explained by these variables. There is some possibility that this is an underestimate of effect because of problems in defining the most appropriate outcome variable and the possibility that some adult ''confounding'' variables which were controlled may indeed have had some mediating role between childhood experiences and adult psychopathology. Thus, we might still cautiously conclude that parent-child separations, at least due to family discord, may predispose to adult psychopathology. If so, what intervening variables are involved in the mediating processes?

Mediators in Childhood

Subsequent Parenting

Parenting problems following any childhood loss would appear to be the most important potential mediator. The available evidence, while confirming the importance of poor parenting as a risk factor for depression generally, does not specifically address its mediating effect between childhood separations and adult depression. There are three retrospective studies of loss and parenting in adults with depression. The first by Brier et al. (1988) failed to show that parental deaths or separations were related to depression. However, in those who had experienced a loss, the relationship with the custodial parent and the stability of home life following loss predicted adult depression. In two similar studies which included normal (no loss) controls, (Harris et al., 1986; Bifulco et al., 1987), loss, per se, did not predict depression in women when parental care was taken into account. Paradoxically, in the latter study, poor parenting had a greater influence on depression in women without loss than in those with early loss. In all three studies, it is not possible to draw clear conclusions about the effects of parenting subsequent to loss since the crucial confounding variable of pre-loss parenting was not controlled. However, from these and other studies, poor parenting appears to be a risk factor for adult depression irrespective of a specific childhood loss. Indeed, these studies show that loss on its own was not an independent risk factor for adult depression.

Four longitudinal studies of divorce have also assessed subsequent parenting (Hess and Camara, 1979; Hetherington et al., 1982; Fergusson et al., 1986; Wallerstein and Kelly, 1980; Wallerstein 1985a,b). All describe an early deterioration in quality of parenting in the first year, and this predicts disturbed behaviors in the child (Hess and Camara, 1979). Similarly, positive parent-child relationships mitigate the adverse emotional effects in children (Hess and Camara, 1979). These behavior problems in the child are also predicted by overt (but not by covert) spouse conflict (Wallerstein and Kelly, 1980; Hetherington et al., 1982). Furthermore, it should be noted that the relationship between parenting problems and disturbed behaviors in the children is reciprocal (Patterson, 1981); this reciprocity is greatest in mother-son interactions. Despite early difficulties, parenting generally improves over time and may eventually be better than that occurring before divorce. The improvement is such that only two years after divorce, behavioral problems may be less severe in divorced families than in stressed but intact families (Hetherington et al., 1982). Indeed, more behavioral disturbances were found in children when their parents were reconciled than when they remained separated (Fergusson et al., 1986). Thus psychopathology in divorced and intact families (especially those in turmoil) may not be as great as imagined; so, for instance, considerable overlap is found in the quality of parenting in divorced and intact families, more variation in parenting is identified within groups than between groups, and parenting factors are found to be far better unique predictors of children's psychological outcome than was actual marital status (Fergusson, 1986; Hess and Camara, 1979).

Arising from this is the critical question of whether it is better for children to remain in intact but stressed families or to face parental separation and its consequences. Wallenstein and Kelly (1980) felt that for boys at least, the continuing conflict in divorced families was more damaging than conflict in intact families, so their evidence would suggest that when divorce leads to a significant reduction in parental conflict, the outcome for children is likely to improve.

Parent-child interactions were found to be more powerful predictors of children's behavior than spouse interactions (Hess and Camara, 1979). This is not surprising although clearly the two are related. It must be born in mind, however, that spouse interaction is likely to be the most important mediator between parent/child conflict and the children's behavior. Evidence from the U.K. National Child Development Study (Whithead, 1979) suggested that separated children were less emotionally disturbed than those where there was an intact family currently in discord. It must be remembered, however, that those separated families may have separated up to seven years previously, so the comparison may not be strictly fair. Nonetheless generally it would appear that, if family discord is continuous, separation is likely to ultimately benefit the children.

Another mediating variable is that of the degree of continuing contact with the father, given fathers are more usually the non custodial parent. There is some evidence that the father's absence in the first five years has some effect on educational attainment, particularly mathematical abilities; these changes are more marked in boys (Shinn, 1978). For girls, father's absence has more effect around puberty, when heterosexual relationships may be disturbed (Heatherington, 1972). The increase in illegitimate births in girls and delinquency in boys seems more due to marital separation and its consequences, not specifically to the father's absence alone, since girls losing their fathers through death are not affected.

Another central factor is the quality of continuing contact with the non-custodial parent, which does predict outcome at six years, especially for boys (Heatherington et al., 1982). The benefit depends, however, on lack of conflict between the parents and appears to be mediated in turn by adequate maternal parenting (Heatherington et al., 1982). Contact with the mother too is important and has some bearing on whether mothers should return to work. Improved maternal parenting is noted when mothers later return to work and finances improve; however, there is a short term adverse effect on children if mothers are forced to return to work in the immediate aftermath of separation (Hetherington et al., 1982).

Finally, when assessed retrospectively in adult life, the quality of parenting in childhood was reported as being no different in separated and non-separated subjects (Parker, 1979). In essence, this evidence demonstrates the positive effects of divorce when there has been preexisting family discord and when divorce leads to a diminution in conflict.

An additional major effect of divorce, of course, is that many children are reared in single-parent families, and there is some evidence to suggest that these children show less satisfactory social and academic development than children raised in conventional two-parent families. (Finer, 1974; Ferri, 1976; Weiss, 1979). These effects are more marked in single-parent families resulting from divorce (Douglas, 1970; Ferri, 1976; Rutter 1981) than in those resulting from widowhood. A confounding variable is however that these divorced families are more likely both to derive from semi- or unskilled groups and to have greater financial hardships. When these influences were accounted for, the effect of single parenthood alone was not great (Ferri, 1976). There was furthermore no substantial difference between mother-headed and father-headed families. Given therefore some adverse correlates of single-parent families, there is some reason to believe remarriage may be beneficial.

Remarriage

On the surface at least, remarriage should provide significant benefits, in that it restores a two care-giver family and economically the family benefits from the presence of the extra income of the stepparent, usually a stepfather. In addition, one might assume somewhat less social stigma in this situation. These factors must, however, be balanced against the negative effects which can include adverse changes in the child's relationship with both the custodial and non-custodial parent and increased friction between parents because of custody issues. Furthermore, the merging of two families of children can significantly disturb the relationship within the new marriage, with a deleterious effect on the children. It is thus not surprising that the empirical evidence does not indicate that remarriage is necessarily good for children.

A review by Longfellow (1979) reports many studies showing no difference between the adjustment of children with no fathers at home and those with stepfathers. A few studies have reported better adjustment, including a small non-random sample of stepsons (Santrock et al., 1982), but more studies, both in the U.S. and U.K. show adverse effects on the children. Douglas (1970) showed increased bedwetting to age 15 years in children in remarried families. There were more anti-social behaviors reported (Herzog and Sudia, 1973; West and Farrington, 1973; McCord et al., 1962; Glueck and Glueck, 1962), low self-esteem and psychosomatic symptoms (Rosenberg, 1965), and being "in need of help" (Zill, 1978). In prospective studies which perhaps provide stronger evidence, the findings are consistent with the above. In a birth cohort study, Fergusson et al. (1986) found a worse outcome in remarried families, and in this same sample some 50 percent had split up again after 3 years. In Heatherington at al.'s (1982) study, worse outcome was also found, with wives in particular not coping with their former husbands remarriage and having increased feeling of depression, anxiety, and anger. Contact with the father usually decreased with his remarriage, especially for his daughters. Problems in the family were greatest between stepfather and stepsons, which was worse if remarriage occurred when the children were older. Problems for sons were identifiable at both 2 and 6 year follow up, but there were no adverse effects on daughters (Heatherington et al., 1982). In general, remarriage cannot be generally recommended from the child's viewpoint.

Institutionalization

Finally, children separated from both parents and institutionalized appear to have a poor psychosocial outcome (Wolkind and Rutter, 1985). It is unclear whether these adverse effects are indeed due to the institutionalization and subsequent experiences, or to genetic and environmental factors preceding it. Nonetheless, women reared in institutions show in later life more personality disorders, criminality, marital discord and separations, and poor parenting skills. Their psychosocial adjustment, however, was as strongly related to their contemporary problems as to patterns of child-rearing (Wolkind and Rutter, 1985). The effect of institutionalization may however be related to social class, since it predicted depression in working-class women but seemed to have no effect on middle class subjects (Harris et al., 1987). This suggests the importance of the social and family environment prior to institutionalization. The adverse effects of such deprived backgrounds, however, seem remediable, for example by a subsequent supportive marital relationship (Rutter, 1985; Parker and Hadzi-Pavlovic, 1984).

Personality

The six studies of early parental death and personality development largely show no effect; in only one are there any positive findings and they are inconsistent (see Tennant et al., 1980). Two other studies have assessed the effect of parent-child separations on personality. Parker (1979) found that while separations were themselves not related to adult depressive symptoms, the duration of separation (probably reflecting poor parenting before loss) correlated with trait depression. Parenting also influenced personality, particularly dependency, in women separated from their mothers (Kennard and Birtchnell, 1982). There is thus no good evidence that parent loss per se influences personality type, although in boys separated from their fathers less masculine sex role behaviors are observed in the short-term, while little or no effect is found in girls (Hetherington et al., 1982; Hess and Camara, 1979; Landy et al., 1969).

It is nonetheless pertinent to bear in mind the indirect evidence relating to the effects of chronic forms of adversity on personality development, as reviewed by Rutter (1984b), in particular those of adaptability, resilience, coping, and self-esteem.

Cognitive Development and Schooling

Cognitive development may also be affected following divorce, but whether it is pre-divorce factors or post-divorce factors which determine this is unclear. In the short-term, performance IQ but not verbal IQ is impaired in single-parent families, and this is more marked for boys (Hetherington et al., 1982). In the short term, less productive working styles are noted (Hess and Camara, 1979). In the intermediate term, some six years after divorce, performance IQ remains impaired in boys but not in girls (Guidubaldi et al., 1983), and ten years after divorce there is noticeable educational and occupational decline in young adults who had originally been referred for counselling following earlier parental divorce (Wallerstein, 1985a). These educational problems are also reflected in higher rates of expulsion and school drop outs.

Social Relationships

Social behaviors are also affected by divorce. Children show less imaginative play, but after two years, differences are only noted in boys, who still show more noxious social behaviors despite some improvement (Hetherington et al., 1982). The school environment also has some influence on these behavior problems; less disturbance is found when the social environment had enforced standards and was predictable (Rutter, 1979, 1985).

Economic Factors

The maintenance of two households clearly leads to economic restrictions, and this is especially true of households headed by women (Ferri, 1976; Finer, 1974; Marsden, 1969; George and Wilding, 1972). Poorer income has a direct negative effect on the children by way of poorer housing, fewer holidays, and the mother being forced to work and so being more often absent from the house.

Mediators in Adolescence and Adult Life

The distinction between childhood mediators and those occurring later in life is of course arbitrary. Furthermore, early mediators may themselves operate by way of later mediators, and there is potentially a cascading effect of intervening variables.

Attitudes to Marriage, and Premarital Pregnancy

Young adults ten years after their parents' divorce remain apprehensive about repeating their parents' mistakes, and women especially are fearful of betrayal in love; this is more marked if divorce occurred later in childhood rather than earlier. Despite this, both sexes express powerful personal commitments to the institution of marriage and fidelity within it (Wallerstein, 1985). Other evidence however is less optimistic, since marital instability in one generation seems to predict it in the next (Pope and Mueller, 1979). Maternal loss and poor maternal care, especially in working class women, predicted pre-marital pregnancy (PMP) which in turn predicts both poor marital support and subsequent depression (Harris et al., 1987). This social class effect was attributed to "entrapment," since more working class women married the father of the child, compared to middle class women. Women with PMP were also "socially entrapped," only one in four were upwardly mobile compared to two thirds of those without. Premarital pregnancy alone, among a wide range of other social variables, was an independent predictor of subsequent depression (Harris et al., 1987).

Marriage, Marital Quality, and Parenting

Poor parenting following loss (but not loss, per se) predicted low self-esteem, premarital pregnancy, marital breakdown, and ultimately depression in working class women in the U.K. (Bifulco et al., 1987). Other reported consequences of separations include earlier pregnancy and poor housing, (Wolkind et al., 1979), and problems with childcare are found in women whose parents divorced and who had a poor subsequent relationship with their fathers (Frommer and O'Sheas, 1973a,b).

In contrast to the above, parental death appears to have no such adverse impact on subsequent marriage. In community samples, parental death in childhood was associated with greater marital closeness, and greater investment in having children (Jacobson and Ryder, 1969) and with lower rates of marital separation and divorce (Kennard and Birtchnell, 1982); the latter study also showed those bereaved in childhood to be no different in their range of marital patterns and affection. The only adverse finding was that early bereaved women were more over-protective of their adolescent children. Childhood bereavement furthermore does not affect the subject's ability to become an effective parent (Frommer and O'Sheas, 1973b). Thus while marital factors and quality of parenting in one generation may affect the next, there is no evidence that loss, per se, has any significant influence. Finally it must be emphasized that these variables, of marital quality, parenting, childrens' emotional problems, and parental depression, are all interrelated.

Vulnerability to Other Life Stressors

It has been argued that early childhood experiences such as loss render subjects more vulnerable to subsequent life stressors (Brown and Harris, 1978). This could occur firstly because such subjects perceive subsequent events as being more stressful; however, this was not confirmed in a study of early bereaved subjects who perceived life events to be no more stressful than controls (Persson, 1980). Secondly, it could occur because these subjects actually experience more acute life events which in turn causes depression. Perris (1983), however, found in depressed patients that those with childhood bereavement experienced similar stressors before their depressive episodes as those who were not bereaved. There is thus no evidence of a relation between parental loss and the frequency of acute life events in later life.

Parenting, as distinct from loss, may however have some relation to later stressful events, particularly in the areas of marriage and childbearing, as discussed. This is confirmed in a study showing that subjects with poor parenting experience more life events overall; poor parenting predicted depression in the presence but not in the absence of such stressors (Bifulco et al., 1987). This study seems to conflict with Perris' (1983) study showing that those depressives with a rejecting mother had fewer life stressors prior to onset of depression than those with non-rejecting mothers. In the first community based study (Bifulco et al., 1987), poor parenting not surprisingly led to a greater risk of life events, perhaps even subject generated, and the two factors together increased the risk of depression. This finding is not however irreconcilable with the second study of depressed patients, where fewer life events were required to precipitate a depression episode in subjects with poor parenting (Perris, 1983).

Conclusion

Parental loss has preoccupied psychiatry for most of this century and has been readily accepted by many as a significant risk factor for adult psychopathology. However, objective scrutiny of the empirical findings reveals their fragility. When loss is refined into that through parental death and that due to parent child separations, there is no evidence that parental death is a significant risk factor for depression; there is, however, some evidence that separations, particularly those occurring in the context of family or parental discord, may contribute to adult depression. These findings, too, are quite brittle, largely because the confounding effects of genetic and environmental factors preceding the loss have not been adequately accounted for. Furthermore, in no study has loss or separation been shown to be a risk factor when subsequent parenting is controlled. One is also forced to heed evidence showing that parental separation is beneficial if it terminates earlier family turmoil; indeed parental reconciliation may be deleterious to the child. The evidence would appear to show that if family breakup occurs and does not seriously affect the quality of parenting in the longer term, then long term psychopathology in the children seems unlikely. While one cannot absolutely conclude, on the available evidence, that prolonged parent-child separation is, per se, not toxic for adult mental health, the case for its toxicity remains to be proved.

This rather negative appraisal of the evidence might be taken as grounds for clinical optimism. However, this is not really the case, since parental child separations occurring in the context of marital disharmony are often indicators of poor earlier parenting and impoverished parenting after the divorce, even if the child-parent separation is itself not pathogenic. This review may also seem pessimistic in the sense that parental loss research has been a fruitless search. This too is not so, as studies of parent loss have generated considerable data on early social risk factors for depression in general. Some of these may ultimately prove to be the mediators in any relation of childhood loss with adult psychopathology, if and when the case for its pathogenicity is proven. Perhaps what emerges most strongly is the importance of parenting as a risk factor and its effect on other risk factors for psychopathology. The evidence is increasing that poor parenting has short, intermediate, and long-term consequences, and its effects are mediated through a diversity of personal, interpersonal, and social consequences until ultimately depression or other psychopathology emerges. For some considerable time now, clinicians have been less obsessed with childhood traumas such as loss, and have focused more on the personal and interpersonal factors alluded to, especially the more contemporaneous factors. Social psychiatric researchers are now following in their steps.

References

Australian Institute of Family Studies, 1987. Implications of Marital Separation for Young Children, compiled by the AIFS from a report of a survey conducted in 1982–83 by Smiley, G.W., Chamberlain, E.R., Dalgleish, L.I. commissioned by the Institute, Working Paper No. 11, Melbourne, Australian Institute of Family Studies.

Bebbington, P., Hurry, J., Tennant, C., Sturt, E., Wing, J.K., 1981a. Epidemiology of mental disorders in Camberwell. *Psychological Medicine*; 11:561–579.

Bebbington, P., Tennant, C., Hurry, J., 1981b. Adversity and the nature of psychiatric disorder in the Community. *Journal of Affective Disorders*; 3:345–366.

Bifulco, A.T., Brown, G.W., Harris, T.O., 1987. Childhood loss of parent, lack of adequate parental care and adult depression: a replication. *Journal of Affective Disorders*; 12:115–128.

Birtchnell, J., 1986. Women whose mothers died in childhood: an outcome study. *Psychological Medicine*; 10:699–713.

Bowlby, J., 1951. *Maternal Care and Mental Health*. Monograph No 2 Geneva: World Health Organization.

Bowlby, J., 1969. *Attachment and Loss*. Vol. 1: *Attachment*. Basic Books, New York.

Brier, A., Kelsoe, J.R., Kirwin, P.D., Beller, S.A., Owen, B.S., Wolkowitz, M.D., 1988. Early parental loss and the development of adult psychopathology. *Archives of General Psychiatry*; 45:987–993.

Brown, G.W., Harris, T., 1978. *Social Origins of Depression: A Study of Psychiatric Disorder in Women*. Tavistock Publications. London.

Cadoret, R., J. O'Gorman, T.W., Troughton, E., Heywood, E., 1985. Alcoholism and antisocial personality. Interrelationships, genetic and environmental factors. *Archives of General Psychiatry*; 42:161–167.

Crook, T., Eliot, J., 1980. Parental death during childhood and adult depression: a critical review of the literature. *Psychological Bulletin*; 87J:252–259.

Douglas, J.W.B., 1970. Broken families and child behaviour. *Journal of the Royal College of Physicians* London; 4: 203–210.

Favarelli, C., Sacchetti, E., Ambonetti, A., Conte, G., Pallanti, S., Vita, A., 1986. Early life events and affective disorder revisited. *British Journal of Psychiatry*; 148:288–295.

Fergusson, D.M., Dimond, M.E., Horwood, L.J., 1986. Childhood family placement history and behaviour problems in 6-year old children. *Journal of Child Psychiatry*; 27:213–226.

Ferri, E., 1976. *Growing up in a One-Parent Family*. NFER Publishing: Windsor.

Finer Report. 1974. *Report of the Committee on One-Parent Families*. Cmnd. 5629. Her Majestys Stationery Office, London.

Frommer, E.A., O'Sheas, G., 1973a. Antenatal identification of women liable to have problems in managing their infants. *British Journal of Psychiatry*; 123:149–156.

Frommer, E.A., O'Sheas, G., 1983b. The importance of childhood experience in relation to problems of marriage and family building. *British Journal of Psychiatry*; 123:157–160.

Furstenberg, F.F. Jr., 1982. Conjugal succession: Reentering marriage after divorce. In: Baltes, P.B., Brim O.G. (eds.). *Life-span Development and Behavior*. Vol. 4. Academic Press. New York.

George, V. and Wilding, P. 1972. *Motherless Families*. Routledge & Kegan Paul. London.

Glueck, S. and Glueck, E.T. 1962. Family Environment and Delinquency, Routledge & Kegan Paul. London.

Guidubaldi, J., Perry, J.D., Cleminshaw, H.D. et al., 1983. The impact of parental divorce on children: Report of the nationwide NASP study. *School Psychology Review*; 12:300–323.

Harris, T., Brown, G.W., Bifulco, A., 1986. Loss of parent in childhood and adult psychiatric disorder: the role of lack of adequate parental care. *Psychological Medicine*; 16:641–659.

Harris, T., Brown, G.W., Bifulco, A., 1987. Loss of parent in childhood and adult psychiatric disorder: the role of social class position and premarital pregnancy. *Psychological Medicine*; 17:163–183.

Hetherington, E.M., 1972. Effects of father absence on personality development in adolescent daughters. *Developmental Psychology*; 7:313–326.

Hetherington, E.M., Cox, M., Cox, R., 1982. Effects of divorce on parents and children. In: Lamb, M.E. (ed.). *Nontraditional Families: Parenting and Child Development*. Hillsdale, Lawrence Erlbaum Associates. New Jersey.

Herzog, E. and Sudia, C.E. 1968. Fatherless homes: a review of research. *Children*; 15, 177–182.

Hess, R.D., and Camara, K.A., 1979. Post-divorce family relationships as mediating factors in the consequences of divorce for children. *Journal of Social Issues*; 35:79–96.

Jacobson, G., Ryder, R.G., 1969. Parental loss and some characteristics of the early marriage relationship. *American Journal of Orthopsychiatry*; 39:779–787.

Kennard, J. and Birtchnell, J., 1982. The mental health of early mother-separated women. *Acta Psychiatrica Scandinavia*; 65:388–402.

Kohlberg, L., La Cross J., and Ricks D. 1972. The predictability of adult mental health from childhood behaviour. In *Manual of Child Psychopathology*. Wolman, B.A. (ed.) McGraw-Hill, New York.

Landy, F., Rosenberg, B.G., Sutton-Smith, B., 1969. The effect of limited father absence on cognitive development. *Child Development*; 40:941–944.

Longfellow, C., 1979. Divorce in context: its impact on children. In Levinger, G. and Moles, O.C. (eds.) *Divorce and Separation*. Basic Books. New York.

Marsden, D. 1969. *Mothers Alone*. London: Allen Lane.

McCord, J., McCord, W., and Thurber E. 1962. Some effects of paternal absence on male children. *Journal of Abnormal & Social Psychology*; 64, 361–369.

Moss, H. and Sussman, E. 1980, Longitudinal study of personality development. In *Constancy and Change in Human Development*. Brim, O.G. and Kagan, J. (eds.) Harvard University Press. Cambridge Mass.

Parker, G., 1979. Parental characteristics in relation to depressive disorders. *British Journal of Psychiatry*; 134:138–147.

Parker, G., 1981. Parental reports of depressives: an investigation of several explanations. *Journal of Affective Disorders*; 3:131–140.

Parker, G., 1983. Parental "affectionless control" as an antecedent to adult depression. *Archives of General Psychiatry*; 40:956–960.

Parker, G. Hadzi-Pavlovic D., 1984. Modification of levels of depression in mother-bereaved women by parental and marital relationships. *Psychological Medicine*; 14:125–135.

Patterson, G.R., 1981. *Mothers: The Unacknowledged Victims*. Monograph of Social Research in Child Development; 46 (whole No. 5).

Perris, H. 1983. Deprivation in childhood and life events in depression. *Archiv für Psychiatrie und Nervenkrankheiten*; 23:489–498.

Perris, C., Holmgren, S., Von Knorring, L., Perris, H. 1982. Parental loss by death in the early childhood of depressed patients and of their healthy siblings. *British Journal of Psychiatry*; 148:165–169.

Perris, C., Perris, H. 1978. Status within the family and early life experiences in patients with affective disorders and cycloid psychosis. *Psychiatry Clinica*; 11:155–162.

Persson, G. 1980. Relation between early parental death and life event ratings among 70 year olds. A test of a sensitization theory. *Acta Psychiatrica Scandinavica*; 62:392–397.

Pope, H., Mueller, C.W. 1979. The intergenerational transmission of marital instability: comparisons of race and sex. In Levinger, G., Moles, O.C. (eds.): *Divorce and Separation: Context, Causes, and Consequences*. Basic Books. New York.

Rosenberg, M. 1965. *Society and the Adolescent Self-Image*. New Jersey: Princeton University Press.

Roy, A. 1978. Vulnerability factors and depression in women. *British Journal of Psychiatry*; 133:106–110.

Roy, A. 1980a. Early parental loss in depressive neurosis compared with other neuroses. *Canadian Journal of Psychiatry*; 25:503–505.

Roy, A. 1980b. Parental loss in childhood and onset of manic-depressive illness. *British Journal of Psychiatry*; 136:86–88.

Roy, A. 1981a. Risk factors and depression in Canadian Women. *Journal of Affective Disorders*; 3:65–70.

Roy, A. 1981b. Vulnerability factors and depression in men. *British Journal of Psychiatry; 138,* 75–77.

Roy, A. 1981c. Role of past loss in depression. *Archives of General Psychiatry;* 38:301–302.

Roy, A. 1983. Early parental death and adult depression. *Psychological Medicine;* 13:861–865.

Roy, A. 1985. Early parental separation and adult depression. Archives of General Psychiatry; 42:987–991.

Rutter, M. 1972. *Maternal Deprivation Reassessed.* Penguin. London.

Rutter, M. 1979. Maternal deprivation, 1972–1978: New Findings, New Concepts, New Approaches. *Child Development;* 50:283–305.

Rutter, M. 1983. Statistical and personal interactions: facets and perspectives in *Human Development: An Interaction Perspective* (D. Magnusson D. and Allen V. (eds.) Academic Press: New York.

Rutter, M., 1984a. Psychopathology and development: 1. Childhood antecedents of adult psychiatric disorder. *Australian & New Zealand Journal of Psychiatry* 18:225–234.

Rutter, M. 1984b. Psychopathology and Development: 11 Childhood experiences and personality development. *Australian & New Zealand Journal of Psychiatry.* 18:314–327.

Rutter, M. 1985. Psychopathology and Development: Links between childhood and adult life. In: *Child & Adolescent Psychiatry.* Chap. 45 Rutter M., Hersov L. (eds.) Blackwell Scientific Publications. London.

Rutter, M., Maughan, B., Mortimore, P., Ouston, J., Smith, A., 1979. *Secondary Schools and their Effects on Children: 15,000 hours.* Open Books. London.

Rutter, M., Cox, A. 1985. Other family influences. In: *Child and Adolescent Psychiatry.* Chap. 4 Butter M., Hersov L. (eds.) Blackwell Scientific Publications. Lond.

Santrock, J.W. and Warshak, R.A., 1979. Father custody and social development in boys and girls. *Journal of Social Issues;* 35:112–125.

Santrock, J.W., Warshak, R., Lindbergh, C., Meadows, L., 1982. Children's and parents' observed social behaviour in stepfather families. *Child Development;* 53:472–480.

Seligman, R., Gleser, G., Raug J., Harris L., 1974. The effect of earlier parental loss in adolescents. *Archives of General Psychiatry;* 31:475–479.

Shinn, M. 1978. Father absence and children's cognitive development. *Psychological Bulletin;* 85:295–324.

Tennant, C., Bebbington, P., Hurry, J., 1980. Parental death in childhood and risk of adult depressive disorders. *Psychological Medicine;* 10:289–299.

Tennant, C., Smith, A., Bebbington, P., Hurry, J., 1981. Parental loss in childhood: relationship to adult psychiatric impairment and contact with psychiatric services. *Archives of General Psychiatry;* 38:309–314.

Tennant, C., Hurry, J., Bebbington, P., 1982a. The relation of childhood separation experiences to adult depressive and anxiety states. *British Journal of Psychiatry;* 141:475–482.

Tennant, C., Bebbington, P., Hurry, J., 1982b. Social Experiences in Childhood and Adult Psychiatric Morbidity—A Multiple Regression Analysis. *Psychological Medicine;* 12:2, 321–327.

Wallerstein, J.S., 1985a. Children of Divorce: Preliminary Report of a Ten Year Follow-up of Older Children and Adolescents. *Journal of American Academy of Child Psychiatry;* 24:545–553.

Wallerstein, J.S., 1985b. Children of Divorce: Emerging Trends. *Psychiatric Clinics of North America*; 8:837–855.

Wallerstein, J.S., Kelly, J.B., 1980. *Surviving the Break-Up: How Children and Parents Cope with Divorce*. London: Grant. McIntyre.

Weiss, R.S. 1979. *Going it Alone: The Family Life and Social Situation of the Single Parent*. Basic Books. New York.

Weissman, M.M., Gammon, G.D., John, K. Merikangas, K.R., Warner, V., Prusoff, B.A., Sholomskas, D., 1987. Children of Depressed Parents. Increased Psychopathology and early onset of Major Depression. *Archives of General Psychiatry*; 44:847–853.

West, D.J. and Farrington, D.P. 1973. *Who Becomes Delinquent?* Heinemann. London.

Whitehead, L., 1979. Sex differences in children's responses to family stress: a re-evaluation. *Journal of Child Psychology & Psychiatry*; 20:247–254.

Wolkind, S.N., Kruk, S., Chaves, L.P., 1976. Childhood separation experiences and psycho-social status in primiparous women: Preliminary findings. *British Journal of Psychiatry*; 128:391–396.

Wolkind, S., Rutter, M., 1985. Separation, loss and family relationships. In: *Child and Adolescent Psychiatry*. Chap. 3 Rutter, M., Hersov, L. (eds.) Blackwell Scientific Publications. London.

Zill, N. 1978. Divorce, marital happiness and the mental health of children. Paper prepared for NIMH workshop on Divorce and Children. Bethesda.

15

Psychiatric Case Registers as Tools for Scientific Investigation

Heinz Häfner

Introduction

Psychiatric case registers are superior to other mental health information systems in four respects. These are: (1) cumulative case-related recording, (2) unduplicated counts, (3) inclusion of contact with all mental health services, and (4) reference to a defined population (Wing 1972a).

The Camberwell Case Register, among the first of its type, was set up at the MRC Social Psychiatry Research Unit in London by Lorna Wing and John Wing on December 31, 1964. From January 1, 1965, information was continuously collected concerning all contacts with psychiatric services made by children and adults, thus including all facilities for the mentally ill and retarded provided for the population of the Camberwell District of South London. The register was set up to serve as a "tool for scientific investigation" as well as an instrument for clinical information and communication. Its functions were "to measure the extent and type of current use of services, to facilitate the examination of patterns of contact over time, to monitor changes accidentally or deliberately introduced, to allow the assignation of future trends, to indicate researchable issues, and to act as a sampling-frame for more intensive studies" (Wing 1972b).

The Camberwell Register served as an extraordinarily fruitful model of evaluative research until its termination in 1984. Two factors operated to its advantage: (1) the "intellectual and professional resources" of the Maudsley and the Bethlem Royal Joint Hospital (Wing 1972b), in particular those of the MRC Social Psychiatry Research Unit, and (2) the "departure from the existing hospital service'' and the setting up of alternative model services and experimental programs in the borough of Camberwell during the register's life. Over the period 1964–71 the register documented increasing hospital admission rates, decreasing long-term residence in hospital, and a new build-up of long-stay patients. The problems and developments which in the following years became evident throughout the U.K. and in other industrialized countries were foreshadowed by these statistics, by studies on psychiatric patients out of contact with services (Leff and Vaughn 1972) and on psychiatric aspects of destitution, and by the contribution of register data to the planning of community psychiatric services and predicting the future need for psychiatric hospital beds (Häfner 1987a).

The early example of the British registers (D.H.S.S. 1971; Hall et al., 1974; Wing and Bransby 1970; Wing and Fryers 1974) illustrated the potential benefits for research and planning. The small circle of researchers involved in studies of case register data in the sixties and seventies has expanded to take in many of those involved in social psychiatry research more broadly defined. This is clearly reflected in the volume *Psychiatric Case Registers in Public Health* (ten Horn et al., 1986). The center of case-register research remains in the United Kingdom and Scandinavia, but new registers have been started throughout Europe, and significant contributions to major issues of mental health service research are being made as a result. The studies published therein nevertheless reveal that we are far from having exhausted the large research potential of case registers. Some promising lines of development are outlined below.

Evaluative Research

The aim of evaluative research is to gain information about needs for mental health care and how these can be met, thus also serving as a basis for planning and administering mental health services. Of no less significance is the investigation of the effectiveness and cost of health services and programs. Since the mental health care system is still subject to the drastic changes documented in the early studies based on the Camberwell Register—the transition from long-term residential care in mental hospitals to extramural care provided by a variety of complementary psychiatric and social services in the community—methods of recording comprehensive and cumulative data for evaluating these changes are of great practical interest. It is still a matter of controversy whether and to what extent services provided by complementary facilities are better and cheaper for psychiatric patients in need of residential care than continued hospital care of good quality (Häfner and an der Heiden, 1989).

The issues in mental health services research that can be tackled on the basis of case registers depend on the coverage, duration and quality of data-collection. The first cumulative psychiatric case register, established by Ödegard in 1936 as a national Norwegian register of psychoses, stored case-related data pertaining to all admissions to psychiatric hospitals in Norway since 1916. Case registers of this type permit the collection of indices of psychiatric in-patient care like first and re-admission rates and length of stay, divided according to diagnostic groups and demographic data. So, for instance, Ödegard analyzed the changing pattern of psychiatric in-patient care in Norway—similar to those observed in other European countries (May, 1976)—on the basis of a continuous evaluation of annual rates. In contrast, Weeke and Strömgren analyzed similar Danish trends by comparing repeated cross-sections made over intermediate periods of time (Ödegard, 1971; Weeke and Strömgren, 1978; Häfner and an der Heiden, 1986b). By measuring changes observed in specific indices, we may obtain some indication of aspects of the quality of in-patient care.

The advantage of case registers over hospital statistics arises from the quality and structure of their data. If hospital admissions are increasing, hospital statistics do not on their own permit us to identify reliably whether this increase is due to an increasing number of *individuals* or of *readmissions* of patients discharged after long-term hospitalization. If national case registers do not exist—and this is the case in almost all countries— the level of data recorded in routine national health statistics can be augmented by local case registers. The interpretation of aggregated data in particular can be improved by the additional use of individual data stored in case registers. Case-register data, diligently collected, can provide the basis for a continued monitoring of mental health care, and contribute to the planning of national mental health services. The Camberwell Register, and later all eight case registers in England and Wales, have often been used for this function (Gibbons et al., 1984).

A central issue has been the consequences of the run-down of mental hospitals. It was illuminated to some extent by the early studies of new long-stay cases accumulating in the comprehensive community mental health services of Camberwell (Wing, 1973) and Salford (Fryers, 1979). The preliminary data collected by Leff (1988) in connection with the ru-down of the Friern and Claybury mental hospitals have confirmed this trend. It is clear that a small number of long-term mentally ill adults with severe disability need continual residential care even with favorable extramural services (Häfner 1987a). Moreover, if the conditions of economic, social, and extramural care in a community are unfavorable, the need for residential care of the chronically mentally ill and disabled increases correspondingly.

Long-term residential care with round-the-clock availability of nurses and physicians may take the form of mental hospitals reduced in size, but providing appropriate facilities for accommodation, leisure-time activities, treatment, and rehabilitation programs (Wing, 1988), or of psychiatric homes with a high level of care. The preferred form should first be decided by the planning authorities. The alternatives should then be assessed in terms of effectiveness, cost, and quality of life on the basis of case-register data and of studies of comparative cost-effectiveness.

Potential Developments in the Use of Psychiatric Case Registers

The simplest way to extend the efficiency of a register is to cooperate with other psychiatric case registers run in the same health care system, register their data under the same conditions of case-finding and apply the same criteria. The advantage of such cooperation is that it furnishes the basis for comparisons and increases the predictive power of the data stored, especially as the demographic and ecological parameters of catchment areas covering a population range of about 80,000 to 600,000 and the system of medical, social, and mental health care provided for it are inevitably subject to variations. This is quite evident from the marked differences in the long term population trends and the socio-demographic indices of the populations resident in the eight British case register areas (Gibbons et al., 1984). A national health care system should therefore run at least two (in larger countries several) cooperating psychiatric case registers.

Further improvement in the efficiency of a case register can be attained if its coverage is extended by including mentally disordered subjects who mainly receive care in sectors other than mental health. An example is furnished by the Camberwell Register itself, which from its very beginning included services for the mentally retarded. Enlarging the range of diagnostic groups and services not only opens the possibility of evaluating the care provided to these groups, but also creates wider opportunities for investigating the epidemiology of these disorders. The studies by Lorna Wing on the prevalence of various grades and forms of mental retardation, on specific retardation profiles, and on the principles of care founded on them, were conceived on the basis of the Camberwell Register and field studies additionally conducted in the catchment area (Wing, 1971; Wing et al., 1972; Wing, 1981; Chap. 6 in this volume).

A further example is provided by the Salford Register (Fryers and Woof, 1989), which included data on contacts with social workers and community psychiatric nurses, thus allowing more detailed comparative research into the nature of the services provided (Woof *et al.*, 1986). In line with demographic changes in the European population, in particular the increase in the very old with their high psychiatric morbidity, the inclusion of the elderly mentally ill in cumulative case registers is of growing interest.

According to a case-register study conducted in Mannheim, only about 1 percent of the persons aged over 65 are admitted to a psychiatric hospital per year (Haas et al., 1982), although the annual prevalence rate amounts to about 24 percent (Cooper, 1986; Bickel, 1987). Four percent of the elderly are accommodated in old people's and nursing homes, but about 20 percent of the deceased elderly have been residents of such homes. The importance of including old people's and nursing homes in case registers is self-evident from these figures. This requires that a reliable psychiatric diagnosis is given and that demographic and health data are recorded. Extension of the register in this way to areas beyond the mental health care system requires psychiatric examination and care of persons who consequently become eligible for inclusion in the register, for example, by a psychiatric consultant. The improvement of psychiatric care in nursing homes and the growing number of psychiatrists in many European countries render such developments possible. It then becomes feasible to evaluate depressive and paranoid syndromes, vascular and Alzheimer-type dementia and their association with somatic disorder and disability continuously over longer periods of time. The developmental psychology of mental disorder is no less significant in old age than in childhood and adolescence. However, the contribution of epidemiological cross-sectional studies is restricted to retrospective data covering limited periods of time. Prospective cohort studies are expensive and restricted to narrow sections of the diagnostic spectrum and can only investigate detailed questions. The importance of a broad monitoring of the course of psychiatric disorders in old age by means of case registers is therefore clear.

The Inclusion of Complementary and Outpatient Services in Case Registers

All adequately comprehensive mental health information systems show an increase in outpatient treatment episodes during the past two to three decades, in some cases by over 100 percent (Kramer, 1986). This may be attributed first to the therapeutic potential of psychotropic drugs and economical methods of social and psychiatric therapy in recent times, and secondly to a concurrent change of public attitudes demanding more freedom and quality of life for the mentally ill and disabled. This means that the pattern of care for the long-term mentally ill with disability can only be determined adequately if complementary care, for example, the care provided in psychiatric homes and group homes, and the psychiatric outpatient or consultant contacts of these patients, is also registered. The extent of the shift in the care of this patient group is evident, for example, in Mannheim, where the number of day-clinic places rose from zero in 1975 to thirty-two in 1985. The number of places in psychiatric homes and group homes increased from 17 in 1975 to 213 in 1985. This signifies that within a short period a new sector of care for the mentally ill and disabled was established, and required to be incorporated in the register. As the Salford psychiatric case register records both data collected by psychiatric consultants in various mental health services and contacts with community psychiatric nurses and social workers (Fryers 1986), it furnishes the prerequisites for a fairly complete detection of this particularly vulnerable group of the long-term ill.

The continuous analysis of the changing pattern of inpatient and complementary care by means of data from the Mannheim case register permitted the need-related planning of complementary services, the establishment of which kept up with the growing need (Häfner and an der Heiden, 1983). It further allowed evaluation of the effectiveness of extramural care and the exact calculation of the cost per case (Häfner and an der Heiden, 1986a). In addition to the routine register data, it was necessary for this purpose to draw from the case register a consecutive sample of admissions of all inhabitants of Mannheim given the diagnosis of schizophrenia and to observe them prospectively over an eighteen-month period. Within this period, all data on care and disorder were collected with standardized methods in three cross-sections. The duration and symptomatology of the disorder on entry into the study, family status, and living conditions were recorded. The result confirmed the hypothesis that regular and intense medical care—most especially the prescription of neuroleptic drugs—constitute the most effective factor in complementary care. This effect is noticeable even among severely disordered patients.

If the length of clinical history at the time of entry into the study is considered, the effect on symptomatology and behavior is most marked in patients living with family; in those living alone the effect was not found at all (Häfner and an der Heiden, 1989).

The mean costs per case—including the costs for hospital readmissions—were about 50 percent lower than the costs for continued hospital care. However, the distribution pattern of case-related costs reveals that the average costs will depend on the proportion of patients receiving extramural care who are severely disordered: 6 percent of the cases provided with extramural care caused costs exceeding those for a one-year in-patient treatment (see Figure 15.1).

Behind this statement stands the fact that the less severely disordered long-stay patients, incurring smaller average costs for extramural psychiatric and social care, are discharged first from the mental hospital. The decrease in the number of long-stay patients in mental hospitals also

FIGURE 15.1
Direct Costs of Community Care
(based on prices in 1980)

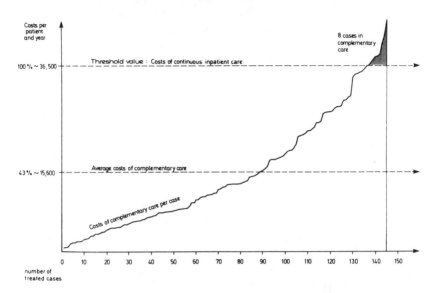

implies that patients with severe behaviour disturbances and disabilities needing a high level of extramural care are increasingly discharged from inpatient care. As a consequence, the average costs for extramural care per case are likely to increase markedly (Häfner and an der Heiden, 1989). This example shows that the results of cost-effectiveness analyses based on sub-populations of psychiatric patients in extramural or intramural care can only be generalized if interpreted in relation to the total group. In our own study, 66 percent of the schizophrenic patients in need of at least a one-year period of residential care were given extramural care. The population-related data on mental health care recorded in a case register may thus furnish the framework for statistical projections based on data collected on a sub-population of the same catchment area. This fact has not yet been considered in studies dealing with the subject.

The Inclusion of Subregisters

By storing attempted suicides in a subregister, the coverage of the Mannheim case register was extended to a psychiatrically relevant group that uses mental health services to a relatively limited extent. All individuals from Mannheim who had been treated in the mental health sector, in the emergency service, or on an inpatient basis in a general hospital for attempted suicide were recorded. Attempted suicide is an event that can be reliably defined even by non-psychiatric physicians. This subregister offered the opportunity to observe trends in the frequency of attempted suicide in relation to age, sex, social data, and ecological distribution over a period of twenty years. We found a distinct period effect, with rates increasing by about 200 percent from 1965-66 to 1976. The increase was steepest for males 15-19 years of age (340 percent), and for females of the same age (300 percent). From 1977 on, the rates for males of all ages decreased by 79 percent, for females by 63 percent (Häfner et al. 1988). The descriptive epidemiological data gave important indications of clusters in small neighbourhoods with peak values of up to twenty times the average value for the city (Welz, 1979). These clusters formed the basis of several studies for testing the imitation hypothesis, until finally we succeeded in furnishing proof of the imitation of a televised suicide model (Schmidtke and Häfner, 1988). The great importance to public health of epidemiological monitoring of attempted suicide emphasizes the value of such subregisters. Without them, significant changes and their causes would remain undiscovered as in most countries there are no other instruments for continuous and comprehensive registration of psychiatrically relevant deviant behavior.

Analytical Epidemiological Research Using Case Registers

Given a sufficient provision of care to the population under study, high utilization rates, and complete registration of contacts with mental health services, case registers provide data on true morbidity that are almost free of distortion. If in the end mental health service research has the purpose of determining "whether the services decrease morbidity or contain it at the lowest possible level" (Wing 1972b), the representativeness of the index population or of the epidemiological basis of service utilization is indeed a prerequisite for generalizing the results of an evaluation study. This principle has been demonstrated in various studies conducted at the MRC Social Psychiatry Research Unit (e.g., Bennett et al., 1972; Wykes, 1982). The simplest contribution of case registers to epidemiological and evaluative research is therefore "to act as a sampling frame for more intensive studies" (Wing 1972b).

Indicators of True Morbidity

Indicators of true morbidity can be obtained from case-register data only if the probability of life-time utilization by a sufferer approaches 1.0

and if the population registered is large enough to support sufficient numbers of patient contacts. For the disease groups of schizophrenia and severe mental subnormality these requirements are met by the national registers of Denmark and Norway covering populations of about 5 and 4 million respectively. Until the publication of the results from the "Determinants-of-Outcome Study" (Sartorius et al., 1986; Jablensky et al., 1990), the first of the transnational schizophrenia studies coordinated by the World Health Organization with the aim of completely identifying first onset schizophrenia in defined populations, case-register data had been the most important basis for transnational comparison of morbidity rates for schizophrenia (Häfner and an der Heiden, 1986b). Comparing the transnational range of about 0.08 to 0.69 per 1000 for annual incidence rates obtained on the basis of case-register data (Häfner and an der Heiden 1986b) with the incidence rates ranging around 0.10 per 1000 obtained by applying standardized methods in the transnational WHO study suggests that differences in diagnostic procedure are a more probable explanation than true differences in morbidity (Häfner 1987b). This assumption is supported by the finding that the marked differences between first admission rates for schizophrenia between Irish and English case registers disappear when an identical procedure of classification, PSE9/CATEGO, is used (Nuallain et al., 1986). It is further supported by a comparison of incidence rates for schizophrenia obtained from the same population (Mannheim) under differing diagnostic definitions and procedures (see Figure 15.2).

Registers can also assist in epidemiological studies of the incidence and characteristics of disorders that are less likely than schizophrenia or severe mental subnormality to lead to contact with specialist services. Mild forms of depression and anxiety are common in the general population, while the more severe forms which are most likely to be studied by specialists are rare. A combination of a register with a community sample provides an opportunity to consider the whole spectrum in epidemiological perspective. (Bebbington et al., 1981).

Epidemiological Monitoring of Long-Term Morbidity Trends

The effects of such sources of error on case-register data as indicators of true morbidity is reduced if, instead of cross-sectional comparisons between different case registers, trend analyses are made on the basis of one case register and over longer periods of time. This requires that the procedure of diagnosis remains similar, and that changes in the age-composition of the population are considered. Case registers operating over longer periods are indeed one of the few sources of information about

FIGURE 15.2
Annual Incidence Rates of Schizophrenia in the Mannheim/Heidelberg Area Assessed
with Different Methods of Identification and Different Diagnostic Definitions

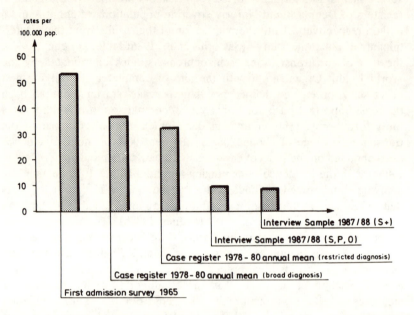

secular changes in psychiatric morbidity (Häfner 1985). Ödegard (1971)
and Astrup (1982), for example, demonstrated on the basis of the Norwegian register of psychoses that age-corrected first-admission rates for
functional non-affective psychoses were almost stable over the period 1926
to 1978. T. Helgason (1975) and L. Helgason (1977) found stable rates of
first contacts for schizophrenia in a comparison of the periods 1926–27,
1956–57, and 1966–67 in Iceland. Ugelstad (1978) reported stable first-
admission rates from the Danish national case register for schizophrenia
in patients aged under 30 years over the period 1957 to 1976. This stability
contradicts the assumption of increasing rates for schizophrenia based on
a comparison between various studies with little reliability or comparability and conducted in different periods of time (Torrey 1980).

Population studies of psychiatric morbidity are toilsome and costly,
especially if low morbidity rates require the examination of a large number
of individuals. For analyzing trends the comparison of studies covering
different periods involves numerous pitfalls, especially if the number of
available studies in comparable populations is too small to apply error-
correcting methods of meta-evaluation. The monitoring of changes in
psychiatric morbidity will rapidly gain significance in the future, as the

populations at risk are subject to major changes in age-composition, and in material and social conditions. The urgency of this issue can already be deduced from the sizeable increases in the morbidity of Alzheimer's disease in countries with high life-expectancy (Henderson, 1983, 1986a, 1986b). It is further reflected in the requirements for reliable projections of morbidity rates and of future needs for care.

The studies conducted by Ödegard on the association between the risk of schizophrenia and migration movements, and on geographical, social and employment factors are an example of the value of case registers in ecological research. By recording the chronological succession of events of geographical, socio-vocational, and personal mobility on the one side and first admission for schizophrenia on the other, Ödegard succeeded in indirectly testing causal hypotheses with data from the Norwegian case register and public statistics (Ödegard, 1932, 1936, 1972, 1973). His findings furnish an essential contribution to the understanding of the interaction between prepsychotic behavior and processes of social and geographical distribution. The considerably lower marriage rate in schizophrenic patients (Ödegard 1946) is found even prior to first admission, and may therefore be attributed to personality traits of the individual later falling ill with schizophrenia, thus supporting selection over the social causation hypothesis. More intensive studies have subsequently confirmed these early findings.

Because of the stream of refugees and foreign workers, transnational migration movements play a major role at present. Monitoring the state of physical and mental health of this population, and providing adequate care for it, is of high humanitarian and political significance. Case registers offer an economical instrument for such monitoring. For example, case-register studies conducted in Mannheim over several years revealed that as a result of their favorable age composition, migratory workers in Germany show lower overall rates for mental disorders than the native German population. When controlling for age, the rates for chronic or recurrent courses of mental disorders are still markedly lower—depending on the length of stay in the host country. The morbidity rates of the national groups with the longest stay in the Federal Republic of Germany are like those of the German population of the same age-group (Häfner 1980).

This finding indicates positive selection of immigrants. Opposed to this, studies conducted among Afro-Caribbean immigrants in the United Kingdom reveal increased rates for example, for schizophrenia, which even in the "second generation" British born exceeded by far the expected value (Ineichen et al., 1984; Harrison et al., 1984; Harrison et al., 1988). The mental health status of emigrants therefore shows very large differences which may be attributed to the selective composition of the emigrant population, and to ecological and psychosocial conditions in the host country.

Cumulative psychiatric case registers are therefore of great theoretical and practical significance as instruments for the continuous indication of the rates of important categories of psychiatric morbidity, and this will increase in the future.

Enlarging Case Registers and Increasing the Detail of the Data Stored

The value of national and large regional case registers as tools for epidemiological research depends on the completeness, reliability and detail of the information stored. The subregister for attempted suicide run at the Mannheim case register has been mentioned previously. To enlarge a case register by setting up a sub-register is often the only way of registering changes in the frequency of serious problems that fall outside the main focus of mental health care, for example, in alcohol- and drug-related disorders or in traffic accidents.

A sufficiently large catchment population, reliable case-identification, complete data-collection, and detailed documentation furnish the basis for the continuous storage of data on rare risks. Mental retardation and deviant behavior in specific chromosomal abnormalities or rare enzyme defects as causes of mental retardation (Dupont, 1981) may serve as examples. A more precise registration of subdiagnoses, or of impairments, disabilities, and other information on additional axes in line with the modern diagnostic systems of ICD 10 and DSM-IV, together with documentation at the level of symptoms have all become possible through the routine use of standardized symptom- and syndrome-scales. The availability of algorithms for the construction and system-transformation of syndrome and disease diagnoses (Olbrich and Maurer, 1988), as well as the enormous enlargement of computer capacity, have considerably increased the potential value of case registers for research.

These more detailed sets of information may serve as the basis of detailed longitudinal studies of the natural history of particular disease categories. If the documentation of treatment and its results and side-effects was standardized, case registers could also contribute to the evaluation of long-term effects and risks of treatment. These detailed longitudinal studies require large and adequately equipped case registers, which would thus become one of the main sources of such therapeutic information.

Linkage with Other Computerized Information Systems

Case-register data become most meaningful when they are continuously related to the socio-demographic characteristics of the population living in the catchment area. Case registers must be notified about deaths so that lethal risks can be studied and data of the deceased deleted to ensure the continuing accuracy of morbidity data (Wing and Hailey 1972).

The linkage of case-register data with public statistics offers a variety of additional opportunities for research, in particular if the register provides access to adequate information on morbidity over long periods of time. Even the association of morbid risks with universal demographic factors has not yet been thoroughly investigated everywhere. For example, the stable epidemiological finding that the mean age at onset of schizophrenia is about five years lower in males has not been sufficiently guarded against artifacts; nor is it known whether the association with gender is direct or the result of confounding (Angermeyer and Kuhn, 1988; Häfner et al., 1989). The same can be said of the consistent finding of an excess of schizophrenic births in winter and spring (Boyd et al., 1986; Häfner et al., 1987). There is some indication, as yet unverified, that a similar pattern of seasonal birth distribution may also be found in other severe disorders (Häfner et al., 1987; Jablensky, 1984). A recent study by Dalen (1988) supports the hypothesis that increased maternal age may explain the findings on season of birth in schizophrenia. For replicating and testing these two hypotheses, case registers linked with the respective data sources are the only practicable research instruments.

The opportunity for evaluating event-related risks by linking case-register data with public statistics has rarely been exploited. Yet it permits the analysis of causal relations in two directions:

1. Where mental health risks follow defined events such as childbirth. The Edinburgh study based on 35729 births over a seven-year period (Kendell et al., 1986), and a recent study by Kastrup (1988) testing the same hypothesis with data from the Danish national case register may serve as examples. The results of these two studies have considerably enlarged our insufficient knowledge of the frequency and type of puerperal psychoses. Comparable epidemiological issues, from which a true increase in clinical knowledge may be expected, include register-linkage studies of the mental health risks of marriage or death among the next of kin. Of special significance is the evaluation of associations of unemployment or job loss with suicide risk through trend analyses or complex indicator models (Brenner, 1973; Häfner, 1988). The results of such studies, which again can only be obtained on the basis of case registers that store data

from large catchment areas over long periods of time, are of great value to social and health policy.

2. Where the causal influence apparently lies in the opposite direction—morbidity and mortality consequent on mental disorders. Studies of this type have primarily been devoted to unnatural causes of death like suicide, or treatment risks. In this context, the excess mortality of psychiatric patients and its composition in relation to exposure to physical risk factors are issues of intensive research (Häfner and Bickel, 1989). One topic of debate is the suicide risk of hospitalized psychiatric patients. Morbidity trends of inpatient suicides can be studied on the basis of large case registers run over a long period of time, by controlling the age composition, the length of stay, and the actual number of persons at risk (Retterstol, 1978; Saugstad and Ödegard, 1979). In most studies of inpatients from selected hospitals, these requirements have been neglected, and the trend towards increasing suicide rates found in them cannot safely be attributed to changes in the hospital regime. This requires the reliable registration of all suicide attempts, and account must also be taken of the trend towards more severe disturbance in patients readmitted as a consequence of shorter previous admissions.

The linkage of case registers with twin and adoption registers has proved extremely useful for population-genetic research on schizophrenia. The elimination of selection biases in identifying twin samples resulted in considerably lower and fairly consistent transnational concordance rates for monozygotic and dizygotic twins (Kringlen, 1987). Studies of adopted persons furnished the precondition for an alternative evaluation of the relative strength of genes and environment in the familial transmission of schizophrenic disorder (Kringlen, 1987). Studies based on linkage of psychiatric case registers with other health information systems like cancer and myocardial infarction registers have to overcome great practical and methodical difficulties. The pioneer work performed in the Oxford record linkage study (Kendell et al., 1981), in which a broad strategy for detecting various risks of somatic disorders was applied, has been successfully continued in a study linking a psychiatric and an obstetric register (Kendell, 1986), and in the transnational WHO study on the incidence of cancer in patients diagnosed as schizophrenic (Dupont et al., 1986). The findings reveal the great potential of these promising efforts. Although most methodological requirements were met, the Danish data show lower cancer rates in schizophrenic patients than in a control population, whereas the Japanese data show the opposite (Nakane and Ohta, 1986). The very large samples needed for studying associations with rare risks constitutes a central problem in schizophrenia research.

Conclusion

Case registers are an excellent tool for epidemiological and evaluative research. Although they require generous financial provision and staffing, case registers are less costly and more practicable for answering many questions than are single studies. This is particularly the case for long-term epidemiology, for example, the recording of indicators of psychiatric morbidity in relation to temporal change in demographic population factors. The same is true of monitoring of utilization, functions, effectiveness, and cost of mental health services and of creating the prerequisites for detailed analyses of these issues. The closer the lifetime utilization rate of the affected population is to 100 percent, the greater the predictive power of a case register.

In many areas of research the opportunities provided by case registers are still at an early stage of development. By setting up case registers and improving methods of data evaluation, we may expect essential knowledge of morbidity and the distribution patterns of mental disorders, of their natural course, of triggering factors and risks of sequelae, and finally of the influence of treatment and care on these variables. For this reason, case register research must be furthered, new registers should be set up and existing ones be enlarged—in spite of the frequently uttered concern that the confidentiality of patient data may not be sufficiently safeguarded. In fact, no single breach of confidentiality to the detriment of patients by any of the numerous case registers has even been known. Strict supervision measures, special training of personnel, and diligent regulations for ensuring data confidentiality provide adequate safeguards against misuse of the confidential information stored in case registers (MRC, 1985).

Despite these arguments, the attitude of the informed public and of politicians in many countries does not favor the existence of psychiatric case registers. In the Federal Republic of Germany all case-related disease registers became illegal following the new data protection law. We were thus forced in 1981 to close the case register at the Central Institute of Mental Health (Häfner and Pfeifer-Kurda, 1986). A similar position in Iceland has been described by Helgason (1986). On several occasions, Wing has argued that case registers are indispensable tools for research, that data confidentiality can be ensured by appropriate safeguards, and that—considering the significance of case registers as instruments for developing better solutions to the health problems of the population—the prohibition or closure of properly run case registers can be seen as unethical (Wing 1986, 1990). One can only hope that this view prevails.

References

Angermeyer, M.C. and Kuhn L. (1988) Gender differences in age at onset of schizophrenia. An overview, *European Archives of Psychiatry and Neurological Sciences,* 237, pp. 351–364.

Astrup, C. (1982) The increase of mental disorders. Unpublished manuscript from the National Case Register of Mental Disorder, Gaustad Hospital, Oslo, Norway.

Bennett, D.H., Birley, J.L.T., Hailey, A.M. and Wing, J.K. (1972). Non-residential services for the mentally ill, 1964–71, in: Wing, J.K. & Hailey, A.M. (eds.) *Evaluating a community psychiatric service. The Camberwell Register 1964–71,* pp. 141–158 (London, New York, Toronto, Oxford University Press).

Bickel, H. (1987) Psychiatric illness and mortality among the elderly: findings of an epidemiological study, in: Cooper, B. (ed.) *Psychiatric epidemiology,* pp. 191–211 (London, Croom Helm).

Boyd, J.H., Pulver, A.E. and Stewart, W. (1986) Season of birth: schizophrenia and bipolar disorder, *Schizophrenia Bulletin,* 12, pp. 173–185.

Brenner, M.H. (1973). *Mental illness and the economy* (Cambridge, Mass., Harvard University Press).

Cooper, B. (1986) Mental illness, disability and social conditions among old people in Mannheim, in: Hafner, H., Moschel, G. and Sartorius, N. (eds.) *Mental health in the elderly,* pp. 35–67 (Berlin-Heidelberg-New York-Tokyo, Springer).

Dalén, P. (1988) Schizophrenia, season of birth, and maternal age, *British Journal of Psychiatry,* 153, pp. 727–733.

Dupont, A. (1981) Definition and identification of severe mental retardation, in: Cooper, B. (ed.) *Assessing the handicaps and needs of mentally retarded children,* pp. 3–12 (London, Academic Press).

Dupont, A., Möller Jenson, O., Strömgren, E. and Jablensky, A. (1986) Incidence of cancer in patients diagnosed as schizophrenic in Denmark, in: ten Horn, G. H.M.M., Giel, R., Gubinat, W.H. and Henderson, J.H. (eds.) *Psychiatric case registers in public health. A worldwide inventory 1960–1985,* pp. 229–239 (Amsterdam-New York-Oxford, Elsevier).

Fryers, T. (1979) Estimation of need on the basis of case register studies: British case register data, in: Häfner, H. (ed.) *Estimating needs for mental health care,* pp. 52–63 (Berlin-Heidelberg-New York: Springer).

Fryers, T. (1986) Administrative and operational research using a psychiatric case register, in: ten Horn, G.H.M.M., Giel, R., Gulbinat, W.H. and Henderson, J.H. (eds.) *Psychiatric case registers in public health,* pp. 101–114 (Amsterdam-New York-Oxford, Elsevier).

Gibbons, J.L., Jennings, C. and Wing, J.K. (eds.) *Psychiatric care in 8 register areas: statistics from eight psychiatric case registers in Great Britain 1976–1981* (Fareham, Hants, Southampton Psychiatric Case Register, Knowle Hospital).

Haas, St., Pfeifer-Kurda, M. and Häfner, H. (1982) Community mental health care for the elderly, in: The Finnish Association for Mental Health (ed.) Book of Proceedings I. 3rd European Symposium on Social Psychiatry, Hanasaari, Sept. 12–15, 1982, pp. 233–251.

Häfner, H. (1980) Psychiatrische Morbidität von Gastarbeitern in Mannheim. Epidemiologische Analyse einer Inanspruchnahmepopulation, *Der Nervenarzt,* 51, pp. 672–683.

Häfner, H. (1985) Are mental disorders increasing over time?, *Psychopathology*, 18, pp. 66–81.

Häfner, H. (1987a) Do we still need beds for psychiatric patients? An analysis of changing patterns of mental health care, *Acta Psychiatrica Scandinavica*, 75, pp. 113–126.

Häfner, H. (1987b) Epidemiology of schizophrenia, in: Häfner, H., Gattaz, W.F. and Janzarik, W. (eds.) *Search for the Causes of Schizophrenia*, pp. 47–74 (Berlin-Heidelberg-Springer).

Häfner, H. (1988) Macht Arbeitslosigkeit krank? Ein Überblick über den Wissensstand zu den Zusammenhängen zwischen Erwerbslosigkeit, körperlichen und seelischen Gesundheitsrisiken, *Fortschritte der Neurologie und Psychiatrie*, 56, pp. 326–343.

Häfner, H. and Bickel, H. (1989) Physical morbidity and mortality in psychiatric patients, in: Öhmann, R., Freeman, H.L., Franck Holmkvist, A. and Nielzen, S. (eds.) *Interaction Between Mental and Physical Illness*, pp. 29–47 (Berlin-Heidelberg, Springer).

Häfner, H., Haas, S., Pfeifer-Kurda, M., Eichhorn, S. and Michitsuji, S. (1987) Abnormal seasonality of schizophrenic births. A specific finding?, *European Archives of Psychiatry and Neurological Sciences*, 236, pp. 333–342.

Haäfner, H. and an der Heiden, W. (1983) The impact of a changing system of care on patterns of utilization by schizophrenics, *Social Psychiatry*, 18, pp. 153–160.

Häfner, H. and an der Heiden, W. (1986a) Organisation, Wirksamkeit und Wirtschaftlichkeit komplementärer Versorgung Schizophrener, *Der Nervenarzt*, 57, pp. 214–226.

Häfner, H. and an der Heiden, W. (1986b) The contribution of European case registers to research on schizophrenia. *Schizophrenia Bulletin*, 12, pp. 26–51.

Hafner, H. and an der Heinden, W. (1989) Effectiveness and cost of community care for schizophrenic patients. *Hospital and Community Psychiatry*, 40, pp. 59–63.

Häfner, H. and Pfeifer-Kurda, M. (1986) The impact of data protection laws on the Mannheim case register, in: ten Horn, G.H.M.M., Giel, R., Gulbinat, W.H. and Henderson, J.H. (eds.) *Psychiatric case registers in public health: A worldwide inventory 1960–1985*, pp. 366–371 (Amsterdam-New York-Oxford, Elsevier).

Häfner, H., Riecher, A., Maurer, K., Löffler, W., Munk-Jörgensen, P. and Strömgren, E. (1989) How does gender influence age at first hospitalization for schizophrenia? A transnational case register study. *Psychological Medicine 19*, 903–918.

Häfner, H., Veiel, H.O.F. and Welz, R. (1988) Epidemiology of suicide and attempted suicide. *Psychiatria Fennica:* yearbook Ed.-in-Chief: Achte, K., Helsinki, 19, pp. 103–123.

Harrison, G., Ineichen B., Smith, J. and Morgan, H.G. (1984) Psychiatric Hospital admissions in Bristol: II. Social and clinical aspects of compulsory admission. *British Journal of Psychiatry*, 145, pp. 605–611.

Harrison, G., Owens, D., Holton, A., Neilson, D. and Boot, D. (1988) A prospective study of severe mental disorder in Afro-Caribbean patients, *Psychological Medicine*, 18, pp. 643–657.

Helgason, L. (1977) Psychiatric services and mental illness in Iceland. *Acta Psychiatrica Scandinavica*, Supplementum 268.

Helgason, T. (1975) *Studies on prevalence and incidence of mental disorders in Iceland with a health questionnaire and a psychiatric case register*, pp. 172–183 (Tromsö Seminar in Medicine, Tromsö).

Henderson, A.S. (1983) The coming epidemic of dementia, *Australian and New Zealand Journal of Psychiatry,* 17, pp. 117–127.

Henderson, A.S. (1986a) The epidemiology of Alzheimer's disease, *British Medical Bulletin,* 42, pp. 3–10.

Henderson, A.S. (1986b) Epidemiology of mental illness, in: Häfner, H., Moschel, G. and Sartorius, N. (eds.) *Mental health in the elderly. A review of the present state of research,* pp. 29–34 (Berlin-Heidelberg-New York-Tokyo, Springer).

ten Horn, G.H.M.M., Giel, R., Gulbinat, W.H. and Henderson J.H. (eds.) (1986) *Psychiatric Case Registers in Public Health: A Worldwide Inventory 1960–1985* (Amsterdam-New York-Oxford, Elsevier).

ten Horn, G.M.H.H. (1986) Inventory of existing psychiatric case registers 1960–1985, in: ten Horn, G.M.H.H., Giel, R., Gulbinat, W.H. and Henderson, J.H. (eds.) *Psychiatric Case Registers in Public Health: A Worldwide Inventory 1960–1985,* pp. 384–426 (Amsterdam-New York-Oxford, Elsevier).

Ineichen, B., Harrison, G., Morgan, H.G. (1984) Psychiatric hospital admissions in Bristol: I. Geographical and ethnic factors. *British Journal of Psychiatry,* 145, pp. 600–604.

Jablensky, A. (1984) Gli studi trans-culturali dell'Organizzazione Mondiale della Sanita sulla schizofrenia: implicazioni teoriche e pratiche, in: Faccincani, C., Fiorio, R., Mignolli, G. and Tansella, M. (eds.) *Le psicosi schizofreniche,* pp. 37–64 (Bologna, Patron).

Jablensky, A., Sartorius, N., Ernberg, G., Anker, M., Korten, A., Cooper, J.E. and Day, R. (1990) Schizophrenia: manifestations, incidence, and course in different cultures. *Psychological Medicine* (in press).

Kastrup, M. (1988) *Epidemiological and therapeutical research in relation to psychiatric registration.* Paper presented at the Fourth European Congress of the Association of European Psychiatrists in Strasbourg, Oct. 19-22, 1988.

Kendell, R.E. (1986) Linkage with an obstetric register, in: ten Horn, G.H.M. M., Giel, R., Gulbinat, W.H. and Henderson, J.H. (eds.) *Psychiatric case registers in public health. A worldwide inventory 1960-1985,* pp. 224–228 (Amsterdam-New York-Oxford, Elsevier). 78–88

Kendell, R.E., Rennie, D., Clarke, J.A., and Dean, C. (1981) The social and obstetric correlates of psychiatric admission in the puerperium. *Psychological Medicine,* 11, pp. 341–350.

Kramer, M. (1986) Use of psychiatric case registers in planning for health for all for the year 2000, in: ten Horn, G.H.M.M., Giel, R., Gulbinat, W.H. and Henderson, J.H. (eds.) *Psychiatric case registers in public health. A worldwide inventory 1960-1985,* pp. 78–88 (Amsterdam-New York-Oxford, Elsevier).

Kringlen, E. (1987) Contribution of genetic studies on schizophrenia, in: Häfner, H., Gattaz, W.F. and Janzarik, W. (eds.) *Search for the causes of schizophrenia,* pp. 123–142 (Berlin-Heidelberg-New York-London-Paris-Tokyo, Springer).

Leff, J. (1988) Evaluating the run-down of two large psychiatric hospitals and the build-up of new community services. Paper presented at the EMRC Workshop on "Reduction of social disablement in severe mental disorders. A rational basis for community care?", London, 10–11 October 1988.

Leff, J. and Vaughn, C. (1972) Psychiatric patients in contact and out of contact with services: a clinical and social assessment, in: Wing, J.K. and Hailey, A.M. (eds.) *Evaluating a community psychiatric service. The Camberwell Register 1964–71,* pp. 259–274 (London-New York-Toronto, Oxford University Press).

May, A.R. (1976) *Mental health services in Europe. A review of data collected in response to a WHO questionnaire* (Geneva, World Health Organization).

Nakane, F. and Ohta, Y. (1986) The example of linkage with a cancer register, in: ten Horn, G.H.M.M., Giel, R., Gulbinat, W.H. and Henderson, J.H. (eds.) *Psychiatric case registers in public health. A worldwide inventory 1960-1985,* pp. 240–245 (Amsterdam-New York-Oxford, Elsevier).

Nuallain, M.N., O'Hare, A., Walsh, D. (1986) Clinical and instrumental diagnosis in schizophrenia compared, in: ten Horn, G.H.M.M., Giel, R., Gulbinat, W.H. and Henderson, J.H. (eds.) *Psychiatric case registers in public health. A worldwide inventory 1960-1985,* pp. 179–185 (Amsterdam-New York-Oxford, Elsevier).

Ödegard, Ö. (1932) Immigration and insanity: a study of mental disease among the Norwegian-born population in Minnesota, *Acta Psychiatrica et Neurologica Scandinavica,* Supplementum 4, pp. 1–206.

Ödegard, Ö. (1936) Emigration and mental health, *Mental Hygiene,* 20, pp. 546–553.

Ödegard, Ö. (1946) Marriage and mental disease, *Journal of Mental Science,* 92, pp. 35–49.

Ödegard, Ö. (1971) Hospitalized psychoses in Norway: time trends 1926-1965, *Social Psychiatry,* 6, pp. 753–58.

Ödegard, Ö. (1972) Epidemiology of the psychoses, in: Kisker, K.P., Meyer, J.E., Müller, C. and Strömgren, E. (eds.) *Psychiatrie der Gegenwart,* 2nd edit, vol. II/1, *Klinische Psychiatrie I.* pp. 213–258 (Berlin-Heidelberg-New York, Springer).

Ödegard, Ö. (1973) Norwegian emigration, re-emigration and internal migration, in: Zwingmann, C. and Pfister-Ammende, M. (eds.) *Uprooting and after. . . . ,* pp. 161–177. (Berlin-Heidelberg-New York, Springer).

Olbrich, R. and Maurer, K. (1988) Zur 10. Revision der Internationalen Klassifikation der Krankheiten (ICD), *Zeitschrift für Nervenheilkunde,* 7, pp. 139–141.

Retterstöl, N. (1979) Suicide in psychiatric hospitals in Norway, *Psychiatria Fennica,* vol. 1978, Supplementum, pp. 89–92.

Sartorius, N., Jablensky, A., Korten, A., Ernberg, G., Anker, M., Cooper, J.E. and Day, R. (1986) Early manifestations and first-contact incidence of schizophrenia in different cultures, *Psychological Medicine,* 16, pp. 909–928.

Saugstad, L. and Ödegard, Ö. (1979) Mortality in psychiatric hospitals in Norway 1950-1974, *Acta Psychiatrica Scandinavica,* 59, pp. 431–447.

Schmidtke, A. and Häfner, H. (1988) The Werther effect after television films: new evidence for an old hypothesis, *Psychological Medicine,* 18, pp. 665–676.

Torrey, E.F. (1980) *Schizophrenia and Civilization* (New York, Aronson).

Ugelstad, E. (1978) *Psykiatriske Langtidspasienter i Psykiatriske Sykehus—Nye Behandlingsforsok* (Oslo, Universitetsforlaget).

Weeke, A. and Strömgren, E. (1978) Fifteen years later. A comparison of patients in Danish psychiatric institutions in 1957, 1962, 1967, and 1972, *Acta Psychiatrica Scandinavica,* 57, pp. 129–144.

Welz, R. (1979) *Selbstmordversuche in städtischen Lebensumwelten. Eine epidemiologische, ökologische und mehrebenenanalytische Untersuchung über Häufigkeit und regionale Verteilung von Selbstmordversuchen in Mannheim* (Weinheim, Beltz-Verlag).

Wing, J.K. (1972a) Principles of evaluation, in: Wing, J.K. and Hailey, A.M. (eds.) *Evaluating a community psychiatric service. The Camberwell Register 1964–71,* pp. 11–39 (London-New York-Toronto, Oxford University Press).

Wing, J.K. (1972b) The Camberwell Register and the development of evaluative research, in: Wing, J.K. and Hailey, A.M. (eds.) *Evaluating a community psychiatric service. The Camberwell Register 1964–71,* pp. 3–9 (London-New York-Toronto, Oxford University Press).

Wing, J.K. (1973) Principles of evaluation, in: Wing, J.K. and Häfner, H. (eds.) *Roots of evaluation,* pp. 3–12 (London-New York-Toronto, Oxford University Press).

Wing, J.K. (1986) Safeguarding the patient and safeguarding research: the U.K. data protection act, in: ten Horn, G.H.M.M., Giel, R., Gulbinat, W.H. and Henderson, J.H. (eds.) *Psychiatric case registers in public health. A worldwide inventory 1960-1985,* pp. 376–380 (Amsterdam-New York-Oxford, Elsevier).

Wing, J.K. (1988) Measurement of need for care and services. Paper presented at the EMRC-Workshop on "Reduction of social disablement in severe mental disorders. A rational basis for community care?", London, 10–11 October 1988.

Wing, J.K. and Hailey, A.M. (1972) *Evaluating a community psychiatric service. The Camberwell Register 1964–71* (London-New York-Toronto, Oxford University Press).

Wing, L. (1971) Severely retarded children in a London area: prevalence and provision of services, *Psychological Medicine,* 2, pp. 405–415.

Wing, L. (1981) A schedule for deriving profiles of handicaps in mentally retarded children, in: Cooper, B. (ed.) *Assessing the handicaps and needs of mentally retarded children,* pp. 133–141 (London, Academic Press).

Wing, L., Corbett, J., Pool, D., Wollen, W. and Yeates, S. (1972) Services for mentally retarded children and adults, in: Wing, J.K. and Hailey, A.M. (eds.) *Evaluating a community psychiatric service. The Camberwell Register 1964–71,* pp. 359–403 (London-New York-Toronto, Oxford University Press).

16

The Evaluation of Reprovision for Psychiatric Hospitals

Julian Leff

Introduction

The Victorians invested large amounts of money in a program of building psychiatric hospitals which began in the middle of the 19th Century and continued into the early years of the 20th century. Most of them were built on large tracts of land outside towns or in the depths of the country, and were intended to be virtually self-sufficient. Many had their own dairy farms, vegetable gardens, water supply, laundries and other facilities required for the support of a thousand or more patients and the staff caring for them. The Victorians were proud of their achievement in providing a public service to replace the private madhouses which had become a scandal.

Unfortunately, once the facilities became available they began to be used as places for the permanent disposal of individuals who were out of step with society, such as unmarried pregnant women, as well as providing long-term asylum for the severely mentally ill. As a result, the growth of their resident population rapidly outstripped the number of places for which they had been designed. For example, Friern Hospital in North London had been built in 1851 for one thousand patients. By 1953 it reached its peak population of nearly 2,400. This gross overcrowding produced slum conditions, with beds forming long lines in spaces that had been intended for recreational activities. It was about this time that books began to appear attacking conditions in psychiatric hospitals and questioning their therapeutic functions. Barton's book, *Institutional Neurosis,* was published in 1959, and Goffman's *Asylums* in 1961.

The national peak in psychiatric bed occupancy was reached in 1954, and since then there has been a steady decline. In some hospitals, the peak occurred earlier; in Claybury Hospital, for instance, it was in 1951. Such forerunners of the national trend demonstrate that the turnaround was not due to the introduction of chlorpromazine, which came into general use in 1955, although it certainly helped to accelerate the move into the community.

Early Research on Psychiatric Institutions

From its earliest days, there was a strong interest in the Social Psychiatry Unit in the nature of psychiatric institutions and their effects on the inmates. The increasing emphasis on rehabilitation of long-stay patients was studied by Wing and Freudenberg (1961). They carried out a controlled trial of active supervision in a workshop setting, and found that not only did patients respond by increasing their output, but that immobility, mannerisms, and restlessness decreased. It was noteworthy that the improvements evident in patients' behavior in the workshops were not seen on the wards. This finding that behavioral changes in schizophrenia are situation-specific presaged the results of behavior therapy introduced many years later.

This early research was followed by a much more ambitious study of 273 long-stay schizophrenic patients in three psychiatric hospitals by Wing and Brown, (1970). They measured the degree of social deprivation in each hospital by a variety of factors, including the amount of time patients spent doing absolutely nothing. They also assessed the negative symptoms of each patient, comprising social withdrawal, flatness of affect, and poverty of speech. They found that there was a strong association between social deprivation and the negative symptoms of schizophrenia, and that the hospital with the most stimulating social environment contained patients with the lowest level of negative symptoms.

During the eight year follow-up period two of the three hospitals showed an initial improvement in the social atmosphere and then a deterioration approximately to the initial level of deprivation. The third hospital continued to improve throughout the eight years. The negative symptoms of the patients in each hospital followed a course which closely paralleled the changes in social environment, whether for better or for worse.

The implication of these two studies that negative symptoms are responsive to the amount of social stimulation present in the environment offers scope to social therapies. However, these findings have not gone unchallenged: in particular, the Northwick Park group headed by Crow maintains that negative symptoms are a manifestation of the brain changes that constitute the schizophrenic pathology, and as such are relatively impervious to manipulation of the social environment. In one study, they found that a sample of 105 schizophrenic patients discharged from hospital five to nine years previously showed a similar level of negative symptoms, as assessed by the Krawiecka scale (Krawiecka et al., 1977), as a sample of 510 chronic schizophrenic inpatients (Johnstone et al., 1981). A much smaller study from India also found negative symptoms to be as common in outpatients as inpatients, although a group of day-patients had lower levels (Mathai and Gopinath, 1985).

The issue remains open of how far the negative symptoms of schizophrenia are induced by institutional practices and to what extent they are a manifestation of irreversible organic cerebral deterioration. This cannot be resolved by cross-sectional studies, but should yield to an experimental approach. A relevant experiment is currently being conducted on a national scale, namely, the run down and closure of a large proportion of the psychiatric hospitals of which the Victorians were so proud. Of course, the politicians involved do not regard this as an experiment, but the lack of any existing evidence for the likely success of this policy makes it imperative that it be considered in this light. Insofar as it is not controlled in the scientific sense, it constitutes a natural experiment, but the breadth of its ambit allows strategies of a scientific nature to be implemented.

Evaluation Strategies

Data collected in order to evaluate a service range from the macrostatistical to the microstatistical. Macrostatistical enquiries are large in scale, but usually limited in depth, while microstatistical studies are small in scale and intense. In macrostatistical studies, data are collected from agencies rather than by interviewing respondents, while the reverse is true of microstatistical studies. An advantage of macrostatistical studies is that the data are relatively easy to collect; however, the material may not be of high reliability since it is derived from secondary sources, for example hospital returns. The collection of data from microstatistical studies is much more arduous, but the effort is compensated for by the high reliability that can be achieved.

The evaluation of a service may be centered on the facilities provided, on the clients receiving the service, or on both. Some examples of the various possible types of evaluation follow.

Macrostatistical Facility-Centered

The number of facilities of different types in a catchment area can be listed, and their distribution between statutory, voluntary, and private organizations. Whether they are based in a hospital or in the community can be recorded. Their accessibility can be expressed in terms of their distance from the catchment population, their hours of opening, the paths of referral, and the refusal rate for referrals. The treatment in a facility can be described in terms of their orientation (e.g., pharmacological, social) and the specific activities offered (e.g., behavioral programs, group therapy).

The number of staff in a facility can be recorded and their various disciplines and the rate of each type per population base. Their main place of work can be determined (e.g., hospital, community facility, clients' homes) and the size of their caseload.

Microstatistical Facility-Centered

A detailed study of one or more particular facilities could determine staff views of the function of the facility. There may well be differences of opinion between staff members, and between their views and the official policy. Research can be directed at determining whether they actually do what they say they do. This would involve detailed time budgets which record the proportion of time spent on each activity (e.g. treatment, managerial, liaison, travel). Enquiries can be made into staff satisfaction with their training and with their job content and conditions. An objective method of checking this is to record time off through sickness, and turnover of staff.

A more experimental approach can be taken by mounting controlled comparisons of different methods of providing care. It is sometimes possible to include randomization of clients to different forms of care, but usually only when the researcher has control over the services being provided (e.g., Paykel et al., 1982, Leff et al., 1989). Otherwise he or she is bound to meet strong resistance to randomization by the providers of the service. More often researchers have to be content with comparison of facilities that have selected their clients (e.g., a day hospital vs. a day center, crisis intervention vs. an acute admission unit). The main problem with this design is the comparability of clients of the facilities being compared. This can be compensated for to some degree by collecting data on client characteristics and checking for closeness of matching.

Macrostatistical Client-Centered

The distribution of clients between statutory, voluntary, and private agencies can be determined from agency returns. There are problems here in that private facilities may be reluctant to divulge information (money buys confidentiality) and voluntary agencies may not keep records comparable with those of statutory services. For inpatients it should be possible to obtain the number of admissions and discharges per unit time, the average length of stay, the length of any waiting list, and the proportion of involuntary admissions. Diagnosis is usually recorded routinely, but may not be very reliable. For outpatients and day patients, the number and frequency of attendances should be available, and for the former the interval between referral and appointment.

As a general index of psychiatric morbidity, the suicide and attempted suicide rates are often recorded, but surveys are necessary to determine other indices of service failure, such as the proportion of mentally ill among prisoners and vagrants.

In this area of enquiry, case registers are invaluable tools, and the Camberwell Register has been used extensively for evaluative studies (Wing and Hailey, 1972).

Microstatistical Client-Centered

This type of research involves interviews with clients and their carers to determine the clinical state and social disabilities of the clients. Additionally, some attempt needs to be made to measure that elusive concept, quality of life. This can be approached in a number of ways, but should include assessment of the standard of the physical environment, the degree of comfort it affords, the availability of leisure facilities, and the number of restrictions on the clients' freedom of choice. The clients' satisfaction with the service should be determined, and if relatives are involved in client care, their views should also be sought, as well as their subjective and objective burden.

Clients can be followed over time in one facility, or changes in the features listed above can be monitored as clients move from one facility to another. The issue of randomization or some other form of control is as important with this type of research as with the facility-centered work.

Combined Client-and Facility-Centered

One example of this will suffice to convey the kind of research possible. Study of the process of rehabilitation in a specific facility might include assessment of staff attitudes to their training, and client attitudes to community vs. hospital care. The content of rehabilitation programs could be determined and the response of individual client's disabilities to treatment could be measured. The effect on public attitudes to the mentally ill of a new rehabilitation facility in their neighbourhood could be studied.

Economic appraisal

In the current financial climate, it is virtually obligatory to build an economic component into any evaluation of a service. The costing of a service should include direct and indirect (e.g., relatives' contribution) costs, and needs to be appraised in relation to any benefits stemming from the service. There are very complex issues involved, which necessitate collaboration with health economists.

The Friern-Claybury Evaluation

The strategies discussed above were considered in the course of deciding how to evaluate the decision of the North East Thames Regional Health Authority (NETRHA) to close Claybury Hospital and partially close Friern Hospital by 1993. This decision was taken in the summer of 1983, allowing ten years for the closure process. Between them, the two hospitals served nine health districts, which were to be responsible for reproviding the services that would disappear with the hospitals. One of the districts served by Friern, West Haringey, borders the hospital and was considered to be sufficiently close to be allocated one third of the extensive hospital grounds, on which to build the necessary facilities. This innovative plan has been described in detail by Wing and Furlong (1986).

The decision to close the two hospitals was clearly in line with long-standing government policy, which had been enunciated in the Mental Health Act of 1959, and reiterated in a number of subsequent White Papers. Although an identical policy had been vigorously pursued in the USA and Italy, neither in those countries nor in the U.K. had a scientific evaluation of the closure of a psychiatric hospital been conducted. The nearest to it was the Worcester Development Project (Wing and Bennett, 1988) which monitored the rundown of Powick Hospital to closure and the establishment of community facilities. However, this research began when the rundown was already well advanced and was consequently limited in scope. A relevant study of the closure of a mental handicap hospital had been mounted in the Unit (see Chap. 17) which provided a useful precedent, but the problems of the psychiatrically ill are qualitatively different, and it is not possible to extrapolate findings from one type of hospital to the other. These arguments persuaded NETRHA to set up a research group, the Team for the Assessment of Psychiatric Services (TAPS), in 1985. Contributions to funding were also obtained from the Department of Health and the Kings Fund.

The first issue facing TAPS was to decide on the priorities for the research, since the potential scope of the project was almost limitless. The populations of the two hospitals were divided reasonably clearly into short-stay patients passing through the acute admission wards, demented patients occupying psychogeriatric beds, and long-stay non-demented patients. The priorities of these groups for reprovision had in fact been set by NETHRA. It was a policy decision to retain the acute admission wards until the last phase of closure, in order to avoid an atmosphere of stasis in the hospitals, which would further lower morale. It was also apparent that it would take some years to provide alternatives for the psychogeriatric patients. The long-stay non-demented population therefore became the first priority for research.

Since we were starting with a cohort of patients who needed to be followed through a change of facilities, this was client-centered rather than facility-centered research. However, it was recognized that some evaluation of the facilities reprovided in the community might also be feasible. Randomisation was considered but rejected on two counts. First, NETHRA had enunciated the policy that patients should move into the community with their friends, and secondly it would have been unacceptable to the community-based teams who were selecting patients for discharge. We soon realized that even the least intrusive research strategy would represent a burden on staff who were severely demoralized by the closure decision. We therefore chose a matched case-control design, which had already been successfully employed in the study of the closure of Darenth Park mental handicap hospital. The aim would be to match as closely as possible each patient being discharged with two others who were likely to stay for at least a year. By finding two matches, we would increase the likelihood that one at least would still be in hospital a year later, when a follow-up was planned. We anticipated that as the pool of remaining patients progressively shrank, we would sooner or later run out of matches. Each discharged patient would then have to act as their own control, a less satisfactory strategy.

In practice for reasons we will explore later, it was rarely possible to find more than one close match for the first year's cohort of leavers, and a small proportion of patients could only be matched very approximately. However, as the aim of matching was to create two *groups* which were closely similar, a small number of mismatched individuals was not disastrous. However, there was another problem generated by the case-control design, and this would also have arisen with random assignment. It was the assumption that the hospital environment was static. The purpose behind the chosen design was to control for the passage of time. Improvements or deteriorations in the patients' condition over a follow-up period might simply reflect the natural history of their illness. The matched patients were intended to control for this. However, they were living in a hospital which was undergoing dramatic changes, so that it would be naive to assume that we were observing the *natural* history of their illness.

It was evident that two major opposing trends were operating in Friern and Claybury Hospitals. On the one hand staff morale had received a hard knock: it became difficult to recruit nursing staff, who saw no future in the posts available. Furthermore, the fabric of the buildings was deteriorating, since there would be no further investment in even essential repairs. What is known as planning blight had cast its shadow over the two hospitals. On the other hand, the plan to discharge all surviving long-stay patients spurred staff on to intensive efforts to rehabilitate them. New wards were organized with the aim of improving the behavioral problems of particularly difficult patients.

It is possible that these two opposing trends might cancel each other out, but if not then any change recorded in the leavers would have to be measured against the shifting baseline of the matched patients who remained.

Choice of Instruments

In selecting a batch of assessment instruments, we had to consider carefully the outcome criteria of greatest relevance to the question which initiated the research; does the policy of hospital closure benefit the patients? It was obvious that we needed to assess the mental state and social disabilities of the patients. We also felt that we should measure their physical ill-health for the following reasons. First, we knew this to be an elderly population with a mean age close to 60. Secondly, their physical health had been closely monitored by the nursing staff and by junior psychiatrists who acted as their general practitioners. We were concerned that, once in the community, patients might not receive the same careful attention to their physical health. Our anxieties had been raised by several preventable deaths from physical illness of discharged long-stay patients.

In addressing the issue of quality of life, we saw the imperative need to ask patients their opinion about the care they received, and to assess the degree of restrictiveness of their environment. Finally, we were concerned to chart the social networks of patients, partly to check whether they were indeed being placed in the community in company with their friends, and partly to determine whether they would develop social links with individuals in the community.

We will describe the instruments chosen for each of these areas of enquiry.

Personal Data and Psychiatric History Schedule (PDPH). This schedule was designed to collect basic data on patients' demographic characteristics, including ethnicity, and factual information about length of stay and previous admissions. The data were collected partly from casenotes and partly from staff. Each patient's primary diagnosis was derived, wherever possible, from the casenotes. However, this had often changed several times in the course of a long admission. Where there was doubt, the patient's consultant was asked to provide a definitive diagnosis.

Present State Examination (PSE). In view of the prominent negative symptoms to be expected in this population, we first used the Krawiecka scale (Krawiecka et al., 1977) in a pilot study. However, in our hands this did not yield satisfactory levels of inter-rater reliability. We therefore chose to use the PSE, particularly as it has been employed in so many studies, both national and international. We were conscious of the problem posed by patients who deny psychotic symptoms in response to the PSE, but are well known by nursing staff to harbor florid delusions or regularly to converse with auditory hallucinations. To accommodate this, we added two items to the PSE which record information from the nursing staff about active psychotic symptoms when the patient denies them.

Physical Health Index (PH). We did not have enough medically qualified research staff to examine each patient physically. Instead we derived information from casenotes and ward staff. The information was collected with respect to seven bodily systems, for each of which two ratings were made: the level of disability and the level of medical and nursing care received. In addition, problems with incontinence, immobility, and dyskinesia were noted, as these are likely to hinder community placement.

Social Behavior Schedule (SBS). We used this schedule, developed in the Unit by Wykes and Sturt (1986) and of established reliability. However, when we began interviewing discharged patients with it, we became aware of some gaps in the schedule. These were mostly to do with areas of self-care, which patients were allowed little or no opportunity to exercise in hospital. We needed to develop a supplementary schedule to cover these areas, but this could not be given to all patients in the hospital cohort, because of the stage at which the deficiency in the SBS was noticed. The additional schedule is known as the Basic Everyday Living Skills (BELS), now in a final form after piloting, but currently undergoing reliability tests. Both schedules rely on information given by staff.

Environmental Index (EI). This schedule was developed from instruments existing in the Unit, and measures the degree of restrictiveness of the patient's environment. In that respect, it reflects institutional practices. We added some questions on the accessibility of a variety of amenities which would be important for patients in the community. These include shops, laundrettes, pubs, parks, and day centers or day hospitals.

Patient Attitude Questionnaire (PAQ). Patients are asked what they like or dislike about their current caring environment. There are also questions about their desire to leave hospital or to stay, and about where they would prefer to live.

Social Network Schedule (SNS). We constructed this questionnaire from scratch, as nothing suitable existed. The enquiry begins with the construction of a time budget that provides the context of activity within which social contacts are made. All the people named by the patient constitute his social universe. Within this he is asked to identify which individuals he talks to regularly, who would be missed if not seen, whom he would visit if they were separated, who is considered to be a friend, and whom he could confide in.

Initially we employed two versions of this schedule, one for patients and one for staff to give information about patients. It soon became evident that staff overestimated the number of friends patients had on the ward and knew little or nothing about social contacts off the ward. Consequently we stopped collecting these data from staff, even though it meant having no SNS information for patients who refused or were unable to complete the interview.

Use of Community Facilities. Information on the use of community facilities, such as day centers, CPNs and GPs was collected for discharged patients to enable the economists to calculate the cost of all the services which were provided to replace the psychiatric hospital.

Collection of the full batch of information occupied about half a day per patient. We began by drawing up a list of patients in the two hospitals who met the criteria for inclusion in the cohort, namely a continuous stay in hospital of more than one year, and no evidence of dementia if aged over sixty-five. We included all patients under sixty-five even if they had dementia, since they would be considered for reprovision alongside the non-demented. The cohort comprised about nine hundred patients at the start of assessments in August 1985, but attrition occurred through the death of more than one hundred of the older patients before they could be interviewed. Assessments were carried out on a total of 770 patients, of which 373 were in Friern (F) and 397 in Claybury (C), and took two years to complete. The cleaning of data and their analysis were also mammoth tasks, as we collected more than five hundred bits of information on each patient.

Material for the population as a whole is not very meaningful, since as yet no comparable data from other psychiatric hospitals have been analysed, though several surveys using TAPS schedule are in progress. Therefore we will present here a comparison of the patients from the two hospitals, summarizing the analysis of data from each schedule in turn.

Comparison of Patient Cohorts from Friern and Claybury Hospitals

PDPH: There were no significant differences in the proportion of men (F.57 percent, C.56 percent), the unmarried (F.66 percent, C.75 percent), or the modal age (F.60-65, C.60-65). When length of stay was analysed in 10-year bands, there was no difference between Friern and Claybury Hospitals. However, following the ascertainment of the baseline cohort of patients on August 1, 1985, we continued to monitor patients who subsequently met our inclusion criteria by remaining in hospital more than one year. We found that patients were accumulating much more rapidly at Friern than at Claybury Hospital. This observation prompted us to examine the number of baseline patients with a one-to-five year duration of stay. It emerged that there were 101 (13 percent) of these in the Friern sample compared with sixty-five (8 percent) in the Claybury sample (p = 0.001). This suggests that the excessive accumulation of patients in Friern Hospital has been occurring from around 1980. This clearly merits further investigation.

There was no difference between the two hospitals in the proportion of patients admitted involuntarily, or currently on a section: 7 percent or less in each hospital. The distribution of number of previous admissions was very similar for the two hospitals.

Schizophrenia was the primary diagnosis for 81 percent of patients in both samples, and neurosis or personality disorder for 4 percent of both. Affective psychosis was diagnosed in a very similar proportion (F.6 percent, C.7 percent), as was organic brain disease (F.3 percent, C.2 percent). The virtually identical distribution of diagnoses in both hospitals is remarkable considering the unreliability of psychiatric diagnosis and the number of clinicians involved in this judgement.

PSE. The full interview can only be conducted with the cooperation of the patient. In the case of mute or uncooperative patients, the sections dealing with observations of behavior, affect, and speech can be filled in. In these instances, the interview is rated as seriously inadequate. This rating was made on a large proportion of patients (F.33 percent, C.25 percent, p = 0.014). The Catego program can be applied to the PSE data to generate classes, which are equivalent to tentative cross-sectional diagnoses (Wing et al., 1974). As with casenote diagnosis, the two hospital populations showed an almost identical distribution of Catego Classes. A broad diagnosis of schizophrenia (Class S+, S?, P+, P?, O+) was assigned to 35 percent of Friern patients and 37 percent of Claybury patients, while doubtful schizophrenia (Class O?) was given to 29 percent of Friern and 26 percent of Claybury patients.

Looking at individual symptoms, delusions were detected in one third of patients in both hospitals, and hallucinations in one quarter. The staff were aware of another sixty-four patients at Friern and 70 at Claybury Hospital who experienced delusions and/or hallucinations which were not detected by the PSE. Florid symptoms were common in patients who had stayed more than 20 years in hospital (delusions—F.26 percent, C.28 percent, hallucinations—F.17 percent, C.20 percent), giving little support to the notion of "burn-out."

PH. For none of the bodily systems did the level of disability differ between the two hospitals. The same was true for the level of medical and nursing care received, with one exception; a higher proportion (18 percent) of Friern patients received daily medication with supervision for gastrointestinal complaints than of Claybury patients (10 percent, $p = 0.001$). Incontinence of urine and/or faeces was significantly ($p < 0.001$) more common in Friern patients (23 percent) than in Claybury patients (12 percent), as was dyskinesia (F.12 percent, C.5 percent, $p < 0.001$). However, the difference in immobility in the two populations was not significant (F.10 percent, C.9 percent).

SBS: Of the twenty specific items of behavior in this schedule, the two cohorts of patients differed significantly on only two: concentration (F.42 percent, C.30 percent, $p < 0.01$) and oddity of speech (F.14 percent, C.25 percent, $p < 0.01$). When the items were ranked in order of frequency, the similarity between the two populations was remarkable. The rank order correlation was 0.93. The commonest problem in both samples was hygiene, affecting more than half, while the least common was suicidal ideas, affecting 1 percent or less.

EI. There were no significant differences between the two hospitals on six of the seven sections of the questionnaire. Access to amenities was significantly worse in Claybury than Friern Hospital, but when this item was excluded the median scores were almost identical.

PAQ. In both hospitals about one third of the men wanted to stay, one third wanted to leave, and one third were uncertain or failed to respond. Among women the distribution was skewed slightly towards those wishing to leave, but the difference between the sexes was not significant.

SNS. As this is a novel questionnaire, the structure of the responses needs to be analyzed, and this is in progress (Leff et al, 1990). However a first level analysis has been conducted and indicates that the median network size was similar in Friern (eight) and Claybury (nine) Hospitals. For one third of the baseline sample we have no SNS data, and of the remaining two thirds, 22 percent of Friern and 21 percent of Claybury patients identified no friends. In both hospitals a similar proportion included no hospital staff (F.66 percent, C.72 percent), and no relatives (F.76 percent, C.72 percent) in their networks. However, a significantly higher proportion of Claybury patients had no confidants and no active relationships, and would miss no-one. Thus a picture has emerged of more intense social activity in the networks of Friern patients.

Summary of Baseline Data Analysis

The outstanding conclusion from this analysis is the remarkable degree of similarity between the two hospital samples on a wide variety of demographic, historical, clinical, and social measures. This suggests that, despite differences in catchment areas and variations in emphasis on rehabilitation over the years, the same kind of patients tends to be left behind by the process of relocation in the community which has been proceeding for 35 years. This formulation may be supported by surveys of the long-stay non-demented populations of other hospitals which are currently in progress and which employ TAPS schedules. This finding means that in addition to being client-centered, this study will allow the comparison of the different types of facility provided by the nine health authorities involved, since they are attempting to care for very similar populations of patients.

Preliminary Findings from Follow-up

The follow-up data have not been analyzed yet, but we can present figures relating to the size of each year's cohort of discharges and the success of follow-up. In addition, we can also assess how representative each year's cohort of movers is in relation to those remaining in hospital.

The number of movers in the first two years and the success of follow-up are presented in Table 16.1. Follow up data were obtained from at least one informant for 90 percent or more of each cohort.

A period of three and a half years elapsed between the announcement of the closure decision and the discharge of the first patients to move to a special reprovision facility. Thus the first year of movers included in the research project included *no* reprovision patients. These discharges represent the tail end of the process that had been continuing since the early 1950s, and the patients were placed in conventional facilities such as hostels and sheltered housing. The costing of the first year of discharges

TABLE 16.1
One Year Follow-up of First and Second Year Cohorts of Movers

	Discharged	Staff and Patient Interviewed	Staff Only	Outstanding	Died	Not seen
First year cohort discharged September 1985–August 1986						
Friern	32	24	6	—	1	1
Claybury	12	10	0	—	1	1
Second year cohort discharged September 1986–August 1987						
Friern	70	48	4	14	1	7
Claybury	46	37	3	2	1	3

has been completed by the team of health economists, with the finding that the cost of caring for these patients was *less* than that of the matched patients who remained in the two hospitals. It would be grossly misleading to extrapolate this finding to subsequent cohorts, for reasons that will soon become evident.

Of the 116 discharges in the second year's cohort, ten were not traced, including a number who were known to have left the country. Virtually all the rest have now been followed up, and were found to have been placed as follows. Sixty-two went to special projects, forty-two to those organized by health authorities and twenty to those set up by voluntary bodies. The special projects consist of ordinary domestic housing which is bought by the organization concerned, and converted into individual flats or multi-occupancy dwellings. Some are staffed during the day only, while others have 24-hour cover, depending on the level of dependency of the clients. Some staff are psychiatric nurses, while others, particularly in the voluntary schemes, have had no psychiatric training. In schemes with high dependency clients, the staff: client ratio is a high as 1:1, equivalent to an acute admission ward. This level of staffing naturally leads to a much higher cost for community care.

The remainder of the cohort went to a variety of placements. Nineteen were placed in private residential care homes, some run by psychiatric nurses as commercial ventures. Five went to hostels, four to council flats, four to adult fostering, and one or two each to other placements, including part III accommodation and a warden-supervised flat. Only a single patient returned to live with relatives, in this instance parents.

Selection of Movers. We anticipated that patients who were easier to place in the community would be the first to be discharged. We tested this prediction by comparing each year's cohort of movers with those remaining. We have already referred above to the patients accumulating after the baseline census date of August 1, 1985. Table 16.2 shows the numbers of baseline and accumulation patients discharged as part of the first three years' cohorts.

Accumulation patients, who have relatively short lengths of stay, form a small proportion of Claybury movers, but a very large proportion of each year's cohort of movers from Friern Hospital: 22 percent, 46 percent and 49 percent consecutively. This clearly reflects the much greater rate of accumulation at Friern than at Claybury Hospital, to which we have drawn attention above.

Data concerning accumulation patients have still to be entered on the computer. However, since such patients form only a small proportion of Claybury movers, it is legitimate to compare the features of the baseline patients in the first three year cohorts of Claybury movers with those remaining in the hospital.

It can be seen from Table 16.3 that there is a progressive rise in mean age, length of stay, and number of severe problems in social behavior with each successive cohort. This not only supports our hypothesis about selective discharge, but indicates that it will not be until the fourth or fifth year of discharge that the movers will approximate in important features to those remaining in hospital. *The important warning that this sounds is that it would be premature to make definitive judgments about either the costs or the benefits of psychiatric hospital closure until the discharge cohorts become representative of the rump of problematic patients remaining in hospital.* It is the ability of the health authorities to provide for this difficult group of patients that constitutes the crucial test of the policy.

TABLE 16.2
Composition of First Three-Year Cohorts of Movers

	Baseline	Accumulation	Total	
First year				
Friern	25	7	32	
Claybury	12	0	12	
			44	Total first year
Second year				
Friern	38	32	70	
Claybury	43	3	46	
			116	Total second year
Third year				
Friern	32	31	63	
Claybury	50	8	58	
			121	Total third year

TABLE 16.3
Comparison of First Three-Year Cohorts of Movers from Claybury with Those
Remaining in Hospital
(Baseline only)

Mean	First year	Second year	Third year	Remaining
Age (years)	54.2	56.1	59.8	62.7
Length of stay (months)	210.1	245.3	317.5	357.4
No. of severe problems in social behavior	1.6	3.4	4.8	6.4

Conclusions

We are still a long way from the goal of our research, but even the preliminary stage of enumerating the patients in the two psychiatric hospitals and assessing them, has given rise to important and intriguing questions. Eventually, we expect to be able to provide evidence as to whether creating a less institutional environment improves the negative symptoms of schizophrenia. Currently we are spending a lot of time and thought on the analysis of patients' social networks. These are acquiring an increasing salience in our understanding of the patients' subculture in an institution, about which Goffman (1961) had a lot to say. Furthermore, from our impressions of the facilities visited for follow-up interviews, we have formed the opinion that patients' abilities to make social bonds exert a major influence on the success of these novel forms of community care. Analysis of the follow-up data will show whether or not we are right.

There is a tendency to look down on health services research as second class science. It is true that the research worker usually has less control over the situation than in more theoretically based studies. However, not only does the health services researcher enjoy the possibility of influencing the care of patients on a wide scale, sometimes nationally, but important theoretical questions can be satisfactorily addressed.

References

Barton, R. (1959). *Institutional Neurosis*. Bristol: John Wright.
Goffman, I. (1961). *Asylums: Essays on the Social Situation of Mental Patients and Other Inmates*. New York: Anchor Books.
Johnstone, E.C., Cummingham Owens, D.G., Gold, A., Crow, T.J. and MacMillan, J. F. (1981). Institutionalization and the defects of schizophrenia. *British Journal of Psychiatry, 139*, 195–203.
Krawiecka, M., Goldberg, D., and Vaughan, M. (1977). Standardized psychiatric

assessment scale for chronic psychotic patients. *Acta Psychiatrica Scandinavica, 55*, 299–308.

Leff, J., Berkowitz, R., Shavit, N., Strachan, A., Glass, I., and Vaughn, C. (1989). A trial of family therapy v. a relatives group for schizophrenia. *British Journal of Psychiatry, 154*, 58–66.

Leff, J., O'Driscoll, D., Dayson, D., Wills, W. and Anderson, J. (1990) The TAPS Project V: The structure of social-network data obtained from long-stay patients. *British Journal of Psychiatry, 157*.

Mathai, P.J. and Gopinath, P.S. (1985). Deficits of chronic schizophrenia in relation to long-term hospitalisation. *British Journal of Psychiatry, 148*, 509–516.

Paykel, E.S., Mangen, S.P., Griffith, J.H., and Burns, T.P. (1982). Community psychiatric nursing for neurotic patients: a controlled trial. *British Journal of Psychiatry, 140*, 573–581.

Wing, J.K. and Bennett, C. (1988). Long-term Care in the Worcester Development Project. Report on Research.

Wing, J.K. and Brown, G.W. (1970). *Institutionalism and Schizophrenia.* Cambridge: Cambridge University Press.

Wing, J.K. and Freudenberg, R.K. (1961). The response of severely ill chronic schizophrenic patients to social stimulation. *American Journal of Psychiatry, 118*, 311–322.

Wing, J.K. and Furlong, R. (1986). A Haven for the severely disabled within the context of a comprehensive psychiatric community service. *British Journal of Psychiatry, 149*, 449–457.

Wing, J.K. and Hailey, A.M. (eds.). (1972). *Evaluating a Community Psychiatric Service.* London: Oxford University Press.

Wykes, T. and Sturt, E. (1986). The measurement of social behaviour in psychiatric patients: An assessment of the reliability and validity of the SBS schedule: *British Journal of Psychiatry, 148*, 1–11.

17

Closing Darenth Park Hospital for Adults with Mental Handicaps

Lorna Wing

Introduction

The story of the evaluation of the effects on the residents of the closure of Darenth Park mental handicap hospital is presented here as an illustration of the problems encountered in such work and our attempts at solving them. The details of the results and the statistical analyses are available elsewhere (Wing, 1989) and will not be given in this chapter, but the general findings will be discussed in relation to the principles of evaluation.

There are two approaches to evaluating services. One is *ideology-centered*. That is, the investigators have an ideal picture of a service and evaluation consists of seeing how far the service under investigation matches the theoretical ideal. The most recent variant of this is the movement for the "normalisation" of the lifestyles of handicapped people (Nirje 1969; Wolfensberger, 1972; Wolfensberger and Glenn, 1975).

The second approach is *client-centered*. Investigators adopting this model attempt first, to understand each individual's underlying impairments, second, to determine what specific methods are available to help minimize these problems and improve the person's lifestyle, and, third, to assess if the service being evaluated makes available to the individuals concerned these methods of helping (Mesibov, 1976; J. K. Wing, 1972). This does not presuppose any theoretical ideal of what a service ought to be like. The aim of making the services "as close to normal as possible" is compatible with this approach whereas "normalization at any cost" is not.

The second approach is the basis of the tradition of evaluative studies carried out in the MRC Social Psychiatry Unit, including that of the closure of Darenth Park Hospital.

Historical Background

Darenth Park was opened in November 1878 as a school for five hundred children with mental retardation, but was soon expanded to accommodate adults. The numbers rose to over two thousand in the first two decades of this century, but slowly declined after this. Darenth had been set up to provide education and occupational training for young people with mental retardation in order to help them avoid the exploitation that was common in the community at that time. As with other similar institutions, there was, over the years, a decline from these original high aims, until the appalling conditions in the community that led to the setting up of the institutions were reproduced within the institutions themselves (Jones, 1975; Korman and Glennerster, 1984).

Public reaction to exposure of such conditions (Cmnd No. 3795, 1969; Cmnd No. 4557, 1971) contributed to a climate of opinion that led to the government policy of running down or closing the mental handicap hospitals and providing alternative residential care in the community.

In the middle 1970's, when there were about fifteen hundred residents, the decision was taken to run down Darenth to eventual closure. At first it was hoped that the Associated Portland Cement Manufacturers would buy the land on which the hospital was built in order to quarry the chalk and that this would provide the finance for building a new type of service. Permission for this sale was refused on environmental grounds in 1978, but the Regional Health Authority decided to continue with the plan to close Darenth using its own financial resources. In parallel with this process, efforts were made to improve life within Darenth, because closure was likely to take a long time.

There was much discussion and disagreement between the health districts involved concerning plans for the provision of alternative residential care. The long, tangled story is told by Korman and Glennerster (1984). It was years before plans were agreed on, and longer still before new buildings or adaptations of existing buildings were completed. During the period before new accommodation was ready, as many residents as could be found places in existing hospitals, hostels, and homes were moved out. In effect, ex-Darenth residents were scattered all over southeast England. It was not until the middle 1980s that most of the residents who moved went to specially planned accommodation.

The MRC Unit's evaluation of the effects of closure on the residents began in August 1980, when there were 893 adult residents aged sixteen and over, and a very few severely or profoundly retarded children living in one ward. The study was confined to the adult residents.

Aims and Hypotheses

The closure of Darenth offered the opportunity of investigating the relationship between patterns of impairments and specific service needs.

The general aims were to study the effect on the Darenth Park residents of moving to different types of residential care, and to derive implications for future closures of other hospitals. The specific aims were to assess the effects of moving on the residents' handicaps, skills, behavior, and lifestyles; to study different types of residential accommodation and, in particular, to compare lifestyles in clusters of living units as opposed to widely separated small houses in ordinary streets; and to examine the effects of the daily programs of care, training, occupation, and leisure within living units.

The study was planned not simply as an exercise in the collection of data but to test three specific hypotheses. The first was that a variety of patterns of impairments could be found among mentally retarded adults. The second was that people with different patterns of impairments and behavior would need different types of environments and programs to minimize behavior problems, develop skills and encourage constructive activities. (For example, the most sociable and capable people would benefit from a low level of supervision, a permissive regime, and opportunities for occupation, leisure, and for making choices. Non-mobile profoundly retarded people would need expert physical care, appropriate types of stimulation, and simple enjoyable experiences. People who were socially impaired and aloof would need a high level of care and supervision given by staff with expert knowledge of this particular pattern of handicaps, a structured organized regime, and appropriate types of occupation and leisure. For this group, the opportunities for making choices would have to be limited to avoid causing distress and confusion.) The third hypothesis was that mixing people with different types of handicaps in the same living units would make it more difficult to provide for the needs of each individual.

Practical Constraints Affecting the Study

When working with human beings and human institutions, certain practical constraints on research are unavoidable, and ways must be found of minimizing their effects. A major problem, already mentioned, was the long delay before planned accommodation was opened and the way in which this biased the selection of residents for moving (see below).

The Social Psychiatry Unit staff engaged in the Darenth study had the positive advantage, from the scientific point of view, of being completely independent observers with no responsibility for any aspect of the running of the hospital, planning its closure or setting up alternative services. They thus avoided the problems inherent in attempts to combine the roles of service provider and evaluator.

Useful though this detached view was, there were also disadvantages. The investigators had no part in decisions concerning which residents should move and where and when they should be placed. It was therefore impossible to arrange for randomized placements of residents with different patterns of impairments in different types of accommodation.

In the early years of the study, moves were arranged by the Darenth consultants with the agreement of the managers or owners of the many hospitals, hostels, and homes receiving the residents, who would not have agreed to accept people chosen by a process of random selection. In the later years, the receiving health districts accepted responsibility for Darenth residents originally admitted from their own areas and would not have been prepared to take people from outside the borders, which would have to have happened if matched pairs or groups were assigned at random to different types of placements. Insisting on such procedures would have meant that the study could not have been undertaken. Apart from these practical problems, there were also serious doubts concerning the ethics of random placement.

In response to these practical problems, two different strategies, both involving matching, were adopted in different parts of the study in order to make valid comparisons, as will be described later.

Techniques of Measurement

Ideally, information on people's behavior and skills and on the pattern of life in a living unit should be obtained from direct observation by more than one observer, as well as from discussions with staff and residents concerned. The scale of the Darenth study made this impossible with the resources available. All data were obtained by interviewing direct care staff, day center staff, relatives, and the residents themselves, supplemented by informal observations made during many visits to living units and day centers to interview informants. Altogether, so many informants were involved that major biases were likely to be corrected. The patterns discerned in the results tended to suggest that a reasonably accurate picture had emerged.

The measures used were designed to examine life within and outside Darenth from two points of view. First, information was recorded on the overall management of each living unit (ward, hostel, or home). Second, ratings were made concerning the handicaps, skills, behavior, and life-styles of each individual selected for assessment. Since the study was concerned with the interaction of patterns of impairment and the lifestyles provided by the services, it was important to see how the overall system of management impinged upon individual residents who differed from each other in their problems and needs.

Past work in the field of evaluation was drawn on when designing the schedules concerned with lifestyles. J. K. Wing and Brown (1961, 1970) found that the degree of environmental poverty was a key factor affecting level of negative symptoms, that is social withdrawal and muteness, in people with chronic ·schizophrenia. In mental handicap hospitals and homes, the degree of autonomy and responsibility given to the person in charge of each living unit have been found to be related to the degree of resident oriented care (King, Raynes, and Tizard, 1971; Raynes, Pratt, and Roses, 1979). The traditional rigid hierarchy in hospitals leaves little room for autonomy at ward level, but Rawlings (1958a, b) noted that an individual head of a ward could, if determined enough, find ways of giving more individualized care. The numbers accommodated within one unit appear to affect the lifestyle of the residents (Baker, Seltzer, and Seltzer, 1977; Felce, deKock, and Repp, 1986; Raynes, Pratt, and Roses 1979). However, there is little evidence concerning the effect on lifestyles of urban versus rural locations, or scattered units in ordinary streets versus units in campuses.

The major difficulty in rating the lifestyles of people with mental retardation is that many of them have insufficient language to express their opinions. Even those who can speak well tend to have difficulty in discussing abstractions, finding it easier to talk on specific, practical issues. In the Darenth study, all residents selected for assessment were interviewed and ratings made for those who could respond, but the major source of information was the direct care staff. It would have been inappropriate to ask them to comment on the abstract concept of quality of life of the residents, so it was decided to follow the practice, used by other workers in the field, of recording details of a range of aspects of daily life.

The idea behind this method is that the degree to which a regime provides various abstract qualities, such as personal dignity, personal independence, freedom of choice, being treated as an individual, permissiveness of the regime, or ease of availability of amenities, can be assessed by combining ratings on a range of specific items. For example, degree of personal independence could be assessed by asking if the person concerned can choose what time they go to bed, if they can watch television when they wish, have visitors of either sex, come in late for a meal which is kept hot, make a cup of tea when they feel like it, wash their own clothes if they want to, put up their own pictures and ornaments, have scissors, matches, and aspirins if they so desire, and so on.

The aim is to provide objective rather than subjective measures of the qualities being assessed, but there are practical limitations on the numbers and types of items that can be used. The choices have to be made on empirical, common-sense grounds in the hope that they represent a general trend in the environment being studied. Such schedules are relevant only in the context of the culture within and for which they were designed, but the general principle could be applied anywhere by workers familiar with the local way of life.

For all the interviews, a pre-coded schedule was designed with detailed guidelines for making ratings. Space was provided for extensive notes as well as the formal codes. The interviews were conducted on semi-structured lines, the interviewer encouraging the informant to talk around the items on the schedule, giving illustrative anecdotes where relevant. Probing questions were asked until the interviewer felt that enough detail had been obtained to make a rating. It should be noted that it was the interviewer who made the ratings, not the informant. Interviews took place in the living unit or day center or, in the case of relatives, in their own homes, in a relaxed and friendly atmosphere in which comment and discussion were encouraged. The importance of convivial tea drinking for facilitating such research should be mentioned.

The research team prepared for the interviews by studying the schedule, discussing each item in detail and sitting in on each others' interviews. Discussions of difficult ratings went on throughout the whole study. The reliability of such instruments depends entirely upon shared knowledge of the purpose and meaning of the items to be rated.

The contents of the schedules, methods of rating, and derivation of scores are given in Wing (1989). Only a brief outline will be presented here.

The Living Unit's Organization Schedule

This schedule was completed by interviewing the person in direct charge of the living unit. The numbers of staff and residents and the types of handicaps of the residents were noted. The degree to which care was individualized, the autonomy of staff and residents in everyday decisions, and degree of privacy available to the residents were rated. Details of formal meetings of staff, whether residents had meetings, opportunities for residents' training, occupation and leisure, and contacts with all kinds of professional staff from outside the living unit were recorded.

In addition to the interviews, the geographical location, and the physical amenities within and outside the living unit were inspected and rated by one of the research team.

Ratings of Individual Residents

The impairments, skills and behavior of residents were assessed by means of the Disability Assessment Schedule (Wing and Gould, 1978). In brief, it is an interview schedule used with the direct care staff and covering self-care, verbal and non-verbal communication, social, practical, domestic and scholastic skills, a wide range of difficult behaviour, and repetitive, stereotyped activities.

The direct care staff were also interviewed concerning residents' life-styles. The schedules used covered much the same ground, with some additional items, as that used for the living unit, but from the point of view of individuals. Details of training and occupation were obtained from the day centre as well as the living unit staff.

Relatives who had contact with residents within the previous year were interviewed in their own homes. On the whole they knew few details of life in Darenth or the new placements, but they were asked their opinions of the physical environment, the care given to their resident, medical and para-medical services, occupation and leisure facilities, the staff attitudes, communication with the staff, how they felt about visiting, and their reaction to the plans for closing Darenth.

A schedule was designed for interviews with residents covering different aspects of life in Darenth and other units, but it was found easier to allow those interviewed to talk as they wished, once launched onto the subject of their experiences of Darenth, the moves and the units in which they had been placed. Notes were made as fully as possible.

Subjects and Procedures

The Phases of the Study

One of the compromises necessary for practical reasons was the division of the study into two phases. The first phase, from August 1980 to December 1985, covered the time when movement was comparatively slow, and most people went to existing accommodation, because only a few of the new planned residences became available during that period.

The types of placements were other hospitals, NHS and social services hostels, privately run hostels, old people's homes, landladies, foster families, and some small houses in ordinary streets. The last named were part of the planned accommodation. Some of the care staff in the small houses were reluctant on ideological grounds to allow any of the research team to visit, so only three such houses could be included in the first phase follow-up.

Altogether, in this phase, 279 people moved out, that is approximately one third of the 893 residents in Darenth at the beginning of the study. Another 136 died, leaving 478 of the total study subjects still in Darenth at the end of 1985. (A few people were admitted after August 1980, but these were not included in the study).

Phase 2, from January 1986 until August 1989, one year after Darenth closed, covered the time when movement occurred more rapidly and when most people went to the new, planned accommodation provided by the health districts.

Different strategies for group comparisons were used in the two phases.

Phase 1: Matching of Movers and Controls

For the first phase, the size of the population remaining in Darenth made it possible to match pairs of individuals comprising one mover and one who would remain in Darenth for at least one year after the partner had left. In the first six months of the study the research team had rated all 893 residents on the Disability Assessment Schedule (DAS) by interviewing direct care staff. These ratings were used for individual matching. The variables selected as of primary importance were sex, mobility, quality of social interaction (aloof, passive, odd, or appropriate for mental age) and ability to communicate. The last three were chosen because they related to the types of impairments considered to be of particular importance in relation to service needs. Age was matched as closely as possible. Other variables taken into account as far as possible were ethnic origin, sensory impairments, epileptic fits, the presence of Down's syndrome, self-help skills, behavior problems, and stereotypies. A computer print-out of the DAS ratings allowed potential matches to be identified. The final choice was made by meeting the mover and possible partners and by discussion with the staff who knew the people concerned.

The process was time consuming, but was considered to be essential to ensure close matching on important variables so as to minimize the scientific disadvantages arising from the inability to select at random which member of the pair was to move and to where. In any case, in Phase 1, the mover out of any closely matched pair was selected because he or she happened to be under the supervision of a particular consultant and not for any reason that could bias the results of the study.

Initial and Follow-up Assessments

Movers were assessed before moving. The DAS was repeated and the various lifestyle schedules completed by interviewing staff, relatives, and the movers themselves. After one year in the new placements, all the interviews were repeated. The matched controls remaining in Darenth were assessed in the same way and followed up a year later, as close as possible in time to their partners who moved.

It was not possible, with the resources available, to assess and follow-up all the movers. During Phase 1, the majority of movers were sociable people. About one third of this group were included, about one half of those with passive or odd social interaction, and almost all of those who were aloof and indifferent to other people. In all, 127 pairs were assessed and followed up.

Results from Phase 1

Full details and tabulations of the results are given in Wing (1989). For this chapter, only the findings that illustrate principles of general interest will be discussed.

Accuracy of the Matching

The individual matching of movers and their controls was achieved with reasonable success, not only on the variables taken into account when choosing pairs (see Table 17.1, 17.2 and 17.3) but also on their lifestyle measures (see Tables 17.4 and 17.5). The only variables on which there was a marked difference was amount of contact with relatives during the preceeding year. Fewer controls than movers had contacts as would be expected from the fact that the possibility of moving closer to involved relatives and pressure from relatives for such a move to occur were factors affecting selection of people to move during Phase 1. Relatives were seen for 65 of the 127 movers and 40 of the 127 controls.

Skills and Behavior

As previously mentioned, most movers in Phase 1 were sociable people. They also tended to be the most able in self care and practical skills (see Table 17.2). Among the 279 moves, only 5 (2 percent) were unable to walk

TABLE 17.1
Movers and Controls: Demographic and Medical Characteristics
(Absolute numbers)

	(Total number)	Movers (127)	Controls (127)
Sex	Male	73	73
	Female	54	54
Ethnic origin of father	U.K.	115	115
	Other	12	12
Medical	Downs	14	14
	Epilepsy	23	33
	Non mobile	6	6
Visual impairment	Severe	7	6
	Minor	11	6
Hearing impairment	Severe	1	2
	Minor	15	12
Age on 31 Dec. 1980 (years)	17–29	33	29
	30–49	39	42
	50–69	46	45
	70–84	9	11
	Range	17–84	18–90
	Mean	45	47

independently at the time of the move, thirty-four (12 percent) were aloof and forty (14 percent) were passive or odd in social interaction. Three quarters of the aloof people who did move were placed in other hospitals, compared with one quarter of the passive or odd people and one fifth of those who were sociable. This emphasizes the difficulties of accommodating the most severely socially impaired people in non-hospital residential care not originally planned to take such people.

The most clearcut finding in the whole study was the contrast between the socially impaired and sociable people in virtually all the variables that were rated. As can be seen from the measures of skills (Table 17.2) and of behavior (Table 17.3), the aloof group had the lowest mean scores, the group comprising both passive and odd people were intermediate, sometimes being nearer the sociable, sometimes nearer the aloof group, and the sociable people had the highest mean scores.

There were no significant changes in mean scores after moving from Darenth, and the differences between the groups remained as before.

The matched controls showed the same pattern of inter-group differences as the movers. For each group the mean scores were closely similar to those of the movers.

TABLE 17.2
Skills (Mean percentages of maximum possible scores)

		ALOOF		PASSIVE/ ODD		SOCIABLE	
		M	C	M	C	M	C
Self care	I	33	31	85	88	97	95
	F	33	31	86	85	95	96
Continence	I	51	48	95	96	97	99
	F	60	55	93	91	96	96
Communication	I	28	23	80	74	90	92
	F	30	22	83	83	91	92
Domestic	I	23	9	53	43	80	82
	F	13	9	61	57	83	84
Literacy	I	4	1	32	29	44	45
	F	0	2	35	35	44	50

Note: The higher the score, the better the skill
  M = Mover
  C = Control
  I = Initial assessment
  F = Follow-up

TABLE 17.3
Behavior (Mean percentages of maximum possible scores)

		ALOOF		PASSIVE/ ODD		SOCIABLE	
		M	C	M	C	M	C
Behavior	I	30	38	70	63	82	83
problems	F	26	32	68	59	72	82
Repetitive	I	42	40	67	60	94	91
stereotyped	F	38	38	62	49	87	91
Abnormal	I	9	12	70	71	92	92
speech	F	10	10	70	75	89	91

Note: The higher the score, the more appropriate the behavior.

Lifestyles

The same pattern was repeated for most of the lifestyle measures. Mean scores for personal independence within and outside the living units, personal possessions, and participating in decisions (see Table 17.4), for having a regular occupation and for amount of leisure time spent in constructive as opposed to stereotyped or no activities (see Table 17.5)

TABLE 17.4
Lifestyle (Mean percentages of maximum possible scores)

		ALOOF		PASSIVE/ ODD		SOCIABLE	
		M	C	M	C	M	C
Independence	I	43	46	59	61	73	74
in unit	F	31	48	62	59	65	75
Independence	I	34	32	63	68	70	76
outside unit	F	31	34	63	69	69	74
Privacy	I	18	22	27	24	36	45
	F	35	28	50	26	60	47
Possessions	I	45	47	59	64	71	75
	F	42	52	62	67	73	75
Decision	I	19	15	29	27	34	40
making	F	11	23	37	24	45	40
Community	I	2	3	2	2	3	2
service use	F	9	1	53	1	55	2

Note: The higher score the better the life-style

were all rated significantly and markedly lower for the aloof socially impaired as compared with the sociable group. The passive plus odd group fell between the other two groups. No significant differences were found after moving, or between movers and controls.

The exceptions to this general picture were personal privacy, using community services (Table 17.4) and taking part in educational activities (Table 17.5). For personal privacy, the mean ratings were significantly and markedly lower for the aloof group both before and after moving. However, all movers had a significant increase in personal privacy after moving out of Darenth, although the differences among the three groups remained as before, the aloof lowest, the passive and odd in the middle, and the sociable group having the highest ratings.

For all the groups, while living in Darenth, there was virtually no use of community medical, para-medical, and personal services, all of these being provided on the campus (Table 17.4). After moving, there was little change for the aloof group, most of whom moved to other hospitals, but the other groups, many of whom went to non-hospital placements, showed a significant and marked increase in the use of the services available to the local community.

Participation in educational activities (Table 17.5) was the only variable which, in Darenth, had a mean rating that was somewhat higher for the aloof group than for the others, though this difference was not significant.

TABLE 17.5
Education, Occupation and Leisure

		ALOOF		PASSIVE/ ODD		SOCIABLE	
		M	C	M	C	M	C
Education	I	39	43	29	38	36	15
	F	57	46	24	48	23	18
Occupation	I	25	32	71	48	74	78
	F	43	25	67	43	56	77
Constructive	I	14	18	42	31	58	59
leisure	F	8	19	40	31	50	58

Notes: Education and occupation scores are the percentages of residents taking part in these activities.

Constructive leisure scores are the mean numbers of hours spent per week in such activities.

After moving, the aloof group had a significantly higher mean rating than the rest. This was again related to the fact that most of the aloof movers went to other hospitals where educational activities were provided on the campus, in contrast to non-hospital placements where opportunities for formal education were limited.

Movers to Small Houses

The effects on the residents (eight sociable people, two passive or odd and one aloof) who moved to small houses in ordinary streets were of particular interest, since this type of placement was, in theory, closest to a normal life. The numbers were too small for statistical analysis, but some trends could be seen. There were no meaningful changes in skills or behavior. The mean ratings for independence within the living unit, partic-ipation in decision making, and for personal possessions rose for this group, whereas, for the other placements, there was a fall or no change. As for all the other units outside Darenth, those in the small houses had a marked increase in privacy and use of community services. On the other hand, the residents of the small houses had no increase in their mean rating for independence outside the unit. In fact the three who were aloof, passive, or odd had somewhat lower ratings for this variable after moving. The ratings for educational activities, having a regular occupation and for using leisure constructively all fell for those in small houses. The drop in educational activities was particularly marked in contrast to the small changes, up or down, for other living units.

The Organization of the Living Units

The physical structure of the units and the numbers of residents affected the amenities for making a personal life and for general comfort and appearance. Darenth and other hospital wards and the privately run hostels tended to have the lowest scores, whereas small ordinary houses came out well on these measures.

The degree of centralization of services and the autonomy of individual living units affected the residents' lifestyles. The hospital wards, with their traditional system of hierarchical organization, scored lowest, while landladies, families and small houses were obviously the least centralized and most autonomous.

The permissiveness of the regime within the unit was rated separately. All the units, even Darenth, came out comparatively high on these items.

These aspects of the living unit organization were, to a large extent, indpendent of each other. They could also vary independently of the handicaps of the residents (Rawlings 1985, a, b; Raynes & Sumption, 1987).

Mean carer to resident ratios were poorest in Darenth and in the old people's homes, and, as would be expected, best in landladies and foster family homes and in the small houses in ordinary streets, which had the fewest residents per living unit.

The Views of the Relatives

Relatives of sixty-five movers and forty control were interviewed, all of whom had had contact with residents within the last year.

Among the relatives of the movers there was a significant overall preference for the new placements, with three quarters saying they liked the new living units better than Darenth. The proportion expressing overall positive feelings were highest for the NHS and social service hostels, followed by other hospitals, then the small houses, private hostels and old people's homes in descending order.

The major reasons for the preferences were the physical appearance and comfort of the new placements, the individual care given to the residents and (slightly) better communication with the staff. These factors helped to make visiting pleasanter for the relatives. Relatives of those in hospitals and in NHS and social service hostels thought that medical and paramedical care was better than at Darenth, but, for other types of living units, no improvement or worsening of these services was reported. Occupation and leisure facilities were rated as improved only in the hospitals.

There was some increase in amount of visiting of the units outside

Darenth. An easier journey appeared to be a major factor affecting visiting patterns.

The Opinions of the Residents

A total of ninety-two movers and seventy controls remaining in Darenth were able to express their opinions sufficiently coherently for the interviewers to record their views. Of these, none was aloof, twelve were passive or odd and the rest (150) were sociable.

Before moving, one third of the movers said they disliked Darenth, one third had mixed feelings and one third said they liked living in the hospital. After moving, just over half liked the new placements, one fifth had mixed feelings and one quarter said they were not happy in the new residences. The NHS and social services hostels and the voluntary homes, landladies and families had the highest proportions of favourable ratings, small houses were in the middle and the private hostels and other hospital wards had the lowest proportions.

The control subjects at first interview were slightly more likely than the movers to say they liked Darenth.

There were certain reasons for preferences that were frequently mentioned by both movers and controls. These were wishing for a private bedroom; wanting to be with friends and within the familiar social network they had established at Darenth; liking good food in sufficient quantity; having a regular, enjoyable occupation; disliking noisy, quarrelsome, or aggressive companions in the living unit; being in pleasant, familiar surroundings indoors and outside. Some of the movers said they missed the large grounds and the countryside around Darenth. None mentioned concern over the stigma of being in a mental handicap hospital, and none spoke of any desire to be part of the normal community, though many were quite clear they wished to remain with the friends they made in Darenth.

The aloof residents interviewed could not express their feelings verbally or non-verbally. It was difficult to know how they responded emotionally to the changes they experienced.

Discussion

All the assessments of individuals and of the living units were made at specific points in time. They represented a series of still pictures from a continuously moving story. What was true at the time of assessment may not have been the case before or since.

Because of the bias in selection and placement of the residents who moved in Phase 1, and the wide variation in the types of placements, the initial hypotheses could not be fully tested.

The first hypothesis, that a variety of patterns of impairments and behavior could be found among the adult residents, was confirmed. The second hypothesis, that people with different patterns of impairments and behavior require different environments and different programs to give each group the best possible lifestyles, could not be properly examined since almost all of the most severely socially impaired went to other hospital wards and not to non-hospital placements, and no special programs had been instituted at the time of follow-up. What is clear is that in all placements the socially aloof residents had markedly poorer ratings on virtually all aspects of lifestyle compared with the sociable groups, and the passive and odd groups fell between the other two. The third hypothesis, concerning the difficulties following from mixing people with different patterns of impairments and skills, was also not tested. However, the sociable residents did comment upon how much they disliked being with those who were noisy, aggressive, destructive, aimlessly wandering, and interfering with other people's possessions. The relatives also disliked such mixing.

Despite the problems inherent in the first phase of the study, some useful findings do emerge.

One of the important points to emphasize is that there is no simple prescription for the best type of residential services for people with mental retardation. There are advantages and disadvantages in all models and, furthermore, the picture changes depending on the point of view.

Looking at the organization of the living units, it was clear that those outside hospitals had the highest levels of autonomy and possibilities for personal privacy. On the other hand, the skills and behavior of the residents did not change, and there were few improvements in individual lifestyle variables, apart from those related to practical issues such as the size and physical amenities of the building, the arrangements made for personal services and the numbers of care staff. It appears that the way in which the management philosophy of a living unit impinges upon the individual residents depends upon their patterns of skills and impairments. Thus if some residents cannot cross a road safely on their own, most care staff take protective measures whatever the theoretical ideal of full independence for all residents. This is the reason for the finding that the organization and philosophy of the living units was to some extent independent of the handicaps of the residents, whereas each individual's lifestyle ratings were heavily dependent upon their pattern of skills, impairments, and behavior. It seems, for example, that it is easier to allow more independence, at least for more capable residents, within a small house, because of the immediate availability of staff, than to permit residents to face the dangers of the streets on their own.

The relatives appreciated the greater comfort, better furnishings and decorations, and more staff provided in many of the living units outside Darenth. They also wanted the resident with whom they were concerned to be safe, well supervised, to have good medical and para-medical care, and plenty of opportunity for constructive occupational and leisure activities. In interviews before the moves had occurred, many relatives expressed their worries concerning safety and supervision. The philosophy of normalization bothered them because they were well aware of the handicaps of the residents and had had past experiences of the problems that could ensue from lack of appropriate supervision. In the event, the majority found they were, on balance, happy with the new accommodation because, in most placements in Phase 1, the idea of normalization, whether or not it was held in theory, had rather little effect in practice. When, in a few cases, normalization was taken seriously, the relatives concerned were upset, even angry, if it seemed to them that their residents lacked the care they needed. For example, a man in his thirties who was sociable but severely retarded was placed in a small house with staff who were dedicated to the ideal of independence for the residents. He did not buy himself new clothes or shoes. His mother found that he had holes in the soles of his outdoor shoes, which he was wearing in the snow. When she protested, she was made to feel that she was interfering and over-protective. In the light of the relatives' views, it is not surprising that they tended to prefer the hospitals outside Darenth and the NHS and social services hostel placements, since, to them, these represented security for the present and the future.

Virtually all the residents who could express their opinions were sociable and comparatively capable. They appreciated privacy, good food, pleasant surroundings, and being with a group of friends. Only just over half felt unequivocally that they were better off in these respects after moving. As with the relatives, the NHS and social services hostels were in general liked, but, unlike the relatives, the residents were least happy with the hospital wards. None was at all concerned with the philosophy of normalization. They were not too happy with the idea of using the normal community services because some (such as hairdressing and transport) had to be paid for.

The major finding from the results of Phase 1 was undoubtedly the dramatic difference in the ratings of skills behavior and lifestyles between the severely socially impaired, aloof people, and the sociable group, and the lack of change in this respect after moving. It was also very evident that the non-hospital placements available in Phase 1 were not geared to the needs of aloof, severely handicapped people and were unable or unwilling to change in order to accept them. The small minority who moved mostly went to other hospitals where they experienced the same lifestyle as in Darenth, but in nicer surroundings indoors. If anything, their freedom of movement outside was even more curtailed, because they no longer had the use of the large grounds surrounding Darenth.

Is it possible to give people in the aloof group a better style of life, in the light of the restrictions imposed by their severe impairments? Rawlings (1985a, b) in a study involving three hospital wards and three small non-hospital units found that, in small well-staffed living units, staff could provide a structured, organized routine and could work with severely socially impaired individuals to guide them in simple self care and domestic tasks and take them out to a range of activities. Good practice in this area requires sufficient staff with experience, dedication, and detailed knowledge of each resident's pattern of skills and impairments. Given the staff and facilities needed, the lifestyles of the aloof group of residents could be significantly improved, though never to the levels achievable for the sociable, more capable people. However, the services required are very expensive.

Implications of the Findings

In evaluating the results of the first phase of the Darenth study, it should be noted that efforts in the 1970s and early 1980s to improve life in the hospital had produced many changes for the better, at least for the more able, sociable residents, if not for the aloof group. Darenth, when the study began, no longer fitted the model of a rigidly run, old-fashioned institution, though many problems still remained, including shortages of staff, physical resources, and money. Thus, the contrasts between life inside and in the alternative placements were not so marked as they might have been for some other less permissive hospitals. If the study had been conducted elsewhere, more significant differences in the ratings after moving might have been found.

When few changes are found in a study of this kind, it is legitimate to ask if the measures were sensitive enough to show changes. They did reveal large differences between the socially impaired and sociable groups that were confirmed by observation. This suggests that meaningful changes, had they occurred, would have been seen in the ratings.

The present study produced no evidence in favor of small units scattered throughout the normal community, as compared with a cluster on a campus. There were indications that living units with small numbers of residents did provide a better lifestyle, but there was nothing to suggest that geographical location was important.

There was strong evidence that, for future hospital closures, plans should be made early on in the process for the placement of the more severely handicapped, aloof, non-communicating residents with poor skills and difficult behavior. If these are left until near closure, the hospital population becomes progressively more handicapped as the sociable, able people are moved out first. Plans for the more severely impaired groups should include training of the staff of non-hospital units in the understanding of the nature of such handicaps and the best ways of helping the people concerned. The philosophy of treating sociable people with mental retardation in the same way as the normal population does have some justification (though it is not without difficulties) but the socially impaired residents need staff with special expertise if their lifestyles are to be improved. Denying the fact of their special handicaps is to deny them their special needs and their human rights.

Phase 2 of the Study

The second phase, from January 1986 until August 1989 (one year after Darenth finally closed) covers the period during which the great majority of movers were placed in new planned placements provided by the district health authorities in Darenth's catchment area. For this part of the study, 150 Darenth residents were selected to represent different patterns of handicaps and types of placements (campuses versus small houses scattered throughout the relevant health districts). Since, in Phase 2, everyone was moved out of Darenth, it was not possible to use individually matched controls remaining in the hospital, so a repeated measures design was employed, with each resident acting as their own control.

At the time of writing, too few of the study subjects have been followed up for results to be given. When completed, the measures used will allow the initial hypotheses to be tested more completely than was possible in Phase 1.

Postscript: The Fall of Darenth Park

Darenth Park hospital closed in August 1988. The former residents are scattered all over southeast England and a few even further afield. The hospital community has been broken up and nothing can ever put it together again. It remains to be seen if the services replacing it will live up to the high hopes with which they were created and if they do, whether they will continue to maintain high standards once the pioneering days are over.

References

Baker, B.L., Seltzer, G.B., and Seltzer, M.M., (1977) *As Close As Possible,* Boston: Litle, Brown.

Cmnd. 3795, (1969) *Report of the Committee of Inquiry into Allegations of Ill-treatment of Patients and Other Irregularities at the Ely Hospital, Cardiff,* London: HMSO.

Cmnd. 4557, (1971) *Report of the Farleigh Committee of Inquiry,* London: HMSO.

Felce, D., de Kock, U., and Repp, A., (1986), An eco-behavioural comparison of small community based houses and traditional large hospitals for severely and profoundly mentally handicapped adults, *Applied Research in Mental Retardation, 7,* 393–408.

Jones, K., (1975) *Opening the Door,* London: Routledge and Kegan Paul.

King, R. D., Raynes, N. V., and Tizard, J., (1971) *Patterns of Residential Care,* London: Routledge and Kegan Paul.

Korman, M. and Glennerster, H., (1984) *The Darenth Park Project: A Narrative of a Hospital Closure,* London: London School of Economics.

Mesibov, G. B., (1976) Alternatives to the principle of normalization, *Mental Retardation, 14,* 30–32.

Nirje, B., (1969) The normalization principle and its human management implication. *In* R.B. Kiegel and W. Wolfensberger (eds.) *Changing Patterns in Residential Services for the Mentally Retarded,* Washington, D.C.: United States Government Printing Office.

Rawlings, S., (1985a) Behaviour and skills of severely retarded adults in hospitals and small residential homes. *British Journal of Psychiatry, 146,* 358–366.

Rawlings, S., (1985b) Life-styles of severely retarded non-communicating adults in hospitals and small residential homes. *British Journal of Social Work, 15,* 281–293.

Raynes, N.V. and Sumpton, R.C., (1987) Differences in the quality of residential provision for mentally handicapped people. *Psychological Medicine, 17,* 999–1008.

Raynes, N.V., Pratt, M.W., and Ross, S., (1979) *Organisational Structure and the Care of the Mentally Retarded,* London: Croom Helm.

Wing, J.K., (1972a) Principles of evaluation. *In* J.K. Wing and A.M. Hailey (eds.), *Evaluating a Community Psychiatric Service,* London: Oxford University Press.

Wing, J.K. and Brown, G., (1961) Social treatment of chronic schizophrenia: a comparative study of three mental hospitals. *Journal of Mental Science, 107,* 847–856.

Wing, J.K. and Brown, G., (1970) *Institutionalism and Schizophrenia.* Cambridge: Cambridge University Press.

Wing, L. (1989) *Hospital Closure and the Resettlement of Residents: The Case of Darenth Park Hospital.* Aldershot: Gower.

Wing, L. and Gould, J., (1978), Systematic recording of behaviours and skills of retarded and psychotic children. *Journal of Autism and Childhood Schizophrenia, 8,* 79–97.

Wing, L. and Gould, J., (1979) Severe impairments of social interaction and associated abnormalities in children: epidemiology and classification. *Journal of Autism and Childhood Schizophrenia, 9,* 11–29.

Wolfensberger, W., (1972) *The Principle of Normalization in Human Services,* Toronto: National Institute on Mental Retardation.

Wolfensberger, W. and Glenn, L., (1975) *Pass 3: A Method for the Quantitative Evaluation of Human Services,* Toronto: National Institute on Mental Retardation.

18

Maintenance Medication for Schizophrenia: Changing Perspectives on Use and Evaluation

Steven Hirsch

Introduction

The practice of trying to prevent relapse by extending the drug treatment of acute schizophrenia to the post recovery period began soon after the introduction of neuroleptics (Shawver et al., 1959). The first double-blind placebo controlled study which specifically looked at maintenance oral medication in patients who had been successfully stabilized after discharge from hospital was conducted by Leff and Wing (1971). Subsequently Hirsch et al., (1973), also working with Wing, carried out the first double-blind placebo study of depot medication for patients well established on treatment. We substituted placebo for active medication randomly in half the sample and studied the subsequent survival rates. Since then more than thirty-eight placebo controlled studies of maintenance medication have been published including more than 3500 patients. Baldessarini's review (1988) of these reports found that during a mean follow-up period of 9.8 (± 1.3) months for different studies, the risk of exacerbation of the psychosis was 55 percent with placebo vs only 14 percent with active medication, a four fold increase in risk on placebo.

The development of research on maintenance medication since the early studies in the MRC Social Psychiatry Unit has demonstrated how multi-facetted the question of efficacy of maintenance treatment can be. The issues raised have included the patients' requirements for treatment, the interaction of drug effects with environmental factors and with psychosocial management, and the criteria used to evaluate efficacy. The so-called side effects of treatment, and the importance of non-schizophrenic symptoms of the illness have become increasingly important. This in turn has focused current interest on alternative strategies of treatment, such as the use of low dose medication and "when required" targeted treatment approaches, giving rise to another cycle of the evaluation process as new treatment and strategies are developed.

Early Evaluation

The Importance of Psychopathology as a Basis for Reliable and Valid Assessments

The use of medication to maintain improvement and prevent relapse reflects a recognition that neuroleptic medication has a suppressant effect, controlling or preventing symptoms, but does not attack the illness at the aetiological level. Pharmacologically, neuroleptics must be influencing a physiological system which is, in turn, being affected by a more fundamental underlying disturbance (Hirsch, 1988).

The earliest attempts to demonstrate the efficacy of maintenance medication suffered from methodological difficulties, such as the lack of double blind placebo controls which are necessary to establish that a treatment is based on a pharmacological effect. Assessments were often unstructured, or used measures such as the BPRS (Overall and Conham, 1962) which do not measure clinically recognized symptoms, or lack specified rating criteria.

The measures of change employed in the MRC Unit's studies employed a hard criterion of relapse: that the physician must be so concerned about the patient's deterioration that they require the patient to be withdrawn from the trial in order to be certain he is receiving active treatment. This was backed up by assessments with the Present State Examination (Wing et al., 1974), which also enabled the patient to be assigned to diagnostic groups and permitted change to be assessed in schizophrenic as well as other symptoms, thereby confirming that the clinical determination of relapse was based on an exacerbation of schizophrenic pathology.

Interpretations of the Results of Trials

The MRC Unit's studies introduced another innovation. By keeping track of the entire cohort of patients initially considered suitable for each trial and examining differences between those accepted for the study and those who the clinician would not enter, it was possible to examine the effect of bias on different groups, enabling the authors to make generalizations about the applicability and limitation of their results (Leff and Wing, 1971).

Other workers carried out so-called "mirror image" studies to examine the effect of depot neuroleptics in reducing the frequency and length of hospitalization (Denham and Adamson, 1971; Johnson and Freeman, 1972). They found that changing to depot neuroleptics from oral or no medication was followed by at least a 50 percent reduction in the number of hospitalizations and total time in hospital, comparing the period since the patient had been on maintenance medication to an equal period of time before.

However, mirror image studies cannot be conclusive because of the sequence effect—the period before going on depot was one in which the relapse was brewing, or the patient would not have been put on depot. Natural changes in the prognosis and course of the illness could not be controlled, nor could ancillary factors such as the quality of support care.

Although almost all thirty-eight placebo controlled studies of maintenance medication have demonstrated much lower relapse rates for patients on active medication than placebo, the rates of psychotic exacerbation with placebo have varied from 18 percent to 97 percent (Baldessarini et al., 1988). This is partly explained by differences in diagnosis and the length of followup, and such factors as whether the patients entered the trial while still acutely ill or when leaving hospital, and whether they had been well stabilized before entering the trial. Other factors which will have a bearing on the observed relapse rates on and off medication are the dose, whether the patients were selected from a low or high risk group, and the criteria used to recognize relapse.

Studies in which patients are randomly withdrawn from active medication and have placebo substituted employ an effective methodology for eliminating the bias which may occur due to the allocation of patients to different treatments, but the results may exaggerate the apparent benefit of treatment if patients have been selected because they had done well on the maintenance treatment—those who were not responsive would have been eliminated. Under these circumstances, if the treatment has been effective, a higher proportion of patients will relapse when the drug is withdrawn than if the cohort included all patients recovered from an acute illness (Leff and Wing, 1971). Taken together, methodological factors can have as great an influence on the magnitude of the observed differences between active and placebo treatment as the pharmacological effects of medication itself (Hirsch, 1986a).

Ethical Problems

In the early days of maintenance medication it seemed that patients might be discouraged from continuing their treatment if, after it had been instituted, they were told that a trial was required to establish its efficacy. Changing attitudes towards patients and improved understanding on their part now make it feasible to obtain their consent for such studies. Ethical committees would normally no longer agree to a study in which patients are not informed that placebo might be substituted for active medication.

Interactions with Other Factors Affecting the Course of the Illness

Life Events and High Expressed Emotion

When the MRC Unit began its investigations of oral and depot treatment in the prevention of schizophrenic relapse, its study to determine whether life events provoke relapse had been recently completed (Brown and Birley, 1968). It was decided to administer the Life Events Schedule to all patients who entered the maintenance medication trials, and repeat it when they relapsed or completed the study. When the Life Event data for both studies were combined it emerged that 89 percent of patients who relapsed on medication had had a life event in the preceding few weeks, compared with about 30 percent of patients who relapsed on drug or were well at the time of the interview (Leff et al., 1973). This observation gave rise to the theory that medication normalises the response of schizophrenic patients to ordinary day to day experience—raising their threshold of susceptibility to relapse, which can nevertheless be exceeded when the patient is stressed by Life Events. Patients on medication are less likely to relapse without a life event (Leff et al., 1973). There has been limited confirmation of this theory since (Jacobs and Myers, 1976), but a prospective trial is in progress (Jolley and Hirsch, personal communication).

As discussed in Chapter 12, Leff and co-workers have shown that patients on medication have a higher risk of relapse if they live in contact with High Expressed Emotion relatives, and that medication reduces the risk of relapse in patients who are exposed to such relatives (Vaughn and Leff, 1976; Chapter 12 in this volume). Depending on the vulnerability of the cohort studied, 60–90 percent of patients who relapsed on medication have had either a life event, lived with a high EE relative or both. (See Hirsch, 1986a, for a summary of the evidence.) Davis (1976) has estimated that medication/no medication accounts for 36 percent of the variance of outcome, whereas Vaughan and Leff (1976) estimated that it explained 15 percent of the variance, while exposure to a high EE environment explained 20 percent of the variance in the clinical trials they reviewed.

The Influence of Psychosocial Treatments

Other Chapters (12 and 19) in this volume review the MRC Unit's success in demonstrating the influence of social factors on the course of schizophrenia. Studies which compare the effectiveness of psychotherapy, behavior therapy and social therapy have been reviewed elsewhere (Hirsch, 1986b). Of the various approaches to treating the patient, Major Role Therapy (MRT) developed by Hogarty and his colleagues was found to confer only a small (14 percent) advantage in lowering the relapse rates of patients who had not relapsed in the first six months (Hogarty and Goldberg, 1973). Unfortunately, Hogarty was unable to replicate this result in a subsequent study (Hogarty et al., 1979). My own conclusion is that there is limited evidence of a response to social treatment which is not of the same order as the response to medication. However, in contrast to these disappointing results, strong evidence emerged from the work in the MRC Unit (Leff et al., 1982) and subsequently elsewhere (Goldstein et al., 1978, Falloon et al., 1982, Hogarty et al., 1986); (See Chap 19, this volume) that treatment of the families of schizophrenic patients aimed at reducing High Expressed Emotion in relatives, or contact with such relatives, has a remarkably powerful effect, reducing the expected relapse rate at one year for patients on medication from 50 percent to 9 percent. This is equal to the effect of maintenance medication, and is complementary to it. Thus we have become aware that the success of medication will depend on environmental factors affecting the patient, and other elements of the treatment. Any assessment needs to be aware of social influences and to consider the extent to which they should be taken into account.

Unwanted Effects of Treatment and Their Influence on Our Approach to Maintenance Medication

As our appreciation of the importance of the side effects of neuroleptic medication has grown, we have become more tentative in their use, but it is the longer term effects which have caused the most concern. Nearly all patients experience extra-pyramidal side effects at some time, but these tend to come and go (Knights et al., 1979).

The persistence of akinesia, with reduced movements in the face and limbs and accompanying greasy skin, can confer mental as well as physical disadvantages, as can akathisia, tremor, hypersalivation and a Parkinsonian stare. Akathisia—motor restlessness and a subjective feeling of motor unease—is increasingly being appreciated as a late and chronic side effect of continuous neuroleptic treatment (Barnes, 1987) which may not respond to treatment. Tardive dyskinesia, and more recently tardive dystonia, have been recognised as the late sequelae of exposure to neuroleptic drugs (Marsden et al., 1986). Kane and Smith (1982) pooled data from nearly 35,000 neuroleptic treated patients, and found the prevalence of bucco-linguo-mastigatory syndrome to be 20 percent, compared with 5 percent

of 11,000 untreated subjects. Though tardive dyskinesia can occur spontaneously, the strongest causal association is with age and exposure to
neuroleptics. The length and cumulative dose of treatment do not appear
to be additive factors. In contrast to all other unwanted effects of neuroleptics, tardive dyskinesia appears to be irreversible in a significant proportion
of patients—possibly up to 30 or 40 percent—but the chance of recovery
relates inversely to age. Tardive dystonia appears to be a variant of tardive
dyskinesia. These unwanted effects must give clinicians pause when they
think of committing patients to lifelong treatment with neuroleptic medication, and urges them to consider alternative approaches to treatment.

A Re-evaluation of the Criteria of Efficacy: Broad vs. Narrow Analysis

The stress on objective criteria of outcome underwrote the methods of
evaluation used by researchers in the 1970s. Total relapse, withdrawal
from blind medication and recrudescence of florid schizophrenic symptoms were the outcome measures typically used in most studies. But
should treatment only be measured in this way? What about the disadvantage of side effects, possible unwanted effects of treatment on the patient's
social demeanour and functioning, and the subjective view of the patients
themselves? Would patients and their families tolerate a higher frequency
of schizophrenic recurrence if they felt better and functioned better
between episodes? Should the total risk of treatment be balanced against
the risk of relapse? How should the risk-benefit equation be structured?
Could the perspective "I wouldn't discontinue maintenance medication
and let my patients risk relapse" be too short-sighted?

With such considerations in mind, a number of workers have examined
the effects of lower dosage and less frequent dosage of maintenance
medication. For example, Caffey et al., (1964) compared treatment on a
daily basis to a three days a week regime, and to treatment withdrawal
(placebo substitution for stabilized chronic outpatients). Within four
months, the relapse rates were 5, 16, and 45 percent, respectively. Capstick (1980) reduced medication gradually by increasing the time between
injections over six months by one week each visit and slowly decreasing
the dose. Medication was eventually discontinued. By the end of 2 years,
80 percent had relapsed, but symptoms quickly remitted when medication
was reintroduced. Kane et al. (1988) carried out a double blind placebo
controlled trial on 126 patients with stable schizophrenia, reducing medication in the experimental group by one tenth (1.25—5mgm) every 2 to 4
weeks. 57 percent relapsed within one year on the low dose and only 7
percent on standard dose, but the social sequelae were minimal in both
groups. Emotional withdrawal, blunted affect, psychomotor retardation,

and tension diminished in the low dose group, raising the possibility that the increased risk of symptom recurrence might be counterbalanced by the advantages of fewer side effects on the lower dose.

Early Signs of Relapse and the Possibility of Intermittent Brief Treatment when They Emerge

The possibility of a revised approach to maintenance treatment emerged after a study by Herz and Melville (1980). They questioned 145 schizophrenic patients and their relatives retrospectively about early signs of relapse. They found that 70 percent of patients and 93% of family members noted mood changes and neurotic symptoms in the patient prior to the onset of relapse, and the study determined the frequency of a long list of symptoms. This was consistent with Knights and Hirsch's (1981) finding that affective symptoms occur in more than 75 percent of acute schizophrenic episodes and remit slowly.

This is consistent with the view that affective symptoms are part and parcel of the schizophrenic syndrome, now confirmed in a number of studies reviewed elsewhere (Hirsch, 1982) most recently in a cohort of unmedicated patients (Leff et al., 1988). The evidence of affective symptoms as part of the schizophrenic syndrome provides empirical support for the scheme of Foulds and Bedford (1975) that psychiatric symptoms can be viewed as a hierarchy from the most common to the most rare, and a patient exhibiting symptoms at any particular level will also tend to show symptoms pertaining to lower levels. From the least to most specific, the levels are: non-specific psychological symptoms, symptoms of neurotic disorders, symptoms of affective psychosis, schizophrenia, and organic brain disease. In the author's view the scheme is only partly accurate, but has heuristic value.

In more than half the cases examined by Herz and Melville (1980), prodromal non-specific symptoms were apparent more than one week prior to relapse. This has led three groups (Carpenter et al., 1987; Herz et al., 1982; and Pietzcker et al., 1986), in addition to our own (Jolley et al., 1989), to examine the use of medication given intermittently and briefly when dysphoric and affective symptoms reappear, as a way of intervening early to prevent relapse. Only preliminary reports have appeared so far. The general finding is of an increased frequency of prodromal episodes triggering brief neuroleptic treatment but less total use of neuroleptics over the first year in the intermittent treatment group. We found a higher rate of symptom recurrence in the experimental group, but no increase in hospitalization in the first year. 73 percent of relapses were preceded by prodromal symptoms. However, by two years the hospitalization rate was significantly higher in the experimental group, without evidence of improved social functioning or improved well being despite a lower incidence of neurological symptoms at the end of the first year (second year result pending). This was disappointing, and suggested that this approach should only be used in special cases.

Perhaps the best approach is that suggested by Marder (1987) in a study of low dose treatment with intermittent augmentation of the neuroleptic dose if prodromal or psychotic symptoms recur. The study lasted one hundred weeks. Using recurrence of symptoms as the criteria for relapse over two years, 69 percent of patients relapsed on low dose (5mgm every two weeks), compared to 36 percent on standard dose (25mgm every 2 weeks). However, using *severe exacerbation or hospitalization* as the criteria of relapse, there was no difference between low and standard dose, as patients with early signs of relapse remitted when the dose was briefly augmented by 10mgm in the low dose group and 50mgm in the standard dose group. Some benefits in terms of a lower incidence of side effects were observed in the first six months, but there were no differences after that point. This study again raises the question of the criteria we should adopt for treatment benefit or failure, and indicates the need for a broader approach.

Whither in Future?

With the recently reported success of clozapine in a multicentered study in the USA (Kane et al., 1988), the way is now open for a new generation of anti-psychotic medication which is more effective and has less side effects than current neuroleptics. Clozapine has long been thought to be a superior drug on the continent, except for the risk of aplastic anaemia. The recent U.S. study showed that 30 percent of patients refractory to standard medication showed a significantly better response to clozapine than chlorpromazine. The risk of blood dyscrasia can be effectively controlled if the patients have a weekly blood count. Clozapine is believed to have less or no risk of tardive dyskinesia, and significantly less extrapyramidal side effects. Pharmaceutical companies are working hard on new drugs which follow the pattern of clozapine, but hopefully will have less associated risks. What we have learned about the evaluation of neuroleptics will no doubt serve us well in coming to grips with these new challenges in the future.

References

Baldessarini, R.J., Cohen, B.M., Teicher, M.H.: (1988). Significance of neuroleptic dose and plasma level in the pharmacological treatment of psychoses. *Archives of General Psychiatry, 45*, 79–91.

Barnes, T.R.E. (1987) The present status of tardive dyskinesia and akathisia in the treatment of schizophrenia. *Psychiatric Developments, 4,* 301–319.

Brown, G.W., Birley, J.T., (1968) Crises and life changes and the onset of schizophrenia. *Journal of Health and Social Behavior. 9,* 203.

Caffey, E.M., Diamond, L.S., Frank, T.V., Grasberger, J.C., Herman, L., Klett, C.J., and Rothstein, R. (1964) Discontinuation or reduction of chemotherapy in chronic schizophrenics. *Journal of Chronic Disease. 17,* 347–359.

Capstick, N. (1980) Long term fluphenazine decanoate. Maintenance dosage requirements of chronic schizophrenic patients. *Acta Psychiatrica Scandinavica. 61,* 256–262.

Carpenter, W., Hendricks, D., Hawton, T. (1987) A comparative trial of pharmacologic strategies in schizophrenia. *American Journal of Psychiatry. 144,* 1466–1470.

Davis, T. (1976) Comparative doses and costs of antipsychotic medication. *Archives of General Psychiatry. 33,* 858–861.

Denham, J. and Adamson, L. (1971) The contribution of fluphenazines enanthate and decanoate in the prevention of readmission of schizophrenic patients. *Acta Psychiatrica Scandinavica. 47,* 420–430.

Falloon, I., Boyd, J., McGill, C., Razani, J., Moss, H., Gilderman, J. (1982). Family management in the prevention of exacerbation of schizophrenia; a controlled study. *New England Journal of Medicine. 306,* 1437–1440.

Foulds, G.A. and Bedford, A. (1975) Hierarchy of classes of personal illness. *Psychological Medicine 5,* 181–192.

Goldstein, M., Rodnich, E., Evans, J., May, P., Steinberg, M. (1978). Drug and family therapy in the aftercare of acute schizophrenics. *Archives of General Psychiatry. 35,* 1169–1177.

Herz, M.I. and Melville, C. (1980) Relapse in schizophrenia. *American Journal of Psychiatry. 137,* 802–805.

Herz, M.I., Szymanski, H.V., Simon, J. (1982) Intermittent medication for stable schizophrenic outpatients: an alternative to maintenance medication. *American Journal of Psychiatry. 139,* 918–922.

Hirsch, S.R. (1982) Depression "Revealed" in Schizophrenia. *British Journal of Psychiatry. 140,* 421–424.

Hirsch, S.R., (1986a). Essential elements in the design of clinical trials. In: Bradley & Hirsch (eds.): *The Psychopharmacology and Treatment of Schizophrenia.* pp. 212–234. Oxford University Press.

Hirsch, S.R. (1986b). Clinical Treatment of Schizophrenia. In: Bradley & Hirsch (eds.): *The Psychopharmacology and Treatment of Schizophrenia.* pp. 324–329. Oxford University Press.

Hirsch, S.R. (1986c). Influence of Social experience and environment on the course of schizophrenia. In: Bradley, P. and Hirsch, S. R. (eds.) *The Psychopharmacology and Treatment of Schizophrenia.* pp. 200–211. Oxford University Press.

Hirsch, S.R. (1988) Essential aspects of the research problem in schizophrenia. *Journal of the Royal Society of Medicine. 81,* 691–697.

Hirsch, S.R., Gaind, R., Rohde, P.D., Stevens, B.C., Wing, J.K. (1973). Outpatient maintenance of chronic schizophrenic patients with long-acting fluphenazine: Double blind placebo trial. *British Medical Journal. i,* 633–637.

Hogarty, G.E., Goldberg, S.C. (1973). Drug and sociotherapy in the aftercare of schizophrenic patients. *Archives of General Psychiatry. 28,* 54–64.

Hogarty, G.E., Schooler, N., Ulrich, R., Mussare, F., Ferro, P., Herron, E. (1979).

Fluphenazine and social therapy in the aftercare of schizophrenia patients. II. 2 year relapse rates. *Archives of General Psychiatry. 31*, 603–608.

Hogarty, G.E., Anderson, C.N., Reiss, D.J., Kornblith, S.J., Greenwald, D.P., Javna, C.D. and Madonia, M.J. (1986). Family psychoeducation, social skills training and maintenance chemotherapy in the aftercare treatment of schizophrenia. *Archives of General Psychiatry. 43*, 633–642.

Jacobs, S., Myers, J. (1976). Recent life events and acute schizophrenic psychosis: a controlled study. *Journal of Nervous and Mental Disorders. 162*, 75–87.

Johnson, D.A.W. and Freeman, H. (1972) Long acting tranquilisers. Practitioner, *208*, 395–400.

Jolley, A., Hirsch, S.R., McRink, A., Manchanda, R., (1989) Trial of brief intermittent neuroleptic prophylaxis for selected schizophrenic outpatients. *British Medical Journal. 298*, 985–90.

Jolley, A., and Hirsch, S.R.: A prospective trial of the interactions between life events, medication, and the susceptibility to develop prodromal symptoms of schizophrenia or relapse. Personal Communication.

Kane, J.M. and Smith, J.M. (1982) Tardive dyskineasia. *Archives of General Psychiatry. 39*, 473–481.

Kane, J., Honigfeld, G., Singer, J., Meltzer, H. and Clozaril Collaborative Study Group. (1988) Clozapine for the treatment-resistant schizophrenic. *Archives of General Psychiatry. 45*, 789–96.

Knights, A., Okasha, M.S., Salih, M. and Hirsch, S.R. (1979) Depressive and extrapyramidal symptoms and clinical effects: a trial of fluphenazine versus flupenthixol in the maintenance of schizophrenic outpatients. *British Journal of Psychiatry. 135*, 514–524.

Knights, A. and Hirsch, S.R. (1981) "Revealed" Depression and treatment for schizophrenia. *Archives of General Psychiatry. 38*, 806–811.

Leff, J.P., and Wing, J.K.: (1971). Trial of maintenance therapy in schizophrenics. *British Medical Journal, iii*, 599–604.

Leff, J., Hirsch, S.R., Rohde, P., Gaind, R., Stevens, B.C. (1973). Life events and maintenance therapy in schizophrenic relapse. *British Journal of Psychiatry. 123*, 659–660.

Leff, J.P., Kuipers, L., Berkowitz, R., Eberlein-Vries, R., and Sturgeon, D. (1982). A controlled trial of social intervention in the families of schizophrenic patients. *British Journal of Psychiatry. 141*, 121–134.

Leff, J., Tress, K. and Edwards, B. (1988) The clinical course of depression symptoms in schizophrenia. Schizophrenia Research, *1*, 25–30.

Marder, S.R., Van Putten, T., Mintz, J., Lebell, M., McKenzie, J., and May, P.R.A. (1987) Low and conventional dose maintenance therapy with fluphenazine decanoate: two year outcome. *Archives of General Psychiatry. 44*, 518–521.

Marsden, C.D., Mindham, R.H.S. and Mackay, A.U.P. (1986) Extrapyramidal movement disorders produced by antipsychotic drugs. In: Bradley, P. and Hirsch, S.R. (eds.) *The Psychopharmacology and Treatment of Schizophrenia.* pp. 340–402. Oxford University Press.

Overall, J.E. and Conham, D.R. (1962) The Brief Psychiatric Rating Scale. *Psychological Reports. 10*, 799–812.

Pietzcker, A., Gaebel, W., Kopcke, M. et al. (1986). A German multicentre study of the neuroleptic long-term therapy of schizophrenic patients. Preliminary Report. *Pharmacopsychiatry, 19*, 161–166.

Shawver, J., Gorham, D.R., Leskin, L.W., Good, W.W., Kabnick, D.E.: (1959)

Comparison of chlorpromazine and reserpine in maintenance drug therapy. *Diseases of the Nervous System, 20,* 452–457.

Vaughn, C., and Leff, J. (1976). The influence of family and social factors on the course of psychiatric illness. *British Journal of Psychiatry. 129,* 125–137.

Wing, J.K., Cooper, J.F. and Sartorius, N.: (1974). *The Measurement and Classification of Psychiatric Symptoms.* Cambridge University Press, Cambridge.

19

Applying Clinical Research in Practice: Meeting the Needs of Long-Term Patients and Their Carers

*It helps to realise that other people have to face
similar problems and that we are not alone.*
—Relative of long term patient.

Liz Kuipers

Introduction

The program of research in the Social Psychiatry Unit has always followed a coherent plan, moving from basic research of theoretical issues, through the testing of clinical applications, to the development and evaluation of new treatments and services. This has nowhere been more apparent than the research on the social influences on schizophrenia. In this chapter, I will describe principles of intervening with patients and carers, which derive from that research and which I have employed to meet the needs of a group of patients with long-standing psychotic illnesses within a routine clinical service.

Those with long-term rather than acute problems do have special features, and the research findings must, in general, be judiciously adapted to accommodate them. In any practice, the process of applying principles derived from research involves having to try them out in new and untested situations. This is part of the interest in developing innovative ways of working. However, it is only fair to point out that in this chapter, I can only present a *model* of the possible ways of applying research ideas to practice with the long-term client group. It is not meant to be either prescriptive or exhaustive, but is an attempt to review methods that might be used with this client group. The approach is based on the objective findings of research interventions, but is colored by the actual experience of conducting them (Leff *et al.*, 1982).

Needs of the Long-Term Group

It is quite clear that long-term psychotic patients and their carers have unique and unenviable problems. Patients have to cope with their vulnerability to relapse and the fact of disabling symptoms; sometimes florid, such as continuing delusions or thought disorder; often the full range of negative symptoms, such as apathy, loss of motivation, self neglect, anhedonia. They may also have to face unemployment, poverty, and a reduced social network (e.g., Henderson, 1980). Insight may be intermittent or absent and, if present, the realization of problems may lead to loss of confidence and depression. The preservation of independence and self-help skills, and the maximization of social functioning may be the most important aspect of surviving in the community for this population. For this to be possible, a range of needs must be met by those who provide services for them. These are listed in Table 19.1.

Of this long-term group—those with a high dependency on services and likely to need day care over many years for their psychiatric illness—nearly half continue to live with relatives (Creer et al., 1982; Brugha, et al., 1988). The relatives faced with this situation appear to be severely burdened, but rarely voice their difficulties, (Gibbons et al., 1984; Fadden et al., 1987a; MacCarthy, 1988). The emotional demands of the support they provide may continue for years with little respite, often at real cost to their own mental health (Fadden et al., 1987b). In the past, psychiatrtic professionals have often blamed or exploited them, without recognizing that they are an important community resource with needs of their own (Kuipers and Bebbington, 1985).

These needs are centered on a requirement for long-term support from, and ready access to, staff who are familiar with their situation and able to offer information, advice, and time to talk (Table 19.1). However, evidence from consumer groups (Hatfield, 1983) and personal clinical experience shows that this continuity and trust are often lacking. Partly because of the likelihood of unpleasant past experience with services, families may be suspicious of professional help and hard to engage in therapeutic endeavours. They may also be so worried and unable to cope with problems that they appear overly demanding (Birley and Hudson, 1983). Staff need to be able to see beyond this initial presentation, and offer

TABLE 19.1
Balancing Needs

Needs of Patients:
Support
Day care—activity and structure
Independence fostered
Self help skills developed, maintained
Practical help
Physical care
Monitoring of symptom levels—medication
Individual counselling

Needs of Relatives:
Continuity
Trust
Collaboration not antagonism
Support
Understanding
Practical help
Shared information

Needs of Staff:
Avoid 'burnout'
Share problems—not individually responsible
See relatives as partners
Interventions must be: feasible
                       acceptable
                       effective

---

understanding and help for the real difficulties and burdens that they experience.

Dealing with this population may also cause problems for professionals (Table 19.1). Long-term psychotic patients have difficulties which continue, and may exacerbate. They may, for instance, need continual prompting and the constant provision of an external structure; demand frequent staff attention and reassurance; or be abusive, aggressive, or totally withdrawn. In consequence, staff "burnout" (Jackson et al., 1986) is likely unless steps are taken to prevent it. Morale is easier to maintain if staff work as a team, rather than having to take individual responsibility for these difficult problems, and new staff with fresh ideas are allowed to become part of any therapeutic effort (Watts and Bennett, 1983).

Given the problems, it is not surprising that staff often do not see it as a priority to engage relatives, particularly if they are seen as difficult or demanding. Moreover, professionals may feel they lack both the time and expertise to deal adequately with families.

In order to surmount these barriers, any model of family intervention has to be feasible, acceptable to staff, not too time-consuming, and effective (that is, worth the effort). The model proposed here relies on the premise that staff should see families, not as a problem, but as partners in a collaborative effort to maintain a patient in the community with as much independence and quality of life as possible, despite residual disabilities.

Research Evidence

There is now considerable research evidence that family atmosphere and the relative's ability to cope with problems has an effect on the outcome of psychotic illness in a variety of cultures (Kuipers and Bebbington, 1988; Leff and Vaughn, 1985; Chapter 12). In particular, families with high levels of criticism or emotional overinvolvement, characterized as high Expressed Emotion (EE) families, are associated with a poor outcome, a relationship which cannot be explained as the effect of variations in medication (Nuechterlein et al., 1986). Several intervention studies with EE families (Leff et al., 1985; Falloon et al., 1985; Hogarty et al., 1986; Tarrier et al., 1988, Leff et al., 1989) now show that it is possible both to reduce EE and to improve relapse rates and social outcome. These interventions have been characterized by several common features (Table 19.2).

First, an educational component has always been included. This has stemmed from evidence (Leff and Vaughn 1985; Brewin et al., 1991) that the poor tolerance of problem behavior shown by highly critical relatives was partly due to their misattribution of its causes. Such relatives tend to blame the patient directly for problems, rather that seeing them as perhaps being outside the patient's own control. Low EE relatives are more likely to understand that there is something "wrong" with the patient, and to be more sympathetic. Successful intervention studies have used the illness model of schizophrenia as a way of trying to help relatives understand the reasons for some of the patient's difficulties, particularly the negative symptoms, which are often otherwise discounted as "laziness" or "bloody-mindedness." This can improve tolerance, and initiate the proc-

TABLE 19.2
Common Features of Successful Outcome Studies

1. Positive attitude to families.
2. Education.
3. Specific problem solving.
4. Medication.

ess of making expectations realistic. It can also help people adjust to a timescale of improvement that stretches over weeks and months rather than days.

There is no assured way of transmitting this information. Studies have offered leaflets, booklets, workshops, and interactive sessions at home (Leff et al., 1982, 1989; Falloon et al., 1982; Hogarty et al., 1986; Smith and Birchwood 1985; Tarrier et al., 1988; MacCarthy et al., 1989a). However, the main value of this education appears to be indirect. Relatives do not necessarily learn many new facts about the illness, but the process by which the professional shares what is known, answers questions freely, and continues to offer information whenever it is requested appears to engender optimism and to engage relatives in subsequent interventions (Smith and Birchwood 1987; Berkowitz et al., 1984).

In the long-term group, most relatives will have received some information about diagnosis. It therefore seems important, not so much to offer facts about schizophrenia or manic depressive illness, but to discuss in detail what is understood by these terms, and their implications for that particular family. This process of providing information also has a broader aspect. It opens the door for relatives to share in decision-making with the team, and makes it possible for both them and the patients to be involved in treatment plans and goals. Relatives often have to bear the effects of decisions by the psychiatric team—sudden discharge, or a change in medication—so it is not surprising that they value being included in the process of making these decisions. A more open, less secretive approach will help to foster the idea of partnership.

A second feature of the recent intervention studies has been a "problem solving" element. Therapeutic effort has focused on selected difficulties of importance to family members, where improvement may be feasible. Effecting a small change, particularly in long-term families where resignation and despair may be prominent features (Creer et al., 1982; MacCarthy, 1988), is often a catalyst for families to think more positively about their situation. The problem solving has typically been directed at particular and limited goals. It is always important to distinguish between the problems that can be solved, and those that, perhaps for the moment, are too difficult. It is particularly necessary for staff to be tolerant of unusual solutions to difficulties that families may have adopted. Some strategies of coping that at first sight seem maladaptive may be very hard to change, and may in fact have a positive function in the family (Tarrier et al., 1988).

Other aspects of the published research emphasize the importance of regular medication, which seems to enhance the patients' resistance to relapse and to general social stresses (Liberman, 1986). This may raise further issues, as the fact of taking medication for many years often requires adaptation. Again, general points about understanding the way medication is used prophylactically, the difference between side effects and negative symptoms, and the possibility that patients may genuinely feel worse when medicated and may resent the obligation to continue taking the drugs, are useful for beginning a family discussion.

The evidence suggests it is possible to offer help to families of psychotic patients, to enhance their coping skills, and to improve the outcome for the patient. In order to adapt these approaches to the long-term group, it may be necessary to offer a less intensive but long lasting intervention that encompasses the range of needs of families and is not merely activated by a crisis (MacCarthy et al., 1989b). Nevertheless, given the burden that most families face when living with long term patients, and the additional problems of stigma and isolation that worsen over the years (MacCarthy, 1988), there are good arguments for offering help to all families in this situation. In this group, diagnosis may be less important than the range of residual disabilities and problems of social performance. There is certainly considerable overlap in the sorts of problems faced by families whether the ill member suffers from depression or from schizophrenia (Kuipers, 1987; Fadden, 1989).

A Model of Intervention with Families of Patients with Long-Standing Mental Illness

In the light of the current research literature, and the adaptations necessary for the needs of the long-term group, a number of possible modes of intervention can be suggested (Table 19.3). Each has advantages and disadvantages, and they may not all be equally easy to implement. They are also not exclusive.

Ideally, patient counselling should always be offered, together with family meetings, a relatives' group, and self help support. In practice, teams are usually restricted in their offers of resources, and by the motivation of clients and families. Patients may reject groups or home visits. It may only be possible to offer one mode at a time. There is evidence that all the interventions can effect change; specifically that education plus family sessions, or relatives' groups, or focused skills training for patients may improve family coping and attitudes and patient outcome.

Whatever the mode adopted, the model works best if it has clear aims which can then form the basis of evaluation. These aims follow from the EE research. Broadly, they are to reduce criticism; to improve tolerance of problems; to reduce over-involvement and to encourage the indepen-

TABLE 19.3
Possible Modes of Intervention for Families of the Long-Term Group

I Education + relatives group	II Education + home visits to family	III Relative only support group	IV Patient counseling
+ low staff cost reduces relatives' isolation offers support	hard to avoid (for family) deals with individual family problems in detail	offers support no staff cost.	Individual problems addressed. standard staff cost.
− some dropouts does not deal with all problems patient may feel excluded	high staff cost isolation not changed	may not enable change.	relatives not offered service.

Note: I–IV not exclusive

TABLE 19.4
Aims of Intervention

1. Reduce criticism.
2. Reduce overinvolvement.
3. Tackle problems.
4. Defuse emotions.
5. Improve patient skills, performance

dence of the patient despite residual disabilities; to tackle real problems; to defuse negative emotions; and to engender optimism for the future.

Methods of Intervention

Each aim is associated with a particular approach to achieving the objectives of improved relative functioning and patient outcome. These methods can be implemented to some extent in any of the modes presented. They are derived from previous work with these families. The techniques employed include a behavioral skills approach, as well as counselling and group facilitation. They are not interpretative or psychodynamic.

Reducing Criticism

Criticism can best be understood as an intolerance of the patient's behavior, a dislike, even a resentment, of things the patient does. At its most extreme (when it is rated as hostility), it includes a frank dislike of the patient as a person (e.g., "He is so awful"), and sometimes an outright rejection (e.g., "I wish he was dead").

Often this intolerance is linked to poor coping skills, in other words all the strategies that a person normally finds successful in interpersonal dealings begin to fail: "I would shout at him but it did no good. He just lay there (in bed)." This combination usually results in feelings of frustration and anger in the carer, and the patient is blamed for the behavior.

In order to change these strong feelings, most interventions have attempted to modify the attributions of blame by offering information or education. Carers are told that the patient's behavior is at least partly explicable as an illness that causes a wide range of both positive and negative symptoms. It is clear from the research findings that negative symptoms are particularly difficult for relatives to understand and attribute correctly (Creer and Wing, 1974; MacCarthy, 1988; Brewin et al. 1991). Providing carers with a different model, that patients are not being "difficult" or "lazy," but are disabled by the effects of a schizophrenic illness, enables them to begin the process of understanding why their relative is behaving so strangely. Sharing this information with a professional also seems to be reassuring, in that at least someone else is aware of their problems, and helps reduce stigma and the sense of isolation. Self-help groups can also provide this information and reassurance.

Once carers can begin to accept this new model, it permits the emergence of a greater tolerance of problems. Part of this process depends on changing carers' expectations of the patient. Carers may have unrealistic beliefs that the patient will "get back to work next week," whereas it almost invariably takes a much longer time to recover, and motivation and interest may have to be fostered, not presumed. Relapse may also be a possibility. If long-term carers can be persuaded that progress may only be apparent over the timespan of, say, a year, it enables a degree of acceptance to emerge. This is important in countering the typical resignation of "nothing ever changes" that many carers adopt. Once realistic targets can be negotiated with the family, small changes can be seen as progress, and it becomes possible for a more optimistic attitude to emerge. Hope for the future is one of the features common to low Expressed Emotion families, reflecting the fact that they have encompassed this long timescale, adjusted to the problems, and discovered ways to cope.

A final aspect of sharing information and understanding is that it is likely to promote co-operation with staff. If carers understand the nature of problems and can see the point of the physical and social treatments that are offered, it is much more likely that they will be able to work constructively with staff on new problems that arise. Issues commonly misunderstood without this sharing are:

1. What is medication for and how does it work?
2. What is my relative experiencing?
3. What is the point of their attending the hospital/day care/workshop.

Even when staff are willing to be clear and open, answering questions and discussing progress with patients and carers, these issues and others like them may sometimes continue to be misunderstood. Without this openness, however, co-operation may be impossible.

Reducing Over-Involvement

As with criticism, it is helpful to start with an understanding of over-involvement and what fuels it. Over-involvement includes elements of over-protection, self sacrifice, upset, worry, and guilt. The term involves unfortunate connotations of blame. This is inappropriate, and although it is useful shorthand for a sort of behavior that may prevent patients from reaching a potential level of functioning, no implication of blame should be conveyed to carers whose situation we can hardly begin to appreciate. Over-involvement is more commonly rated in parents than in spouses. It involves treating patients, not as independent adults, but as children who continue to need extensive protection and decisions to be made for them. This issue of independence seems to be central; the dilemma is real, given that these long-term patients often cannot function entirely autonomously. The over-involved carer leans towards assuming that very little independence is possible; the style then becomes very similar to an "enmeshed" family (Minuchin, 1974).

Long term patients may remain vulnerable, and are often disabled by both positive and negative symptoms. They may require considerable assistance and prompting, and their relatives may indeed have to take over some of the roles normally assumed by adults in order for them to survive in the community. However, all this has to be balanced against the fact that *too much* of this care can be counterproductive. Over-involvement essentially reflects an inappropriate level of protection, care, and the taking over of tasks or roles. With these psychotic illnesses, it is also the case that care that might be appropriate in an acute stage can easily be continued into the recovery phase,when it may become unhelpful.

These distinctions are complex, and it may be premature to discuss them with a carer who has just agreed with you that the patient has an illness and thus merits care rather than blame. It is useful to regard it as an issue of degree. It is also worth remembering that over-involvement is often a very long standing style that predates onset (i.e., a parental style), and may be very slow or unamenable to change.

As an approach to changing over-involvement, it has been found useful to discuss it with carers in terms of independence. Emphasising the adult features of the patient—their age and past skills—can be used as the starting point for a discussion of the gradual return to independence. This may, however, lead to arguments if it is obvious that the patient is currently very disabled and cannot function without a great deal of help. Although this may have arisen partly because of the lost skills and confidence, and the lack of practice at living independently that over-involved carers may exacerbate, there is normally an underlying vulnerability and loss of judgement that has been correctly identified by the carer. There may also be some very basic fears of the worst outcome if this level of care is not continued, i.e., the house will be burnt down because the patient would leave a gas ring unattended. A parallel approach is to emphasize the carer's own need for an independent life. It is important to suggest that it can be caring to leave the patient alone some of the time. Enmeshed parents typically cannot leave the house without worrying what will happen, and they may have given up outside work, interests, and friends in order to look after the patient. Giving carers "permission" to start leading an independent life also relieves them of guilt. Similarly it can allow the beginning of a process whereby the carer can feel less resentful of the tie and develop outside support and interests. Outside activity then gives perspective to problems that may otherwise seem overwhelming.

Limit setting is something that these carers may be particularly poor at—how can you negotiate a limit to disruptive or embarrassing behavior if the patient is ill? This issue can often lead to quite complex arguments about responsibility and the ability of the mentally ill to control their own behavior. There is a particular problem because a person suffering from longstanding psychotic illness may be very unpredictable, and show fluctuating impairment of insight. Discussing with carers how to negotiate and agree on realistic limits with patients, and then to adhere to them consistently, helps both to assert the carers' right to their own view and independent life, and to demonstrate that patients can take responsibility for some of their own behavior even while "mad."

Aiming at adult individuation usually involves a mixture of task setting and time spent in independent activity. It may also imply that patients need to learn new skills to cope with these new roles and environments.

For patients who have become very withdrawn and inactive, encouraging social skills, social activity, and communication can, itself, improve and extend role performance. Often it is very helpful to include day care in this, as by definition it provides a setting where independence can be fostered in a structured and meaningful way. Work based activities may be particularly important both for their social meaning and ability to generate a separate income, and because they can increase confidence and the number of roles available to a patient.

Patients and carers in the most over-involved relationships are often those least able to separate, and it may therefore be difficult to get the patient to engage in individual activities such as attending for day care. The fears and worries associated with extreme over-involvement in carers, and the child-like behavior of the patients who live with them will tend to prevent engagement. Unless the carers and patients have been enlisted in the therapeutic effort and can see the point of it, interventions are likely to be sabotaged. Thus with the most over-dependent families it is sensible to aim for a very gradual separation of function. Clinically it has proved impossible to deal with over-involvement by directly encouraging patient and carer to spend less time together—until the emotional worries have been dealt with, such attempts will be rejected or traduced (thus confirming the family as uncooperative and difficult).

Tackling Problems

In addition to an educational component involving the free exchange of information between patients, carers, and professionals, the successful intervention studies have all been characterized by a focus on problem solving. Although the links are still tentative, it seems likely that high EE families are also poorly equipped to cope with the problems that they face (Kuipers and Bebbington, 1988). Certainly, poor coping in relatives is associated with a worse outcome in schizophrenic patients (Birchwood and Smith, 1986), and high EE is associated with higher levels of stress, tension and strain, as well as less adequate coping (Bledin et al., 1990).

It is particularly important to help carers of the long-term group to tackle problems, as it is possible thus to begin to counteract the resignation and hopelessness characteristic of many. However, because of their lack of success in the past, it is common to find a persistent pessimism that may take many months to overcome. Typically, when a range of possible solutions are discussed, all are rejected because "we've tried that" (Berkowitz et al., 1984). This unwillingness to try again and *persist* with problem solving seems related to the admission that if the problems *do* turn out to be soluble, the carers could and should have done more;

criticism is seen as implicit in the professional's optimism. If the insolubility of the problems can be maintained (no one could do better, and it is therefore not the carer's fault), the situation although bad is at least known, and has the potential at least to elicit sympathy from professionals and others.

Changing these long standing patterns cannot be easily managed. In order to risk the attempt to solve them, carers have to feel that their problems are not being minimised, nor they belittled. The process of change is in any case genuinely risky—problems may, after all, get worse. One way to begin is deliberately to aim for slow but tangible progress. Carers typically present problems in non-specific terms—"he's just lazy, he's never been any good at anything." It is then essential to focus down on to a single specific issue—for instance, not getting out of bed in the morning. Attempts to modify this are then broken down into small steps that can be accomplished. It is important that targets are realistic and negotiated rather than imposed (aiming perhaps to get the patient to rise by lunchtime, not 8:00 am). It is also necessary to work to a long time scale (months, not days), and to ensure that success is perceived and acknowledged by the carer (instead of "Oh yes, he gets up now, but he's still lazy").

Focusing on one problem at a time and gradually bringing about change by getting the carer to respond in a feasible, consistent, and negotiated manner towards the patient will help the family acknowledge the possibility of a more optimistic approach. Sometimes, a very small change in a single area will have a disproportionately large effect on improving morale and hope.

It may also be essential to decide with the family what is in fact insoluble. The possibility of failing again because the chosen problem is immoveable may have to be recognized, and it helps the family if professionals acknowledge this and try another area. Some long standing problems may often only be amenable to change when a carer dies, or when another drastic life change forces some action.

The ability to listen is another skill that may be very poorly developed, particularly in high EE family members (Kuipers et al., 1983). The therapist may have to take steps to enhance communication between relative and patient. This often includes fostering a situation in which family members, particularly the patient, can have their problems considered equally. Even relatively simple matters like allowing other members a turn in the conversation may need to be tackled. Dealing with communication difficulties of this type may need to be one of the first targets of the therapist, and is often one of the most important.

Helping relatives to solve problems of whatever type depends crucially on the professional being prepared to take those problems seriously. The relatives must never be left with the impression that their views or efforts are being belittled. This seriousness of approach is central to engaging families in the business of practical change.

Defusing Emotions

It is implicit in the previous sections that therapeutic effort is at least partly aimed at emotional processing (Rachmann, 1980; Raphael, 1986). Carers and patients may feel a wide variety of powerful and upsetting emotions. They range from guilt, grief, fear of the future, anger, and rejection of the patient, to worries about the patient's vulnerability to relapse or exploitation by others. There is also the remaining stigma of mental illness, particularly difficult to discuss with friends and neighbours because patients usually look reasonably "normal," and the resulting isolation and loneliness that may affect carer and patient alike. Frustration with professionals, their lack of consultation, and their inability to cure the disorder may be great.

It is increasingly clear that the burdens of care adversely affect the relatives' own mental health (MacCarthy et al., 1989b); the increased levels of distress, anxiety, and despair are clinically measurable, and above those found in the general population (Fadden et al., 1987b). With long term carers, the burdens are likely to have been carried for many years, usually without much professional help, and often without respite.

One of the obvious ways of dealing with these emotions, and also of reducing stigma and isolation, is to encourage relatives to talk to each other, either through facilitated or self-help groups. The realization of common experience and the ability to share it was one of the most important positive factors in a recently evaluated relatives' group (MacCarthy et al., 1989; Kuipers et al., 1989). Other important functions include being able to meet others who have coped with difficulties and survived, and being in contact at non-crisis times with staff, who will thus be in a position to spot problems before they develop.

It is equally important for staff to be able to "allow" the negative emotions, including those about themselves, and to accept and work with them as a normal and expected response of carers.

A crucial aspect of working in the long-term field is the need for staff to stay around: patients and carers can get very used to nothing changing but the membership of the clinical team. Even if staff members are indeed going to move from time to time, and this may well be desirable for training purposes and to avoid staff institutionalization (Watts and Bennet, 1983), it is sensible for there to be at least a continuity in the philosophy and way of working of staff. Otherwise, carers will not feel support and encouragement, but confusion and the frustration of starting again with another professional. This is not the way to help carers deal with the emotional problems of their situation.

Helping the Patient to Cope more Effectively

While engaging the whole family is an ideal, relatives will sometimes not accept intervention, and patients may not allow staff to "bother" the relatives. There is still a considerable amount that can be done to enhance the patient's coping skills, both within the family setting and in other difficult environments. It seems eminently obvious, particularly with long-term problems, that helping patients manage their difficulties better should be a basic part of any individual treatment program. In the family intervention studies, good results have been obtained merely by improving the social skills of patients (Hogarty et al., 1986).

In long-term care, a patient has a number of basic needs such as shelter or accommodation, daytime activity including use of leisure time, control of positive and negative symptoms, physical care and nutrition, and individual help with problems. These are discussed at length by Wing (1987). Day care may offer access to a number of other essentials— structure, a social network, specialized behavior programs, and the monitoring of symptom levels and medication. Individual counselling can provide specific help with residual problems, goal setting to improve confidence and performance, and discussion or information to improve insight into the illness and to allow patients to take maximum control of their remaining symptoms and disabilities. The aim again is to enhance the patient's independence and quality of life during and after recovery from acute episodes.

Other Aspects

It can be appreciated from the above discussion that there may be considerable overlap between the various methods that should be considered. Often a single intervention has multiple effects. For instance, problem solving might increase tolerance and reduce criticism as the problem improves. Defusing emotions may allow a start to be made in dealing with a particular problem. Encouraging the patient's independence is a double edged process; unless a patient can be helped to be more capable, and can show improvements in at least some aspects of activity and social performance, it may be impossible to reduce the carer's over-involvement. An increase in the patient's skills may obviate the need for such high levels of care and involvement by the relative, but it may take considerable time for both sides to adjust to such changes.

The London group (Leff et al., 1982; 1985; 1989) have in the past been criticized for placing too much emphasis on separation. This was as a result of early ideas that a reduction in the amount of time spent together (low "face-to-face" contact) in a difficult home atmosphere was associated with better outcome (Vaughn and Leff, 1976). We now know that reducing unhelpful contact is not easily achieved without reducing the emotional worry that is its cause. If this worry can indeed be mitigated, there is then less need for a physical separation that may not be either possible or desirable. Patients who live alone may be exposed to loneliness and problems of negative symptoms such as self neglect, which may worsen without considerable levels of support. On the other hand, in the long-term group in particular, one needs to remain flexible about what represents a good outcome. In some cases, living apart may actually mean more family and social contact, with all its implications of normality, that continuing to live in an impossibly difficult or demanding family setting.

It must also be remembered that many patients and families have multiple problems. This can be overwhelming for both staff and clients. The focussing techniques previously discussed do not guarantee success. Not all problems have a solution; many will have to be lived with, rather than removed. Improving the coping skills of both relatives and patients may well turn out to be the most appropriate way of offering help to these families (Birchwood and Smith, 1987; MacCarthy et al., 1989a).

Summary

Long-term psychotic patients have particular needs and problems. Many of these are shared by their relatives. Staff involved in offering services to clients have to be aware of these needs, and of the importance of offering a collaborative, rather than an antagonistic, relationship. Interventions with this group can benefit from ideas gained from research with more acutely ill psychotic patients and their families, but they have to be adapted so that they are seen by staff as feasible, acceptable and not too costly in terms of professional time and effort. Staff need for cohesiveness, consistency, high morale, and achievement must also be considered, or such interventions will not be given priority.

The model presented here incorporates elements of education, problem solving, and counselling as possible approaches to these families. Several strategies are suggested which may overlap, and should often be used together.

The problems encountered and particular difficulties of heavy users of services have been discussed. The model has been formally evaluated and it appears useful for this group, as it can change attitudes in relationships (MacCarthy et al., 1989b; Kuipers et al., 1989). Given the nature of the difficulties and problems that long-term patients and their carers are subject to, any interventions which can show positive effects must be seriously considered. From this starting point, it is to be hoped that other approaches will develop which might improve the outlook for this severely disabled population and their families.

References

Berkowitz, R., Eberlein-Fries, R., Kuipers, L., and Leff, J. (1984). Educating relatives about schizophrenia. *Schizophrenia Bulleting. 10* 418–429.

Birchwood, M., and Smith, J. (1987). Schizophrenia. In: J. Orford (ed.). *Coping with Disorder in the Family*. London, Croom Helm.

Birley, J., and Hudson, B. (1983). The family, the social network and rehabilitation. In: F.N. Watts and D.H. Bennett (eds.). *Theory and Practice of Psychiatric Rehabilitation* Chichester, John Wiley and Sons.

Bledin, K., MacCarthy, B., Kuipers, L., and Wood, R. (1990). Daughters of people with dementia. Expressed Emotion, strain and coping. *British Journal of Psychiatry. 157* 221–227.

Brewin, C. R., MacCarthy, B., Duda, K. and Vaughn, C. E. (1991) Attribution and Expressed Emotion in the relatives of patients with schizophrenia. *Journal of Abnormal Psychology* (in press).

Brugha, T.S., Wing, J.K., Brewin, C.R., MacCarthy, B., Mangen, S., LeSage, A., and Mumford, J. (1988). The problems of people in long-term psychiatric day care: An introduction to the Camberwell High Contact Survey. *Psychological Medicine. 18* 443–456.

Creer, C., Sturt, E., and Wykes, T. (1982). The role of relatives. In: J.K. Wing (ed.). *Long Term Community Care: Experience in a London Borough. Psychological Medicine Monograph Supplement 2.*

Fadden, G. (1989). Pity the spouse: depression within marriage. *Stress Medicine. 5* 99–107.

Fadden, G., Bebbington, P., and Kuipers, L. (1987a). The burden of care: the impact of functional psychiatric illness on the patient's family. *British Journal of Psychiatry. 150* 285–292.

Fadden, G., Kuipers, L., and Bebbington, P. (1987b). Caring and its burdens: a study of the spouses of depressed patients. *British Journal of Psychiatry. 151.* 660–667.

Falloon, I.R.H., Boyd, J.L., McGill, C.W., Razani, J., Moss, H.B., and Gilderman, A.M. (1982). Family management in the prevention of exacerbations of schizophrenia: A controlled study. *New England Journal of Medicine. 306,* 1437–40.

Falloon, I., Boyd, J.L., McGill, C.W., Williamson, M., Razani, J., Moss, H.B., Gilderman, A.M., and Simpson, G.M. (1985). Family management in the prevention of morbidity of schizophrenia. Clinical outcome of a two-year longitudinal study. *Archives of General Psychiatry. 42* 887–896.

Folkman, S., and Lazarus, R.S. (1985). If it changes it must be a process: a study of emotion and coping during three stages of a college examination. *Journal of Personality and Social Psychology. 48* 150–170.

Gibbons, J.S., Horn, S.H., Powell, J.M., and Gibbons, J.L. (1984). Schizophrenic patients and their families. A survey in a psychiatric service based on a DGH Unit. *British Journal of Psychiatry. 144* 70–77.

Hatfield, A.B. (1983). What families want of family therapists. In: W.R. McFarlane (ed.). *Family Therapy in Schizophrenia.* Guildford.

Henderson, S. (1980). Personal networks and the schizophrenias. *Australian and N Z Journal of Psychiatry. 14* 255–259.

Hogarty, G.E., Anderson, C.M., Reiss, D.J., Kornblith, S.J., Greenwald, D.P., Javna, C.D., and Madoniz, M.J. (1986). Family psychoeducation, social skills training and maintenance chemotherapy in the aftercare treatment of schizophrenia. *Archives of General Psychiatry. 43.* 644–642.

Jackson, S.E., Schwab, R.L. and Schulter, R.S. (1986). Towards an understanding of the burnout phenomenon. *Journal of Applied Psychology, 71,* 630–640.

Kuipers, L. (1987). Depression in the family. In: J. Orford (ed.) *Coping with Disorder in the Family.* London. Croon Helm.

Kuipers, L., and Bebbington, P.E. (1985). Relatives as a resource in the management of functional illness. *British Journal of Psychiatry. 147* 465–471.

Kuipers, L., and Bebbington, P.E. (1988). Expressed Emotion research in schizophrenia. Theoretical and clinical implications. *Psychological Medicine, 18,* 893–909.

Kuipers, L., MacCarthy, B., Hurry, J., and Harper, R. (1989). Counselling the relatives of the long-term mentally ill: A low-cost supportive model. *British Journal of Psychiatry. 154* 775–782.

Leff, J.P., Kuipers, L., Berkowitz, R., Eberlein-Vries, R., and Sturgeon, D. (1982). A controlled trial of social intervention in the families of schizophrenic patients. *British Journal of Psychiatry. 141* 121–134.

Leff, J.P., Kuipers, L., Berkowitz, R., and Sturgeon, D. (1985). A controlled trial of social intervention in the families of schizophrenic patients: 2 year follow up. *British Journal of Psychiatry. 146* 594–600.

Leff, J., and Vaughn, C.E. (1985). *Expressed Emotion in Families.* The Guilford Press.

Leff, J., Berkowitz, R., Sharit, N., Strachan, A., Glass, I., and Vaughn, C. (1989). A trial of family therapy v. a relatives' group for schizophrenia. *British Journal of Psychiatry, 154,* 58–6.

Liberman, R.P. (1986). Coping and competence as protective factors in the vulnerability—stress model of schizophrenia. In: M. J. Goldstein, I. Hand and K. Hahlweg (eds.). *Treatment of Schizophrenia: Family Assessment and Intervention.* Berlin, Springer-Verlag.

MacCarthy, B. (1988). The role of relatives. In: *Community Care in Practice.* (eds.) A. Lavender and F. Holloway. Chichester, John Wiley & Sons.

MacCarthy, B., Kuipers, L., Hurry, J., Harper, R. and Lesage, A. (1989a). Counselling the relatives of the long term mentally ill. In: Evaluation. *British Journal of Psychiatry, 154,* 768–775.

MacCarthy, B., Lesage, A., Brewin, C.R., Brugha, T.S., Mangen, S. and Wing, J.K. (1989b). Needs for care among the relatives of long term users of day care. *Psychological Medicine 19,* 725–736.

Minuchin, S. (1974). *Families and Family Therapy,* London, Tavistock press.

Nuechterlein, K.H., Snyder, K.S., Dawson, M.E., Rappe, S., Gitlin, M. and

Fogelson, D. (1986). Expressed Emotion, fixed-dose fluphenazine decanoate maintenance, and relapse in recent onset schizophrenia. *Psychopharmacology Bulletin, 22*, 633–639.

Rachman, S.J. (1980). Emotional processing. *Behaviour Research and Therapy, 18,* 51–60.

Raphael, B. (1986). *When Disaster Strikes,* Hutchinson.

Smith, J.V., and Birchwood, M.J. (1985). *Understanding Schizophrenia.* Health Promotion Unit, West Birmingham Health Authority. Mental Health Series.

Smith, J.V., and Birchwood, M.J. (1987). Specific and non-specific effects of educational interventions with families of schizophrenic patients. *British Journal of Psychiatry. 150* 645–652.

Tarrier, N., Barrowclough, C., Vaughn, C., Bamrah, J.S., Porceddu, K., Watts, S., and Freeman, H. (1988). The community management of schizophrenia: A controlled trial of behavioural intervention with families to reduce relapse. *British Journal of Psychiatry, 153,* 532–542.

Vaughn, C.E., and Leff, J.P. (1976). The influence of family and social factors on the course of psychiatric illness. *British Journal of Psychiatry. 129* 125–137.

Watts, F., and Bennett, D., (1983). *Theory and Practice of Psychiatric Rehabilitation.* Chichester, John Wiley and Sons.

Wing, J.K. (1987). Psychosocial factors affecting the long term course of schizophrenia. In: J. Strauss, W. Böker, and H. Brenner. (eds.). *Psychosocial Treatment of Schizophrenia,* Stuttgart, Hans Huber.

Contributors

BEBBINGTON, DR. PAUL E. M.A., Ph.D., MRCP, MRCPsych, Reader in Social and Epidemiological Psychiatry, University of London.

BIRLEY, DR. J. L. T. FRCPsych., FRCP, DPM, Emeritus Psychiatrist, Bethlehem Royal and Maudsley Hospitals, Past President, Royal College of Psychiatrists.

BREWIN, DR. CHRIS R. B.A., M.Sc., Ph.D., Senior Scientist, MRC Social and Community Psychiatry Unit.

BROWN, PROFESSOR GEORGE W. Ph.D., FBA., Professor of Sociology, University of London and External Scientific Staff, Medical Research Council.

CLARKE, PROFESSOR RON. V. M.A., Ph.D., Professor and Dean of Criminal Justice, Rutgers University, New Jersey, USA.

FRITH, DR. CHRISTOPHER D. Ph.D. Clinical Research Centre, Harrow.

FRITH, DR. UTA. Ph.D., MRC Cognitive Development Unit, London.

GIEL, PROFESSOR R. M.D., Professor of Social Psychiatry, University Hospital, Groningen, Netherlands.

HÄFNER, PROFESSOR H. M.D., Ph.D., Professor of Psychiatry, Head, Central Institute of Mental Health, Mannheim, W. Germany.

HIRSH, PROFESSOR STEVEN R. B.A., M.D., MPhil., FRCP, FRCPsych. Professor of Psychiatry, Charing Cross and Westminster Medical School, London.

HURRY, DR. JANE. B.A., M.A., Ph.D., Thomas Coran Research Unit, University of London.

KUIPERS, DR. LIZ. B.Sc., M.Sc., Ph.D., AFBPs., Senior Lecturer in Psychology, Institute of Psychiatry, London.

LEFF, PROFESSOR JULIAN P. B.Sc., M.D., FRCPsych., MRCP., Professor of Social and Cultural Psychiatry, University of London, Director MRC Social and Community Psyhciatric Unit, London.

MANGEN, DR. S. P. Ph.D., Lecturer in European Social Policy, London School of Economics and Political Sciences.

MECHANIC, PROFESSOR DAVID. Ph.D., Rene Dubos, Professor of Behavioural Science and Director, Institute for Health, Health Care Policy and Aging Research, Rutgers University, New Jersey, USA.

SINCLAIR, PROFESSOR IAN. Ph.D., Professor of Social Work, University of York.

TENNANT, PROFESSOR C. M.D., MPH., MRCPsych., FRANZCP, Head, Department of Psychiatry, University of Sydney.

WING, PROFESSOR JOHN K. M.D., Ph.D., Emeritus Professor of Psychiatry, Institute of Psychiatry, London.

WING, DR. LORNA. M.D. FRCPsych. Retired, late of MRC Social Psychiatry Unit.

WYKES, DR. T. MPhil., DPhil., Lecturer and Clinical Psychologist, Institute of Psychiatry, London.

Index